T0226610

Interface Between Pediatrics and Children's Mental Health

Guest Editors

SANDRA L. FRITSCH, MD
HARSH K. TRIVEDI, MD

PEDIATRIC CLINICS
OF NORTH AMERICA

www.pediatric.theclinics.com

August 2011 • Volume 58 • Number 4

SAUNDERS an imprint of ELSEVIER, Inc.

W.B. SAUNDERS COMPANY
A Division of Elsevier Inc.

1600 John F. Kennedy Boulevard ● Suite 1800 ● Philadelphia, Pennsylvania 19103-2899

http://www.theclinics.com

THE PEDIATRIC CLINICS OF NORTH AMERICA Volume 58, Number 4
August 2011 ISSN 0031-3955, ISBN-13: 978-1-4557-1229-8

Editor: Kerry Holland

© **2011 Elsevier Inc. All rights reserved.**

This journal and the individual contributions contained in it are protected under copyright by Elsevier, and the following terms and conditions apply to their use:

Photocopying
Single photocopies of single articles may be made for personal use as allowed by national copyright laws. Permission of the Publisher and payment of a fee is required for all other photocopying, including multiple or systematic copying, copying for advertising or promotional purposes, resale, and all forms of document delivery. Special rates are available for educational institutions that wish to make photocopies for non-profit educational classroom use. For information on how to seek permission visit www.elsevier.com/permissions or call: (+44) 1865 843830 (UK)/(+1) 215 239 3804 (USA).

Derivative Works
Subscribers may reproduce tables of contents or prepare lists of articles including abstracts for internal circulation within their institutions. Permission of the Publisher is required for resale or distribution outside the institution. Permission of the Publisher is required for all other derivative works, including compilations and translations (please consult www.elsevier.com/permissions).

Electronic Storage or Usage
Permission of the Publisher is required to store or use electronically any material contained in this journal, including any article or part of an article (please consult www.elsevier.com/permissions). Except as outlined above, no part of this publication may be reproduced, stored in a retrieval system or transmitted in any form or by any means, electronic, mechanical, photocopying, recording or otherwise, without prior written permission of the Publisher.

Notice
No responsibility is assumed by the Publisher for any injury and/or damage to persons or property as a matter of products liability, negligence or otherwise, or from any use or operation of any methods, products, instructions or ideas contained in the material herein. Because of rapid advances in the medical sciences, in particular, independent verification of diagnoses and drug dosages should be made.

Although all advertising material is expected to conform to ethical (medical) standards, inclusion in this publication does not constitute a guarantee or endorsement of the quality or value of such product or of the claims made of it by its manufacturer.

The Pediatric Clinics of North America (ISSN 0031-3955) is published bimonthly by Elsevier Inc., 360 Park Avenue South, New York, NY 10010-1710. Months of issue are February, April, June, August, October, and December. Periodicals postage paid at New York, NY and additional mailing offices. Subscription prices are $179.00 per year (US individuals), $423.00 per year (US institutions), $243.00 per year (Canadian individuals), $563.00 per year (Canadian institutions), $289.00 per year (international individuals), $563.00 per year (international institutions), $87.00 per year (US students and residents), and $149.00 per year (international and Canadian residents and students). To receive students/resident rare, orders must be accompanied by name of affiliated institution, date of term, and the signature of program/residency coordinator on institution letterhead. Orders will be billed at individual rate until proof of status is received. Foreign air speed delivery is included in all *Clinics* subscription prices. All prices are subject to change without notice. **POSTMASTER:** Send address changes to *The Pediatric Clinics of North America*, Elsevier Health Sciences Division, Subscription Customer Service, 3251 Riverport Lane, Maryland Heights, MO 63043. **Customer Service: 1-800-654-2452 (US and Canada). From outside of the US and Canada: 1-314-447-8871. Fax: 1-314-447-8029. For print support, E-mail: JournalsCustomerService-usa@elsevier.com. For online support, E-mail: JournalsOnlineSupport-usa@elsevier.com.**

Reprints. For copies of 100 or more, of articles in this publication, please contact the Commercial Reprints Department, Elsevier Inc., 360 Park Avenue South, New York, NY 10010-1710. Tel.: 212-633-3812; Fax: 212-462-1935; E-mail: reprints@elsevier.com.

The Pediatric Clinics of North America is also published in Spanish by McGraw-Hill Inter-americana Editores S.A., Mexico City, Mexico; in Portuguese by Riechmann and Affonso Editores, Rua Comandante Coelho 1085, CEP 21250, Rio de Janeiro, Brazil; and in Greek by Althayia SA, Athens, Greece.

The Pediatric Clinics of North America is covered in *MEDLINE/PubMed (Index Medicus), Excerpta Medica, Current Contents, Current Contents/Clinical Medicine, Science Citation Index, ASCA, ISI/BIOMED,* and *BIOSIS.*

Printed and bound by CPI Group (UK) Ltd, Croydon, CR0 4YY

Transferred to Digital Print 2011

GOAL STATEMENT

The goal of the *Pediatric Clinics of North America* is to keep practicing physicians and residents up to date with current clinical practice in pediatrics by providing timely articles reviewing the state-of-the-art in patient care.

ACCREDITATION

The *Pediatric Clinics of North America* is planned and implemented in accordance with the Essential Areas and Policies of the Accreditation Council for Continuing Medical Education (ACCME) through the joint sponsorship of the University Of Virginia School Of Medicine and Elsevier. The University Of Virginia School of Medicine is accredited by the ACCME to provide continuing medical education for physicians.

The University of Virginia School of Medicine designates this enduring material for a maximum of 15 *AMA PRA Category 1 Credit*(s)™ for each issue, 90 credits per year. Physicians should only claim credit commensurate with the extent of their participation in the activity.

The American Medical Association has determined that physicians not licensed in the US who participate in this CME activity are eligible for a maximum of 15 *AMA PRA Category 1 Credit*(s)™ for each issue, 90 credits per year.

Credit can be earned by reading the text material, taking the CME examination online at http://www.theclinics.com/home/cme, and completing the evaluation. After taking the test, you will be required to review any and all incorrect answers. Following completion of the test and evaluation, your credit will be awarded and you may print your certificate.

FACULTY DISCLOSURE/CONFLICT OF INTEREST

The University of Virginia School of Medicine, as an ACCME accredited provider, endorses and strives to comply with the Accreditation Council for Continuing Medical Education (ACCME) Standards of Commercial Support, Commonwealth of Virginia statutes, University of Virginia policies and procedures, and associated federal and private regulations and guidelines on the need for disclosure and monitoring of proprietary and financial interests that may affect the scientific integrity and balance of content delivered in continuing medical education activities under our auspices.

The University of Virginia School of Medicine requires that all CME activities accredited through this institution be developed independently and be scientifically rigorous, balanced and objective in the presentation/discussion of its content, theories and practices.

All authors/editors participating in an accredited CME activity are expected to disclose to the readers relevant financial relationships with commercial entities occurring within the past 12 months (such as grants or research support, employee, consultant, stock holder, member of speakers bureau, etc.). The University of Virginia School of Medicine will employ appropriate mechanisms to resolve potential conflicts of interest to maintain the standards of fair and balanced education to the reader. Questions about specific strategies can be directed to the Office of Continuing Medical Education, University of Virginia School of Medicine, Charlottesville, Virginia.

The faculty and staff of the University of Virginia Office of Continuing Medical Education have no financial affiliations to disclose.

The authors/editors listed below have identified no financial or professional relationships for themselves or their spouse/partner:

Tami D. Benton, MD; Rebecca Brown, Mdiv; I. Simona Bujoreanu, PhD; David Ray DeMaso, MD; Michelle M. Ernst, PhD; Sandra L. Fritsch, MD (Guest Editor); M. Elena Garralda, MD, MPhil, FRCPsych, FRCPCH, DPM; Alka Goyal, MD; Barbara Hastie, PhD; Carla Holloway, (Acquisitions Editor); Patricia Ibeziako, MD; Mark C. Johnson, MD; Caprice Knapp, PhD; Brian P. Kurtz, MD; Vanessa Madden, BSc; Ann E. Maloney, MD; Laura McLafferty, BS; Lourival Baptista Neto, MD; Mark W. Overton, MD; Nancy A. Pattison, MD; Todd E. Peters, MD; Karen Rheuban, MD (Test Author); Douglas R. Robbins, MD; Matthew S. Siegel, MD; Margaert L. Stuber, MD; Harsh K. Trivedi, MD (Guest Editor); and Douglas Vanderbilt, MD.

The authors/editors listed below identified the following professional or financial affiliations for themselves or their spouse/partner:

Annah N. Abrams, MD's spouse is employed by Advanced Practice Strategies.
Daniel Button, MS, LCSW, ACHP-SW is employed by Hope Hospice and Community Services.
Gregory K. Fritz, MD edits a newsletter for John Wiley & Sons Inc (publishers).
Mary Margaret Gleason, MD owns stock in Merck Pharmaceuticals.
Wendy E. Smith, MD is an industry funded research/investigator for Hyperion Therapeutics, Inc and Genzyme Therapeutics.
Lori J. Stark, PhD receives grant support from the CF Foundation.
Eva Szigethy, MD, PhD authored a book on CBT for American Psychiatry Publishing.

Disclosure of Discussion of Non-FDA Approved Uses for Pharmaceutical Products and/or Medical Devices

The University of Virginia School of Medicine, as an ACCME provider, requires that all faculty presenters identify and disclose any off-label uses for pharmaceutical and medical device products. The University of Virginia School of Medicine recommends that each physician fully review all the available data on new products or procedures prior to clinical use.

TO ENROLL

To enroll in the Pediatric Clinics of North America Continuing Medical Education program, call customer service at 1-800-654-2452 or visit us online at www.theclinics.com/home/cme. The CME program is available to subscribers for an additional fee of $223.00.

Contributors

GUEST EDITORS

SANDRA L. FRITSCH, MD
Training Director, Child and Adolescent Psychiatry; Clinical Associate Professor, University of Vermont College of Medicine; Associate Clinical Professor, Tufts University School of Medicine, Maine Medical Center, Portland, Maine

HARSH K. TRIVEDI, MD
Executive Medical Director and Chief-of-Staff, Vanderbilt Psychiatric Hospital; Associate Professor of Psychiatry, Vanderbilt Medical School, Nashville, Tennessee

AUTHORS

ANNAH N. ABRAMS, MD
Assistant Professor, Harvard Medical School; Staff, Child Psychiatry Consultation Liaison Service, Department of Child and Adolescent Psychiatry; Child Psychiatrist, Department of Pediatric Hematology Oncology, Massachusetts General Hospital, Boston, Massachusetts

TAMI D. BENTON, MD
Assistant Professor of Psychiatry, University of Pennsylvania School of Medicine; Director of Psychiatric Education, The Children's Hospital of Philadelphia, Philadelphia, Pennsylvania

REBECCA BROWN, MDiv
Department of Pediatrics, University of Florida, Gainesville, Florida

I. SIMONA BUJOREANU, PhD
Assistant in Psychology, Department of Psychiatry, Children's Hospital Boston; Instructor in Psychology, Harvard Medical School, Boston, Massachusetts

DANIEL BUTTON, MS, LCSW, ACHP-SW
Department of Epidemiology and Health Policy Research, University of Florida, Gainesville, Florida

DAVID RAY DEMASO, MD
Senior Associate in Psychiatry and Cardiology, Department of Psychiatry, Children's Hospital Boston; Professor of Psychiatry and Pediatrics, Harvard Medical School, Boston, Massachusetts

MICHELLE M. ERNST, PhD
Assistant Professor, Division of Behavioral Medicine and Clinical Psychology; Department of Pediatrics, Cincinnati Children's Hospital Medical Center, University of Cincinnati College of Medicine, Cincinnati, Ohio

SANDRA L. FRITSCH, MD
Training Director, Child and Adolescent Psychiatry; Clinical Associate Professor, University of Vermont College of Medicine; Associate Clinical Professor, Tufts University School of Medicine, Maine Medical Center, Portland, Maine

GREGORY K. FRITZ, MD
Professor and Director, Division of Child and Adolescent Psychiatry, Alpert Medical School of Brown University, Providence; Academic Director, E.P. Bradley Hospital, East Providence; Associate Chief and Director of Child Psychiatry, Rhode Island Hospital/ Hasbro Children's Hospital; Bradley Hasbro Children's Research Center, Providence, Rhode Island

M. ELENA GARRALDA, MD, MPhil, FRCPsych, FRCPCH, DPM
Professor of Child and Adolescent Psychiatry, Academic Unit of Child and Adolescent Psychiatry, Imperial College London St Mary's Campus, London, United Kingdom

MARY MARGARET GLEASON, MD
Assistant Professor, Departments of Psychiatry and Behavioral Sciences and Pediatrics, Tulane Institute of Infant and Early Childhood Mental Health, New Orleans, Louisiana

ALKA GOYAL, MD
Assistant Professor of Pediatrics, Division of Pediatric Gastroenterology, Children's Hospital of Pittsburgh, Pittsburgh, Pennsylvania

BARBARA HASTIE, PhD
Assistant Professor, Department of Community Dentistry and Behavioral Science, University of Florida, Gainesville, Florida

PATRICIA IBEZIAKO, MD
Assistant in Psychiatry, Department of Psychiatry, Children's Hospital Boston; Instructor in Psychiatry, Harvard Medical School, Boston, Massachusetts

MARK C. JOHNSON, MD
Assistant Professor, Division of Child and Adolescent Psychiatry, Department of Pediatrics, Cincinnati Children's Hospital Medical Center, University of Cincinnati College of Medicine, Cincinnati, Ohio

CAPRICE KNAPP, PhD
Assistant Research Professor, Departments of Epidemiology and Health Policy Research, University of Florida, Gainesville, Florida

BRIAN P. KURTZ, MD
Department of Psychiatry, Division of Pediatric Psychiatry, Tufts Medical Center and Floating Hospital for Children at Tufts Medical Center, Boston MA

VANESSA MADDEN, BSc
Department of Epidemiology and Health Policy Research, University of Florida, Gainesville, Florida

ANN E. MALONEY, MD
Formerly, Clinical Assistant Professor, Child and Adolescent Psychiatry, University of Vermont College of Medicine; and currently, Assistant Professor, Center for Clinical Translational Research, Maine Medical Center Research Institute, Portland, Maine, Assistant Professor of Psychiatry, Tufts University Medical Center, Boston, and Assistant Professor, Department of Psychiatry, Child and Adolescent NeuroDevelopment Initiative, University of Massachusetts Medical School, Worcester, Massachusetts

LAURA MCLAFFERTY, BS
Department of Psychiatry, University of Pittsburgh School of Medicine, Pittsburgh, Pennsylvania

LOURIVAL BAPTISTA NETO, MD
Assistant Clinical Professor of Psychiatry, Division of Child and Adolescent Psychiatry, Department of Psychiatry, Columbia University; Director of Clinical Services in Pediatric Psychiatry, New York Presbyterian Hospital, Columbia University Medical Center, New York, New York

MARK W. OVERTON, MD
Fellow, Child and Adolescent Psychiatry Fellowship, Maine Medical Center, Portland, Maine

NANCY A. PATTISON, MD, FAAP
Post Pediatric Psychiatric Portal Resident, Department of Psychiatry, Maine Medical Center, Portland, Maine

TODD E. PETERS, MD
Division of Child and Adolescent Psychiatry, Alpert Medical School of Brown University, Providence, Rhode Island

DOUGLAS R. ROBBINS, MD
Clinical Professor, University of Vermont College of Medicine; Chair, The Glickman Family Center for Child and Adolescent Psychiatry; Division Chief, Child and Adolescent Psychiatry, Maine Medical Center, Portland, Maine

MATTHEW S. SIEGEL, MD
Assistant Professor, Department of Psychiatry, Tufts University School of Medicine, Boston, Massachusetts; Medical Director, Developmental Disorders Program, Spring Harbor Hospital, Westbrook, Maine; Department of Psychiatry, Division of Child Psychiatry, Maine Medical Center, Portland, Maine

WENDY E. SMITH, MD
Director, Division of Genetics, Department of Pediatrics, The Barbara Bush Children's Hospital, Maine Medical Center; Maine Medical Partners, Pediatric Specialty Care, Portland, Maine

LORI J. STARK, PhD
Professor, Director, Division of Behavioral Medicine and Clinical Psychology, Department of Pediatrics, Cincinnati Children's Hospital Medical Center, University of Cincinnati College of Medicine, Cincinnati, Ohio

MARGARET L. STUBER, MD
Jane and Marc Nathanson Professor of Psychiatry, Department of Psychiatry and Biobehavioral Sciences, Semel Institute, David Geffen School of Medicine at University of California, Los Angeles, Los Angeles, California

EVA SZIGETHY, MD, PhD
Associate Professor of Psychiatry, Department of Psychiatry, University of Pittsburgh School of Medicine; Director, Medical Coping Clinic, Division of Pediatric Gastroenterology, Children's Hospital of Pittsburgh, Pittsburgh, Pennsylvania

HARSH K. TRIVEDI, MD
Executive Medical Director and Chief-of-Staff, Vanderbilt Psychiatric Hospital; Associate Professor of Psychiatry, Vanderbilt Medical School, Nashville, Tennessee

DOUGLAS VANDERBILT, MD
Assistant Professor of Clinical Pediatrics, Keck School of Medicine at the University of Southern California; Developmental-Behavioral Pediatrics, Children's Hospital Los Angeles, Los Angeles, California

Contents

> Neurodevelopmental disorders with identified genetic etiologies present a unique opportunity to study gene-brain-behavior connections in child psychiatry. Parsing complex human behavior into dissociable components is facilitated by examining a relatively homogenous genetic population. As children with developmental delay carry a greater burden of mental illness than the general population, familiarity with the most common genetic disorders will serve practitioners seeing a general child population. In this article, basic genetic testing and 11 of the most common genetic disorders are reviewed, including the evidence base for treatment. Based on their training in child development, family systems, and multimodal treatment, child psychiatrists are well positioned to integrate cognitive, behavioral, social, psychiatric, and physical phenotypes, with a focus on functional impairment.

> Cystic fibrosis (CF) is a multisystemic life-limiting genetic disorder, primarily affecting respiratory functioning. Most patients with CF are diagnosed by 2 years of age, and the current median predicted survival rate is 37.4 years old, with 95% of patients dying from complications related to pulmonary infection. Given the chronic, progressive, and disabling nature of CF, multiple treatments are prescribed, most on a daily basis. Thus, this illness requires children, with the aid of their families, to adopt multiple health-related behaviors in addition to managing more typical developmental demands. The morbidity and mortality factors pose cognitive, emotional, and behavioral challenges for many children with CF and their families. This article applies a developmental perspective to describing the psychosocial factors affecting psychological adjustment and health-related behaviors relevant to infants, preschool and school-age children, and adolescents with CF. Topics particularly pertinent to developmental periods and medical milestones are noted, with clinical implications highlighted.

> Solid organ transplantation has become the first line of treatment for a growing number of life-threatening pediatric illnesses. With improved survival, research into the long-term outcome of transplant recipients has become important to clinicians. Adherence to medical instructions remains a challenge, particularly in the adolescent population. New immunosuppressant approaches promise to expand organ transplantation in additional directions. Extension of transplantation into replacement of organs such as faces and hands raises complex ethical issues.

> This article reviews the etiology, clinical characteristics, and treatment of inflammatory bowel disease (IBD) and associated psychological sequelae

in children and adolescents with this lifelong disease. Pediatric-onset IBD, consisting of Crohn's disease and ulcerative colitis, has significant medical morbidity and in many young persons is also associated with psychological and psychosocial challenges. Depression and anxiety are particularly prevalent and have a multifaceted etiology, including IBD-related factors such as cytokines and steroids used to treat IBD and psychosocial stress. A growing number of empirically supported interventions, such as cognitive behavioral therapy, hypnosis, and educational resources, help youth and their parents cope with IBD as well as the psychological and psychosocial sequelae. While there is convincing evidence that such interventions can help improve anxiety, depression, and health-related quality of life, their effects on IBD severity and course await further study.

Asthma, the most common chronic disease in children and adolescents in industrialized countries, is typified by airway inflammation and obstruction leading to wheezing, dyspnea, and cough. However, the effect of asthma does not end with pulmonary changes. Research has shown a direct link between asthma and stress and psychiatric illness, which if untreated results in heightened morbidity and effects on society. The link between asthma and psychiatric illness, however, is often underappreciated by many pediatric and child mental health professionals. This article reviews the diagnosis and treatment of asthma as well as the correlation between asthma and psychiatric illness in children in an effort to improve management and treatment strategies for this prevalent disease.

Diabetes mellitus is a common childhood illness, and its management is often complicated by mental health challenges. Psychiatric comorbidities are common, including anxiety, depression, and eating disorders. The illness can profoundly affect the developing brain and family functioning and have lifelong consequences. The child mental health provider can provide valuable assistance to support the child and family and assessment and treatment of comorbid mental health problems and to promote positive family functioning and normal developmental progress.

Child and adolescent psychiatrists frequently encounter children who are obese in their practices and may be asked to work alongside primary care physicians and other specialists who treat youngsters with obesity. To offer expert consultation, they must understand all aspects of the pediatric obesity epidemic. By summarizing the relevant endocrinology, cardiology, nutrition, exercise science, and public health literature, this review of pediatric obesity assesses the epidemic's background, delineates the challenges of clinical care, and appraises the therapeutic recommendations for this population of patients and their families.

> Pediatric epilepsy is a common, chronic, and challenging physical illness for children and their families. This article provides a medical overview and discusses the cognitive functioning and psychosocial adjustment as well as the psychiatric management for children and adolescents with pediatric epilepsy. The management of these children involves establishing a collaborative health care approach, evaluating academic functioning, considering psychotherapy, and managing psychopharmacologic treatment. A thorough understanding of the biopsychosocial concerns in pediatric epilepsy can enable medical providers and mental health clinicians to promote resiliency and adaptation in children and their families facing troubling seizure disorders.

> The psychosocial impact of human immunodeficiency virus (HIV) disease has been recognized since the beginning of the epidemic for affected adults, but there has been less focus on the impact of HIV on young people. Among HIV-positive (HIV+) adults, high levels of distress, psychiatric symptoms, and their associations with worse health outcomes were recognized early in the epidemic. Subsequently, many studies have focused on understanding the prevalence of psychiatric symptoms among HIV+ adults and on identifying effective treatments for these symptoms. Fewer studies have examined these symptoms and their treatments among HIV+ children and adolescents. This article reviews what is known about psychiatric syndromes among HIV+ youths, their treatments, and other psychosocial factors of concern to the psychiatrist when treating children and adolescents with HIV disease.

> The diagnosis and treatment of children and adolescents with cancer has a tremendous and lasting effect on the patients, their families, and other individuals in their social network. It carries a host of psychological and behavioral ramifications, from questions of mortality to changes in levels of functioning in multiple domains. In this review the authors address the psychosocial and treatment-related issues that arise in children with cancer, with attention to the adjustment to cancer at different developmental stages, mood and anxiety issues, treatment-related psychiatric sequelae, and the challenges faced by childhood cancer survivors.

> Children with life-threatening illnesses and their families may face physical, emotional, psychosocial, and spiritual challenges throughout the children's course of illness. Pediatric palliative care is designed to meet such

challenges. Given the psychosocial and emotional needs of children and their families it is clear that psychiatrists can, and do, play a role in delivering pediatric palliative care. In this article the partnership between pediatric palliative care and psychiatry is explored. The authors present an overview of pediatric palliative care followed by a summary of some of the roles for psychiatry. Two innovative pediatric palliative care programs that psychiatrists may or may not be aware of are described. Finally, some challenges that are faced in further developing this partnership and suggestions for future research are discussed.

THE CLINICS ARE NOW AVAILABLE ONLINE!

Access your subscription at:
www.theclinics.com

Preface

It's All Connected: Mental Health and Primary Care

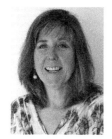 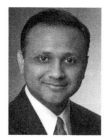

Sandra L. Fritsch, MD   Harsh K. Trivedi, MD
Guest Editors

There has long been a struggle, both in the medical profession and in the general public, about the interplay between the mind and the body. The notion that one's mental health can be so inextricably linked to one's physical health is often discounted or overlooked. Take, for example, the patient with asthma who is on prednisone and develops an altered mental status with hallucinations. A critical corollary to this is the notion that one's mental health care provider needs to work collaboratively with one's primary care provider. Indeed, this is all too often not the case and as the saying goes "never the twain shall meet." This phenomenon is also present in the healthcare industry as mental health carve-outs are used to manage mental health and substance abuse benefits.

With the recent passage of mental health parity legislation and health care reform, integration of mental health and physical health will be key. The Mental Health Parity and Addiction Equity Act passed by the US Congress ensures that coverage for mental health and substance abuse benefits will be equitable to medical and surgical benefits for group health plans with more than 50 employees. The Patient Protection and Affordable Care Act establishes accountable care organizations and creates a substrate for better integration of all care. The opportunity to improve children's health at this critical juncture should not be missed.

—From Harsh K. Trivedi, MD, Consulting Editor,
Child and Adolescent Pyschiatric Clinics of North America

Pediatr Clin N Am 58 (2011) xv–xvii
doi:10.1016/j.pcl.2011.06.015   **pediatric.theclinics.com**
0031-3955/11/$ – see front matter © 2011 Elsevier Inc. All rights reserved.

"Health is a state of complete physical, mental and social well-being, and not merely the absence of disease or infirmity."
— *World Health Organization, 1948*

As we enter the era of health care reform, "accountable care" organizations, and patient- and family-centered medical home models, never has the interface of pediatric health care and child mental health needs been more necessary. This edition was originally published in the *Child and Adolescent Psychiatry Clinics of North America* to help child and adolescent psychiatrists gain basic understanding of common pediatric illnesses, both to understand the health care challenges of their own patient in the office and to have a common language with primary care clinicians. The goal of this issue is to provide the reader a basic understanding of common chronic illnesses beginning in childhood (even at the time of conception); an understanding of the role of development, the family, and mental health issues, and how they may affect treatment adherence; and challenges faced when transitioning to adulthood.

The issue begins with an overview on the Pediatric Medical Home. Drs Trivedi's, Pattison's, and Neto's article provides a historical overview and defines basic concepts, constructs, and credentialing issues to become a Medical Home. Professor Garralda's article on unexplained physical complaints greatly underscores the need for a Pediatric Medical Home and the expertise of child mental health providers. She also reports on two chronic health conditions: recurrent abdominal pain and chronic fatigue syndrome; recent advances in evidence-based treatments for the conditions and mixed findings on the etiology of chronic fatigue syndrome.

The next series of articles focuses on the psychosocial challenges of the very premature infant, behavioral and psychiatric concerns for the neurodevelopmentally challenged child, and the developmental perspective of the child and family with cystic fibrosis. Drs Vanderbilt and Gleason address the mental health concerns of the very premature infant throughout the lifespan from attachment concerns in infancy, to attentional and learning issues in the school-age child, to risk for psychopathology in the teen and young adult. My colleagues, Drs Siegel and Smith, have written a concise, yet thorough article on phenotypic and behavioral manifestations of major genetically based syndromes. In addition they provide a primer on basic genetic testing. Our colleagues from Cincinnati Children's Hospital have written an elegant article addressing the developmental and psychosocial issues of the newborn to the transitioning young adult with cystic fibrosis. Their article could serve as a treatise on normal development and the impact of a chronic illness in the context of development. In addition the authors note the increasing social isolation for children and teens with cystic fibrosis, social isolation that is required to prevent/lessen infectious disease complications and novel Internet programs to address that isolation. One potential sequelae of cystic fibrosis is organ transplantation and our next article in the series is Dr Stuber's article on Psychiatric Issues in Pediatric Transplant. Included are a historical overview, family and psychological considerations pretransplant, pregnancy following transplant, and a brief note on the emerging field of face and hand transplants.

The next group of articles in the series includes potentially lifelong chronic illnesses including inflammatory bowel disease, asthma, diabetes mellitus, obesity, and epilepsy. Szigethy and colleagues educate us about the rapid advances in defining the genetics and development of treatments for the two major conditions of inflammatory bowel disease: Crohn's disease and ulcerative colitis. In addition, they underscore quality-of-life issues and comorbid mental health considerations lending to further treatment challenges. Peters and Fritz provide an overview of the medical and treatment aspects of asthma, linkages of psychosocial stressors and exacerbation of illness, the mental health conditions associated with asthma, and the essential work with the patient and family on symptom perception. The next article in the series focuses on diabetes mellitus, predominately insulin-dependent diabetes mellitus, but makes note of the increasing incidence of type 2 diabetes and metabolic syndrome. In addition to focusing on neuropsychological consequences of hypo- and hyperglycemia, the article also broadens our understanding of family factors, comorbid psychiatric conditions, and the notion of "assent" for treatment of the developing child. An overview of pediatric obesity is provided by Dr Maloney, which underscores the public health crisis and the need for policy reform and education to address this crisis. Our colleagues from Children's Hospital of Boston advance understanding of pediatric epilepsy and psychiatric concerns. They underscore the need for collaborative care models, involvement with schools, and factors to promote resiliency.

The final portion of the issue addresses potential life-threatening illnesses, including HIV and oncologic illnesses, and finishes with an article on palliative care. Dr Benton's article on pediatric HIV reports a chilling trend of increasing cases of HIV infection in teens, a preventable illness! She underscores the need to address mental health issues, which may lead to increased risk for infection as well as treatment adherence challenges of the HIV-infected person. Kurtz and Abrams write about the psychiatric issues associated with pediatric cancer, including the impact of the developmental level of the child and family at the time of diagnosis, the changing landscape, with an increasing number of children surviving cancer and factors aiding successful transition to adulthood, and the overall role of child mental health providers working with children, adolescents, and family members receiving treatment for pediatric cancer. Our issue ends with an informative overview of palliative care issues for children and families. Knapp and colleagues describe two innovative programs in Florida and provide a roadmap for mental health collaboration in pediatric palliative care.

The authors in this issue are to be commended for the valued contribution they each made under a deadline that was challenging. I must personally thank Sarah Barth at Elsevier for her support, guidance, and clear thinking during times of potential chaos or disaster and her recommendation to consider publishing the complete original edition in *Pediatric Clinics of North America*. Thanks must also be given to Kerry Holland at Elsevier for publishing the "Interface between Pediatrics and Children's Mental Health" in this issue of the *Pediatric Clinics of North America*. Thank you.

Sandra L. Fritsch, MD
Child and Adolescent Psychiatry
Maine Medical Center
Tufts University School of Medicine
22 Bramhall Street
Portland, ME 04102, USA

Harsh K. Trivedi, MD
Vanderbilt Psychiatric Hospital
1601 23rd Avenue South
Nashville, TN 37212, USA

E-mail addresses:
FRITSS@mmc.org (S.L. Fritsch)
harsh.k.trivedi@Vanderbilt.edu (H.K. Trivedi)

Pediatric Medical Home: Foundations, Challenges, and Future Directions

Harsh K. Trivedi, MD[a,b,*], Nancy A. Pattison, MD[c],
Lourival Baptista Neto, MD[d,e]

KEYWORDS

- Primary care • Medical home
- Child and adolescent psychiatry • History • Challenges
- Future directions • Health care delivery/access • Health policy

FOUNDATIONS AND EVOLUTION OF THE MEDICAL HOME

The term "medical home" first appeared in the 1967 American Academy of Pediatrics (AAP) publication *Standards of Child Health Care*. It was originally coined to delineate a central location that would serve as a repository for a child's medical records. The impetus for its creation was to ensure that neither gaps in care nor duplication of services occurred for children with special health care needs (CSHCN) who were commonly being treated by multiple providers.[1]

The AAP Council on Pediatric Practice further broadened the term in 1974 to include a broader vision for function, inclusivity, and nomenclature. It was proposed that pediatricians would become the advocates for continuity of care without regard for financial or social constraints. Likewise, this iteration included the concept that "every child deserves a medical home." It also included a more controversial notion: to eliminate all

A version of this article was previously published in the *Child and Adolescent Psychiatric Clinics of North America, 19:2.*
This work was not supported by any grant.
[a] Vanderbilt Medical School, 21st Avenue South, Nashville, TN 37232, USA
[b] Vanderbilt Psychiatric Hospital, 1601 23rd Avenue South, 1157, Nashville, TN 37212, USA
[c] Department of Psychiatry, Maine Medical Center, 22 Bramhall Street, Portland, ME 04102, USA
[d] Division of Child and Adolescent Psychiatry, Department of Psychiatry, Columbia University/ NYSPI, Unit 78, 1051 Riverside Drive, New York, NY 10032, USA
[e] New York Presbyterian Hospital, Columbia University Medical Center, 622 West 168th Street, New York, NY 10032, USA
* Corresponding author. Vanderbilt Psychiatric Hospital, 1601 23rd Avenue South 1157, Nashville, TN 37212.
E-mail address: harsh.k.trivedi@vanderbilt.edu

mention of pediatrician, family physician, and related terms in favor of exclusively using medical home. This last provision delayed adoption of medical home in an official policy of the AAP until 1979, when the central location and provision of continuity of care were accepted as central tenets.[1]

Attempts were then made for adoption of medical home models across multiple states. A review of early Every Child Deserves a Medical Home Training Programs found that pediatricians had difficulty in understanding the medical home concept. It was also difficult to communicate and manage care coordination across multiple systems. A key issue was the difficulty of securing reimbursement for this potentially time- and labor-intensive model of health care delivery.[2] After gaining federal grant support from the Maternal and Child Health Bureau and legislative victories for improved reimbursement via state legislatures and through Medicaid's Early and Periodic Screening, Diagnosis, and Treatment (EPSDT), the medical home model was applied to multiple states primarily for CSHCN.[1] **Box 1** reviews AAP's first official policy defining the medical home from 1992.[3]

During the 1990s, the medical home was further disseminated by inclusion as a core element in the Community Access to Child Health (CATCH) program, by creation of a national Medical Home Training Project, and by establishment of a National Center of Medical Home Initiatives for Children with Special Needs.[1] During this time, the Institute of Medicine (IOM) released a report entitled Crossing the quality chasm: a new health system for the 21st century. The report highlighted concerns regarding

---

Box 1
Major components of AAP medical home policy statement from 1992

- Medical care of infants, children, and adolescents ideally should be accessible, continuous, comprehensive, family centered, coordinated, and compassionate

- Delivered or directed by well-trained physicians who are able to manage or facilitate essentially all aspects of pediatric care

- Physician should be known to the child and family

- Physician should be able to develop mutually responsible and trusting relationship with patient and family

- Acknowledges that attainment of medical home is unobtainable for many children because of geographic barriers, personnel constraints, practice patterns, and economic and social forces

- Comprehensive health care should include provision of preventive care, assurance of care for acute illnesses, provision of care for an extended period of time to enhance continuity, identification and referral for subspecialty consultation, interaction with school and community agencies regarding special health needs, and maintenance of a central record that is accessible and confidential

- Potential for provision of such care as listed above at other venues including hospital outpatient clinics, school-based and school-linked clinics, community health centers, health department clinics, and others

- Potential for provision of such care as listed above by physicians or other health care providers under physician direction, such as nurses, nurse practitioners, and physician assistants

- Whether physically present or not, physician acts as child's advocate and assume control and ultimate responsibility for care provided.

Data from American Academy of Pediatrics ad hoc task force on definition of the medical home: the medical home. Pediatrics 1992;90:774.

safety and quality in the health care system, inability to translate research knowledge into clinical practice, inefficient and duplicative use of services, lack of application of information technology (IT) solutions, inability to shift to a model of managing chronic conditions, and patient experiences of difficulty in navigating this fragmented health care system. It then presented 6 major aims for a quality health care system; that the system should be safe, effective, patient-centered, timely, efficient, and equitable.[4]

The most recent iteration of AAP medical home policy focuses on creating an operational definition. An initial read of the medical home as the first stop for obtaining health care for all ages may seem like a resurrection of the gatekeeper mandate from 20 years ago. In that system, the patient was obligated to see the primary care physician for every aspect of medical care and without which approval would not be granted for referral to consultation or subspecialty care. The medical home is in actuality a team approach in which the multiple needs of the patient and family are addressed by the medical home team (consisting of the physician, physician extenders, nurses, care managers, and others) working collaboratively with specialists, the patient, and the family. The model works well for children and adolescents, especially those with complex medical issues. The medical home is a place, such as a physician's office, community health center, or a school-based student health service; and a process, a change in the health care system by which patients are provided high-quality, cost-effective medical care.[5]

Specific recommendations in the 2002 AAP medical home policy[6] include that "primary, pediatric medical subspecialty, and surgical specialty care providers should collaborate to establish shared management plans in partnership with the child and family and to formulate a clear articulation of each other's role"; and the "provision of care coordination service in which the family, the physician, and other service providers work to implement a specific care plan as an organized team." It also further delineated family centered care; provided for the discussion of unbiased information with the family about available services; and included the provision of culturally sensitive care. A list of desirable characteristics of the medical home is provided in **Box 2**.

In March 2007, the American Academy of Family Physicians, the AAP, the American College of Physicians, and the American Osteopathic Association issued *Joint principles of the patient-centered medical home*. These principles include patients having a personal physician in a physician-directed medical practice that is accessible, that is whole-person oriented, that provides coordinated care, that is concerned about patient quality and safety, and that receives payment that recognizes the added value provided to patients.[7]

Efforts have similarly been made to quantify how well a particular practice is meeting the qualities of being a medical home. Although many models exist, only 2 of the major assessment programs are described in this article. The National Committee for Quality Assurance (Physician Practice Connections–Patient-Centered Medical Home, http://www.ncqa.org) has created one such tool, which is endorsed by the AAP. It stresses safety and quality of care, coordinated care, whole-person orientation, physician-directed medical practice, and each patient having an ongoing relationship with a personal physician. It encourages access and adequate reimbursement as a result of the extra resources necessary to provide a medical home. By using a self-reporting Web-based rating system, it results in 3 levels of recognition. Increasing level of complexity and providing more aspects of the medical home model yield elevation to higher levels of the scale. For example, basic IT requirements at Level 1 mandate an electronic practice management system; Level 2 requires more IT, such as an electronic health record (EHR) or e-prescribing capability; and Level 3 requires

---

Box 2
Desirable characteristics of a medical home

Accessible

    Care is provided in the child's or youth's community

    All insurance, including Medicaid, is accepted

    Changes in insurance are accommodated

    Practice is accessible by public transportation, where available

    Families or youth are able to speak directly to the physician when needed

    The practice is physically accessible and meets Americans With Disabilities Act[10] requirements

Family centered

    The medical home physician is known to the child or youth and family

    Mutual responsibility and trust exist between the patient and family and the medical home physician

    The family is recognized as the principal caregiver and center of strength and support for the child

    Clear, unbiased, and complete information and options are shared on an ongoing basis with the family

    Families and youth are supported to play a central role in care coordination

    Families, youth, and physicians share responsibility in decision making

    The family is recognized as the expert in their child's care, and youth are recognized as the experts in their own care

Continuous

    The same primary pediatric health care professionals are available from infancy through adolescence and young adulthood

    Assistance with transitions, in the form of developmentally appropriate health assessments and counseling, is available to the child or youth and family

    The medical home physician participates to the fullest extent allowed in care and discharge planning when the child is hospitalized or care is provided at another facility or by another provider

Comprehensive

    Care is delivered or directed by a well-trained physician who is able to manage and facilitate essentially all aspects of care

    Ambulatory and inpatient care for ongoing and acute illnesses is ensured, 24 hours a day, 7 days a week, 52 weeks a year

    Preventive care is provided that includes immunizations, growth and development assessments, appropriate screenings, health care supervision, and patient and parent counseling about health, safety, nutrition, parenting, and psychosocial issues

    Preventive, primary, and tertiary care needs are addressed

    The physician advocates for the child, youth, and family in obtaining comprehensive care and shares responsibility for the care that is provided

    The child's or youth's and family's medical, educational, developmental, psychosocial, and other service needs are identified and addressed

    Information is made available about private insurance and public resources, including Supplemental Security Income, Medicaid, the State Children's Health Insurance Program, waivers, early intervention programs, and Title V State Programs for Children With Special Health Care Needs

Extra time for an office visit is scheduled for children with special health care needs, when indicated

Coordinated

A plan of care is developed by the physician, child or youth, and family and is shared with other providers, agencies, and organizations involved with the care of the patient

Care among multiple providers is coordinated through the medical home

A central record or database containing all pertinent medical information, including hospitalizations and specialty care, is maintained at the practice. The record is accessible, but confidentiality is preserved

The medical home physician shares information among the child or youth, family, and consultant and provides specific reasons for referral to appropriate pediatric medical subspecialists, surgical specialists, and mental health/developmental professionals

Families are linked to family support groups, parent-to-parent groups, and other family resources

When a child or youth is referred for a consultation or additional care, the medical home physician assists the child, youth, and family in communicating clinical issues

The medical home physician evaluates and interprets the consultant's recommendations for the child or youth and family and, in consultation with them and subspecialists, implements recommendations that are indicated and appropriate

The plan of care is coordinated with educational and other community organizations to ensure that special health needs of the individual child are addressed

Compassionate

Concern for the well-being of the child or youth and family is expressed and demonstrated in verbal and nonverbal interactions. Efforts are made to understand and empathize with the feelings and perspectives of the family as well as the child or youth

Culturally effective

The child's or youth's and family's cultural background, including beliefs, rituals, and customs, are recognized, valued, respected, and incorporated into the care plan

All efforts are made to ensure that the child or youth and family understand the results of the medical encounter and the care plan, including the provision of (para)professional translators or interpreters, as needed

Written materials are provided in the family's primary language

Physicians should strive to provide these services and incorporate these values into the way they deliver care to all children. (Note: pediatricians, pediatric medical subspecialists, pediatric surgical specialists, and family practitioners are included in the definition of physician.)

From The medical home. American Academy of Pediatrics, Medical Home Initiatives for Children with Special Needs Project Advisory Committee. Pediatrics 2002;110(1):184–6; with permission.

interoperable IT capabilities. For a practice to be recognized as a medical home, a certain number of points and certain mandated features must be in place.

The Accreditation Association for Ambulatory Health Care (AAAHC, http://www.aaahc.org) published its first set of standards on assessing a medical practice as a medical home in 2009. Any outpatient medical facility may seek accreditation by AAAHC. During an on-site accreditation survey, the extra qualities or standards that make a medical practice a medical home are assessed. This tool additionally assesses the age ranges that can be served by the medical home model in that practice. For example, in a group practice seeking accreditation as a medical home for all ages, if pediatrics is not covered 24/7, then that practice might opt to only seek accreditation as a medical home for adults and geriatrics. This would not necessarily affect their ability to be accredited as a medical facility overall. Regardless of which program is used, being accredited as a medical home is a symbol of quality. Likewise, as more practices meet medical home standards it is feasible to envision that such accreditation may become mandatory, that it may be a distinction of a superior practice, or that it may ultimately lead to greater reimbursement from payers.

CHALLENGES OF THE MEDICAL HOME

Pediatric mental health is a major public health issue. Approximately 1 in 4 pediatric primary care visits involve behavioral, emotional, or developmental issues.[8] A report published in 2009 by the IOM and the National Research Council, showed that 14% to 20% of adolescents experience mental, emotional, or behavioral disorders at any given time, with the first symptoms of these disorders occurring 2 to 4 years before the onset of a full-blown disorder.[9] Aligning well with this need, public mental health policies have long endorsed organized systems of care as critical in improving the quality of care. As the health care debate has evolved, strong emphasis has been placed on medical homes as high-quality, cost-effective health care delivery systems. Collaborative-care models, such as medical homes, have been found to be effective in treating mental illness in more than 35 randomized controlled trials.[10] As logical as it seems to shift to a medical home model, early experiences during its development as well as recent research findings point to significant potential barriers to its successful adoption and implementation.

Patient/Family Factors

As much as the medical home model supports the notion of working with a primary care physician who is known to the patient and the family, it is not uncommon for parents to avoid discussing mental health concerns with the pediatrician. Briggs-Gowan and colleagues[11] studied the prevalence of psychiatric disorders among 5- to 9-year-olds presenting to general pediatric practices as well as factors associated with parents' use of pediatricians as resources concerning emotional/behavioral issues. The study found that the prevalence of any disorder was 16.8% when using a standardized instrument, the Diagnostic Interview Schedule for Children (DISC-R). Most parents (55%) who reported concerns about their child also stated not discussing behavioral/emotional concerns with their pediatrician. Additional research needs to be conducted regarding the replicability of these findings as well as better understanding of the patient/family factors that prevent more forthright reporting of concerns to providers.

One such factor that may prevent parents from seeking help is the stigma of mental illness. In the first nationally representative study of public response to child mental health problems, Pescosolido and colleagues[12] studied public knowledge and assessment of child mental health problems in the National Stigma Study - Children. Of nearly 1400 participants, only 58.5% correctly identified depression and 41.9% correctly identified attention-deficit hyperactivity disorder (ADHD) in children. Surprisingly, a substantial group of participants who correctly identified the presence of a psychiatric disorder rejected the mental illness label (19.1% for ADHD and 12.8% for depression). The study concluded "Unless systematically addressed, the public's lack of knowledge, skepticism, and misinformed beliefs signal continuing problems for providers, as well as for caregivers and children seeking treatment."

In those parents willing to seek care, the effect of maternal or caregiver mental health issues on the ability to access care for the child as well as its effect on the child's symptomatology and functioning cannot be understated. For example, in a recent study of more than 9500 mother-child dyads, maternal mental health was significantly associated with the presence of ADHD in school-aged children supporting a link between maternal mental health and behavioral outcomes in children.[13] This is in addition to a long-standing body of evidence regarding the effects of maternal depression on infant attachment,[14] behavioral problems,[15] and psychopathology.[16] Consider, in addition, the effects of socioeconomic status,[17] language and racial disparities,[18] geographic issues,[19] and other related factors that affect access.

Provider Factors

Although there is support at an organizational level for the medical home model, there is significant variability regarding pediatrician attitudes to being responsible for managing and treating mental health problems. Stein and colleagues[20] recently studied whether practicing pediatricians broadly accepted responsibility for identification of emotional issues in their patients and whether they think their responsibility should be to treat or refer problems that they identify. Through the AAP Periodic Survey of Members, they found that less than one-third agreed that it is their responsibility to treat/manage such problems, except for children with ADHD. **Table 1** presents specific data divided by broad psychiatric diagnostic categories. Pediatricians were not asked about more severe psychopathology such as bipolar disorder, psychosis, or pervasive developmental disorders. Inclusion of these diagnoses would likely have yielded even lower outcomes for responsibility to identify and/or treat. In addition, as the investigators point out, "it is striking that the overwhelming majority think that it is their responsibility to refer most conditions, rather than to treat them. This is a major concern because a recent report by Rushton and colleagues[21] indicates that only 1

Table 1
Pediatrician agreement about being responsible based on child's condition/problem

Child's Problem/ Condition	Agree Pediatricians Should be Responsible for:		
	Identification, n (Weighted %)	Treating/Managing, n (Weighted %)	Referring, n (Weighted %)
Attention-deficit/ hyperactivity disorder	595 (91)	452 (70)	352 (54)
Child/adolescent depression	577 (88)	158 (25)	560 (86)
Behavior management problems	552 (85)	136 (21)	551 (85)
Learning disabilities	382 (59)	101 (16)	581 (89)
Anxiety disorders	536 (83)	180 (29)	509 (79)
Substance abuse	576 (88)	133 (21)	584 (90)
Eating disorders	597 (91)	204 (32)	551 (85)

Data from Stein REK, Horwitz SM, Storfer-Isser A, et al. Do pediatricians think they are responsible for identification and management of child mental health problems? Results of the AAP periodic survey. Ambul Pediatr 2008;8(1):11–17.

in 5 children with a psychosocial problem is referred outside the practice, suggesting that few pediatricians are actually doing what they say in terms of referral."

In an interesting corollary study, the same researchers conducted a smaller survey of primary care pediatricians and child and adolescent psychiatrists in 7 counties surrounding Cleveland, Ohio. They examined whether the 2 physician groups agreed about the pediatrician's role in identification, referral, and treatment of childhood mental health disorders; and whether they agreed about the barriers to the identification, referral, and treatment of childhood mental health disorders. Aside from ADHD, both physician groups agreed that pediatricians should be responsible for identifying and referring, but not treating child mental health conditions (**Table 2**). With regard to

Table 2
Primary care pediatrician and child and adolescent psychiatrist agreement with pediatrician responsibility for identifying, treating, and referring child mental health problems

Agree that Pediatricians Should be Responsible for	PCPs (n = 132)		CAPs (n = 31)		P Value
	N	Weighted %	N	Weighted %	
ADHD					
Identifying	117	90.1	23	73.3	0.01
Treating	110	85.6	18	57.0	0.005
Referring	46	35.6	17	56.8	0.04
Child/Adolescent Depression					
Identifying	111	84.7	19	62.6	0.008
Treating	17	13.3	3	9.2	0.52
Referring	110	83.8	23	84.7	0.91
Behavioral Problems					
Identifying	107	82.0	25	78.7	0.68
Treating	21	17.2	4	13.8	0.66
Referring	104	79.6	22	77.5	0.80
Learning Disabilities					
Identifying	77	58.4	20	61.3	0.77
Treating	14	11.1	5	18.4	0.30
Referring	120	91.6	24	82.8	0.16
Anxiety Disorders					
Identifying	112	85.0	22	68.2	0.04
Treating	21	16.5	2	7.7	0.26
Referring	106	80.9	25	88.6	0.30
Child Substance Abuse					
Identifying	113	86.3	25	81.6	0.51
Treating	15	11.7	2	7.7	0.55
Referring	120	91.9	25	84.7	0.26
Child Eating Disorders					
Identifying	115	89.2	27	87.4	0.77
Treating	20	15.5	3	10.3	0.49
Referring	114	86.8	24	82.0	0.52

Data from Heneghan A, Garner AS, Storfer-Isser A, et al. Pediatricians' role in providing mental health care for children and adolescents: do pediatricians and child and adolescent psychiatrists agree? J Dev Behav Pediatr 2008;29(4):262–9.

barriers, both agreed about the lack of mental health services. Child and adolescent psychiatrists identified pediatrician's lack of training in identifying child mental health problems as a barrier, whereas pediatricians cited poor confidence in their ability to treat child mental health problems with counseling, long waiting periods to see mental health providers, family failure to follow through on referrals, and billing/reimbursement issues.[22]

Systemic Factors

Although patient/family and provider factors are significant, the greatest impediments to successful adoption of the medical home lies within systemic factors. Current systemic issues include lack of standardized definitions, presence of administrative and financial barriers to its adoption, lack of technological interoperability and confidentiality concerns, lack of adequate training of medical professionals, relative supply/demand of specific types of providers, and a lack of evidence of large-scale feasibility and population-level improvement in health outcomes.

Although the medical home model exists and attempts have been made to create operational definitions of how this should form the basis of a medical practice, there are currently several stakeholders, each with varying views. A few rhetorical questions are included to illustrate how complicated the nuances can be. Should a pediatric medical home located in the outpatient clinic of a major tertiary care Children's Hospital in New York City look and function exactly the same as a pediatric medical home located in a rural family practitioner's office 75 miles from Missoula, Montana? Should a general pediatrician be expected to evaluate, manage, and treat the same level of patient severity as a developmental-behavioral pediatrician in the same medical home practice? How will the medical home model equilibrate with regard to varying expectations of providers and patients about when to refer patients to specialty providers, for which conditions, and after how much clinical intervention has occurred at the medical home site? How will patient outcomes be measured to ensure that each provider is functioning according to the medical home model and using optimal decision making to maximize medical home gains? Which assessment tool(s) will become universally accepted for evaluating medical home practices? Will accreditation become necessary to engage in medical practice or will it be the higher bar that only certain practices will meet? Will payers uniformly pay a premium for patients receiving care in these medical home sites? These and many additional questions will need to be figured out as the medical home is rolled out.

With our fragmented system of health care, there are also significant administrative and financial barriers to successful adoption of the medical home. The American Academy of Child and Adolescent Psychiatry (AACAP) Health Care Access and Economics Committee and the AAP Mental Health Task Force recently published a white paper for reducing administrative and financial barriers to access and collaboration as a method to improve mental health services in primary care.[23] Administrative barriers cited by this group include mental health intake procedures that bypass the primary care clinician, limited access to effective psychosocial interventions, lack of procedural and diagnostic parity in mental health and physical health benefits, inadequate communication and comanagement mechanisms, lack of coverage for recommended assessment and treatment services, and limited or no coverage for out-of-network providers (even when in-network providers are not able to see new clients). Financial barriers include lack of payment for visits with parents only (without child present as identified patient), lack of payment for other non–face-to-face components of care and consultation, insufficient payment for mental health services including management of emerging problems or symptoms not meeting a diagnostic threshold, insurance plan policies precluding payment to primary care clinicians when mental health diagnostic codes are reported, high out-of-pocket expenses for certain medications, and application of "incident to" payment methodology to prevent coverage of colocated services.

Although there has been a significant push recently for the adoption of meaningful use IT solutions in health care, several significant concerns remain unaddressed. Although many practices are beginning to use EHRs and e-prescribing, interoperability of different software platforms drastically impedes the ability of medical homes to effectively and efficiently collaborate with other providers.[5] Anecdotally, some physicians have found that even when newer versions of the same software programs are rolled out within the same practice, vendors are disallowing access to data in the previous software version out of concerns about liability if the newer software either omits or erroneously migrates the wrong information. Likewise, as medicine shifts to IT solutions, the potential for breach of confidentiality also increases. Because of the stigma of mental illness, this is of particular concern to the mental health community.

Even if these concerns could be addressed, there are also fundamental issues in the training of physicians to care for psychiatric illnesses. Nationally, there has been a trend to decrease the length of psychiatry rotations in medical schools[24] with many offering little to no exposure to child psychiatry. It can easily be said that a first year house officer in Psychiatry is more likely to know how to appropriately diagnose and manage asthma or diabetes; than a first year Pediatrics resident is likely to know how to appropriately diagnose and manage ADHD or first break psychosis. When these medical students graduate and enter a pediatrics residency, the Accreditation Council for Graduate Medical Education Residency Review Committee (RRC) training requirements do not mandate any mental health training thus leading to minimal development of knowledge base and clinical management of psychiatric illnesses. How then can primary care pediatricians be expected to safely and effectively diagnose, manage, and refer all children walking into their primary care pediatric practices with mental health problems?

Even for those medical home practices that are keen to adopt mental health diagnosis and management, there is the problem of supply/demand of providers. Although screening has been shown to be feasible in pediatric practices,[25] a common problem is where to refer the patients who are severely ill and require specialty care. Children's mental health faces a significant shortage of all levels of providers. For example, in child and adolescent psychiatry, 7000 are in practice although there is currently a need for 30,000.[26] Imbalances also exist on the primary care end of this equation. In a commentary regarding whether everyone can have a medical home, Pan[27] notes that the growth in the number of general pediatricians will greatly exceed the growth of the pediatric population by 2020. Likewise, this growth is expected to exceed sufficiency and create a competitive situation where there may not be enough pediatric patients for primary care pediatricians and family practitioners. Pan suggests "Family medicine could partially or wholly withdraw from the care of children and focus on the aging population, or they could compete directly with pediatrics for the primary care of children and adolescents. An alternative to these options is for family medicine and pediatrics to collaborate in providing medical homes for all children and their families. Collaboration is an important option for the future."

On the issue of an evidence base, although studies have been done to elucidate the effectiveness of medical homes for CSHCN, significant data are lacking as to whether the medical home model can be justified for nonmedically complicated children. Homer and colleagues[28] looked at the evidence for medical homes for children with special health care needs. After reviewing more than 30 studies, they found that there is moderate support for the conclusion that "medical homes provide improved health related outcomes for children with special health care needs," however, "more research encompassing all or most of the attributes of the medical home need to be undertaken." In an era of health care reform and concerns about the ballooning cost of health care, robust data are needed on clinically significant improvements in health, actual cost-effectiveness of this health care delivery model, as well as, data justifying expansion of the medical home model to include all comers.

FUTURE DIRECTIONS

The argument in favor of increasing access to high-quality mental health care by promoting primary care–mental health integration is compelling. Using the medical home as a platform makes sense and could decrease costs in the long-term. This could be achieved by focusing on prevention and health promotion, which could lead to less frequent emergency room visits or hospitalizations. The current health care debate has the potential to push health care delivery toward the medical home model.

Child psychiatry and pediatric primary care providers have a great opportunity to use the medical home model as a platform to further integrate mental health and primary care. Pediatric primary care providers can provide additional mental health care through incorporating screenings and directly treating less severely mentally ill patients. Pediatric mental health providers can support primary care providers through a combination of colocation, consultation and enhanced collaboration. The concept of less fragmented and better-coordinated care system models needs to be universal and must include mental health. Successful adoption of the medical home model will require a comprehensive plan to address the challenges reviewed more than. Specific action items to aid in the adoption of the medical home are discussed in the following paragraphs.

One of the largest barriers to overcome is stigma. Australia and New Zealand have focused extensively in destigmatizing mental illness. Like Minds Like Mine (http://www.likeminds.govt.nz) is a high-profile national campaign funded by the Ministry of Health in New Zealand. This program has won a prestigious advertising award and has featured well-known New Zealanders talking about their experience of mental illness. Those featured include athletes, musicians, business people, and others with prominence in the community. The general public would benefit from a more open environment to discuss their mental health concerns as well as a better understanding of fundamental concepts, such as the fact that mental illness is just as real as heart disease or cancer; and that it is quite treatable.

Next comes the issue of developing a greater knowledge base and improved clinical acumen in the provider community. Improved psychiatric education in medical schools and in postgraduate residency training is a fundamental step in that process. Mental health needs to be taught as a common problem in routine medical visits. Greater emphasis needs to be placed on psychiatry, and more specifically, child psychiatry as a core medical school rotation. In 2009, the AAP published a policy statement on Mental Health Competencies for Pediatric Primary Care.[29] The statement suggests strategies for mental health education, describes the many challenges and states, "attainment of the mental health competencies proposed is a future goal, not a current expectation." Currently, pediatric residents have limited exposure to mental health during their training and even when it happens, it is often an elective rotation and not considered an important aspect of their training as a physician. The RRC needs to mandate exposure to child psychiatry into pediatric residency training.

For those providers who are already in practice, significant efforts need to be put in place to retool their skill set. One innovative method is through the use of standardized assessment and treatment algorithms.[30] By beginning with the most common chief complaints presenting to a pediatric primary care office, the use of a programmed text can allow providers to input clinical information to ascertain the next steps in the diagnosis and treatment of common child mental health conditions. With time, as these algorithms are used repeatedly, pediatric primary care providers would become more accomplished in incorporating best practices into their management of psychiatric conditions. A key aspect of such a resource is the inclusion of a primer on how to restructure a primary care practice to efficiently treat and manage youth and families dealing with mental health problems; how to incorporate the standard use of pediatric rating scales[31] and screening tools,[32] such as the pediatric symptom checklist, within routine primary care appointments; and incorporation of when to refer criteria so that primary care providers are not left managing cases that are beyond their level of expertise.[30]

The next major hurdle comes in the form of creating viable practice models. One such method is to colocate pediatric mental health providers with primary care providers. This would allow for greater provision of direct patient care in the primary care setting; perhaps including assessment and treatment of more complex patients by mental health providers; serve as an in-house consultation service to primary care providers; and can allow for greater collaboration for shared cases. Colocation would also improve access to mental health care to patients with other serious or chronic illnesses, such as diabetes or heart conditions, whose medical course and recovery are impaired by a coexisting mental health disorder, such as depression. In addition, improved behavioral outcomes that affect overall wellness in children, such as obesity, can be addressed in collaboration between the mental health and primary care provider.

Colocation also allows for greater access to appropriate treatment of mild or moderate mental health disorders by either direct service from the mental health provider or through treatment provided directly by the primary care provider as a result of easier consultation. For more complex cases, improved referral and linkage to mental health specialty care is advantageous. This health care delivery model can only be successful if coding and billing limitations are addressed to make it financially viable. More broadly, administrative and financial barriers identified in the Joint AACAP/AAP white paper[23] also need to be addressed.

In 2006, in a landmark decision with national implications, the US District Court in Springfield, MA, ruled that the Commonwealth of Massachusetts was violating the federal Medicaid Act by failing to provide home-based mental health services to an estimated 15,000 children with serious emotional disturbance. The class lawsuit was known as Rosie D versus Romney and was based on the broad interpretation of the federal Medicaid Act, in particular the EPSDT mandate. Attorneys for the plaintiff class contended that state officials violated the Medicaid Act by failing to comply with its EPSDT mandate. As a result, Massachusetts has greatly enhanced their requirements for screening and treatment of developmental and mental health issues for children and adolescents.

The Massachusetts Child Psychiatry Access Program (MCPAP) is a collaborative-care model that focuses on expanding the role of the mental health provider as a consultant to pediatric primary care offices. As opposed to a straight colocation model, MCPAP provides pediatricians with immediate access to telephone consultation, outpatient evaluation, care coordination, and educational resources to support the provision of care for children in the primary care setting. Instead of simply accepting consults, MCPAP clinicians help to educate primary care providers about appropriate next steps and may eliminate the need for a referral to a child psychiatry specialist for uncomplicated patients. For more complex cases, MCPAP provides care coordination to facilitate referral to a child and adolescent psychiatrist for treatment. Pediatric practices participating in MCPAP agree to maintain appropriate involvement in the monitoring and coordination of care for children with mental health problems.

Perhaps, a more immediate and attainable intervention is the promotion of mental health education through Collaborative Office Rounds (COR). COR have been established in various communities for the purpose of enhancing mental health knowledge and skills of primary care providers and their communication with mental health specialists.[33–35] It has typically been done through a 1- to 2-hour session per month that involves psychiatrists and/or developmental-behavioral pediatricians and primary care providers in a case-based discussion. COR could be considered as 1 starting point to developing relationships between mental health specialists and primary care providers that would then develop into more formalized consultation systems. Financing and sustaining a COR program can sometimes pose a significant obstacle. In some places, COR programs have been funded through grants. Innovative programs funded by public and private payers to support COR would be beneficial. Likewise, investment in developing and researching collaborative models of care between child psychiatry and primary care is needed to further elucidate best practices.

True improvement in child mental health will not occur without a significant increase in the availability of child mental health providers. Passage of the Child Health Care Crisis Relief Act[36] in Congress to provide loan forgiveness and scholarships to individuals who study in graduate and medical programs in child mental health is crucial to the success of the medical home.

There is a significant need to show improved outcomes for children within medical homes, particularly when using the broader definition to include all children. Because of economic realities in health care, it will also be imperative to show long-term cost savings to gain broader acceptance from private ensurers. There is currently a medical home demonstration project being conducted by the Center for Medicare and Medicaid Services to investigate the value of the medical home for care of adults with chronic conditions.[5] It will be important to have such a study for children as well as in the general population for those without chronic medical conditions.

A great opportunity to incorporate the medical home model as a health care delivery platform is currently on the horizon to improve mental health care by further integrating mental health and primary care. Significant resources will be needed to address the multitude of challenges present in preventing its successful adoption. The presence of a robust evidence base to support its adoption will be key.

REFERENCES

1. Sia C, Tonniges T, Osterhus E, et al. History of the medical home concept. Pediatrics 2004;113:1473–8.
2. Moore B, Tonniges T. The "every child deserves a medical home" training program: more than a traditional continuing medical education course. Pediatrics 2004;113(Suppl):1479–84.
3. American Academy of Pediatrics ad hoc task force on definition of the medical home: the medical home. Pediatrics 1992;90:774.

4. Institute of Medicine. Crossing the chasm: a new health system for the 21st century. Washington, DC: National academy Press; 2001.

5. Wegner S, Antonelli R, Turchi R. The medical home – improving quality of primary care for children. Pediatr Clin North Am 2009;56:953–64.

6. American Academy of Pediatrics, Medical Home Initiatives for Children with Special Needs Project Advisory Committee. The medical home. Pediatrics 2002;110(1):184–6, Reaffirmed Pediatrics 2008;122(2):450.

7. Joint principles of the patient-centered medical home. March 2007. Available at: http://www.aafp.org/online/etc/medialib/aafp_org/documents/policy/fed/jointprinciplespcmh0207.Par.0001.File.tmp/022107medicalhome.pdf. Accessed February 8, 2010.

8. Cooper S, Valleley RJ, Polaha J, et al. Running out of time: physician management of behavioral health concerns in rural pediatric primary care. Pediatrics 2006;118:132–8.

9. The National Research Council and the Institute of Medicine. Preventing mental health, emotional and behavioral disorders among young people: progress and possibilities. Washington, DC: National Academies Press; 2009.

10. Thielke S, Vannoy S, Unutzer J. Integrating mental health and primary care. Clinics in Office Practice. Prim Care 2007;34:571–92.

11. Briggs-Gowan MJ, Horowitz SM, Schwab-Stone ME, et al. Mental health in pediatric settings: distribution of disorders and factors related to service use. J Am Acad Child Adolesc Psychiatry 2000;39(7):841–9.

12. Pescosolido BA, Jensen PS, Martin JK, et al. Public knowledge and assessment of child mental health problems: findings from the National Stigma Study-Children. J Am Acad Child Adolesc Psychiatry 2008;47(3):339–49.

13. Lesesne CA, Visser SN, White CP. Attention-deficit/hyperactivity disorder in school-aged children: association with maternal mental health and use of health care resources. Pediatrics 2003;111:1232–7.

14. Lyons-Ruth K, Connell DB, Grunebaum HU. Infants at social risk: maternal depression and family support services as mediators of infant development and security of attachment. Child Dev 1990;61:85–98.

15. Webster-Stratton C, Hammond M. Maternal depression and its relationship to life stress, perceptions of child behavior problems, parenting behaviors, and child conduct problems. J Abnorm Child Psychol 1988;16:299–315.

16. Beardslee WR, Bemporad J, Keller MB, et al. Children of parents with a major affective disorder: a review. Am J Psychiatry 1983;140:825–32.

17. Lasser KE, Himmelstein DU, Woolhandler S. Access to care, health status, and health disparities in the United States and Canada: results of a cross-national population-based survey. Am J Public Health 2006;96(7):1–8.

18. Flores G, Tomany-Korman SC. The language spoken at home and disparities in medical and dental health, access to care, and use of services in US children. Pediatrics 2008;121:e1703–14.

19. Gopal KS, Strickland BB, Ghandour RM, et al. Geographic disparities in access to the medical home among US CSHCN. Pediatrics 2009;124:S352–60.

20. Stein REK, Horwitz SM, Storfer-Isser A, et al. Do pediatricians think they are responsible for identification and management of child mental health problems? Results of the AAP periodic survey. Ambul Pediatr 2008;8:11–7.

21. Rushton J, Bruckman D, Kelleher K. Primary care referral of children with psychosocial problems. Arch Pediatr Adolesc Med 2002;156:592–8.

22. Heneghan A, Garner AS, Storfer-Isser A, et al. Pediatricians' role in providing mental health care for children and adolescents: do pediatricians and child and adolescent psychiatrists agree? J Dev Behav Pediatr 2008;29:262–9.
23. American Academy of Child and Adolescent Psychiatry Committee on Health Care Access and Economics and American Academy of Pediatrics Task Force of Mental Health. Improving mental health services in primary care: reducing administrative and financial barriers to access and collaboration. Pediatrics 2009;123:1248–51.
24. Serby M, Schmeidler J, Smith J. Length of psychiatry clerkships: recent changes and the relationship to recruitment. Acad Psychiatry 2002;26:102–4.
25. Zuckerbrot RA, Maxon L, Pagar D, et al. Adolescent depression screening in primary care: feasibility and acceptability. Pediatrics 2007;119:101–8.
26. Kim WJ, Enzer N, Bechtold D, et al. Meeting the mental health needs of children and adolescents: addressing the problems of access to care. Report of the Task Force on Workforce Needs. Washington, DC: American Academy of Child and Adolescent Psychiatry; 2001.
27. Pan RJ. A Jacobian future: can everyone have a medical home? Pediatrics 2006; 118:1254–6.
28. Homer CJ, Klatka K, Romm D, et al. A review of the evidence for the medical home for children with special health care needs. Pediatrics 2008;122(4): e922–37.
29. American Academy of Pediatrics Committee on Psychosocial Aspects of Child and Family Health Task Force on Mental Health. The future of pediatrics: mental health competencies for pediatric primary care. Pediatrics 2009;124:410–21.
30. Trivedi HK, Kershner JD. Practical child and adolescent psychiatry for pediatrics and primary care. Cambridge (UK): Hogrefe and Huber; 2009.
31. Navon M, Nelson D, Pagano M, et al. Use of the Pediatric Symptom Checklist in strategies to improve preventative behavioral healthcare. Psychiatr Serv 2001;52: 800–4.
32. Stancin T, Palermo TM. A review of the behavioral screening practices in pediatric settings: do they pass the test? J Dev Behav Pediatr 1997;18:183–93.
33. DeMaso DR, Knight JR, editors. Collaboration essentials for pediatric and child and adolescent psychiatric residents: working together to treat the child. American Academy of Child and Adolescent Psychiatry and American Academy of Pediatrics. Boston: Children's Hospital Boston; 2004.
34. Fishman ME, Kessel W, Heppel DE, et al. Collaborative office rounds: continuing education in the psychosocial/developmental aspects of child health. Pediatrics 1997;99(4):e5.
35. Connor DF, McLaughlin TJ, Jeffers-Terry M, et al. Targeted child psychiatric services: a new model of pediatric primary care clinician—child psychiatry collaborative care. Clin Pediatr 2006;45:423–34.
36. Child Health Care Crisis Relief Act of 2009. HR 1932, 11th Cong, 1st session. 2009. Available at: http://www.thomas.gov. Accessed February 8, 2010.

Unexplained Physical Complaints

M. Elena Garralda, MD, MPhil, FRCPsych, FRCPCH, DPM

KEYWORDS

• Physical complaints • Somatization • Somatoform disorders

Physical complaints tend not to feature prominently in the everyday work of child and adolescent psychiatrists or child and youth mental health clinics. These problems are more likely to be referred to the local pediatric clinic. As a result, expertise in the assessment and management of the psychiatric aspects of such problems varies considerably and can be limited. An exception are psychiatric pediatric liaison teams as they deal primarily with problems at the interface between physical and mental health problems, which include medically unexplained symptoms. Nevertheless, family engagement in assessment and treatment can be problematic even for specialist liaison teams.

Whether children and families engage with and benefit from psychiatric services depends to a large extent on whether families appreciate the link between physical and psychiatric symptoms, and wish to work on the comorbid psychopathology such as anxiety disorders or on the contributing psychosocial problems such as family disruption or school difficulties. Benefit may also depend on the joint expertise of pediatric and child and adolescent mental health teams in attending to these types of problems.

DEFINITIONS AND GENERAL CLINICAL ISSUES

Physical complaints or somatic symptoms are common in children and adolescents, and the majority will have a physiologic explanation rather than one deriving from a diagnosable medical illness. Nevertheless, they often lead to pediatric visits. General population surveys show that young people report a mean of 2 somatic symptoms being present "a lot" in the 2 weeks before assessment; the most common being headaches, low energy, sore muscles, nausea and upset stomach, back pains, and stomach pains.[1] Many of these symptoms will be mild but for a minority they will be recurrent and impairing. About 1 in 10 children report recurrent impairing aches and pains, and a comparable number have distressing somatic symptoms or are regarded by their parents as "sickly."

The way complaints are managed relies on how they are understood; if parents or young people see them as a likely expression of medical illness, they will either visit

A version of this article was previously published in the *Child and Adolescent Psychiatric Clinics of North America, 19:2.*
Academic Unit of Child and Adolescent Psychiatry, Imperial College London St Mary's Campus, Norfolk Place, London W2 1PG, UK
E-mail address: e.garralda@imperial.ac.uk

Pediatr Clin N Am 58 (2011) 803–813
doi:10.1016/j.pcl.2011.06.002
0031-3955/11/$ – see front matter © 2011 Elsevier Inc. All rights reserved.

their doctor or handle the problem themselves using their personal medical knowledge and experience. On the other hand, they may be of the opinion that the symptoms are temporary and unlikely to indicate illness, such as when a child's abdominal symptoms are linked to certain foods "not agreeing" with them. Alternatively, they can have a psychological or social explanation, for example, symptoms exacerbated by stress such as worries about school, the child complaining in order to be comforted and to avoid going to school, or a particularly feared lesson. Common and effective parental reactions to dealing with symptoms thought to be psychosocially influenced are to "play down" the importance of the symptom so that the child learns to cope, or to comfort the child and try to find the cause of the distress.

There are times, however, when symptoms become marked and persistent, remain unexplained after pediatric examination, and cause considerable distress and impairment. There may also be indications of ongoing stress or associated psychiatric symptoms; however, these are not always obvious and parents and doctors may be at a loss to explain the severity and impairment. A psychiatric opinion is helpful to assist with differential diagnosis and confirm or exclude the presence of somatization, or of a somatoform disorder or another primary or comorbid psychiatric disorder amenable to psychiatric intervention. It is also helpful to identify psychosocial factors likely to be playing a part in symptom maintenance even when a definite psychiatric disorder is not present, and in medically informed psychosocial rehabilitation.

Somatization and Somatoform Disorders

For many children coming into contact with medical services with unexplained physical complaints, there will be evidence of somatization. This term describes a constellation of clinical and behavioral features indicating a tendency to experience and communicate distress through somatic symptoms unaccounted for by pathologic findings, and for these symptoms nevertheless to be attributed to physical illness, thus leading the patient to seek medical help. Somatization is a crucial feature of several ICD-10 (*International Classification of Diseases*, tenth revision) and DSM-IV (*Diagnostic and Statistical Manual of Mental Disorders*, fourth edition) somatoform disorders of which the most commonly seen in children and adolescents are persistent somatoform pain disorder, dissociative/conversion disorder, and—even though not part of DSM-IV and referred to as "neurasthenia" in ICD-10—chronic fatigue syndrome (CFS). Mental factors are assumed to have major significance as either precipitating or maintenance influences in these disorders.

Unexplained physical complaints become a clinical problem when, in addition to severe, recurrent, and impairing, they lead to repeated medical contacts with expectations of medical treatment. It is common by that stage for parents and children to hold the belief that there is some medical problem their doctor may be missing; this leads on the one hand to excessive special investigations determined more by the principle of not leaving any stone unturned than by sound clinical indication, and on the other to a reluctance to seek or accept a referral for psychiatric evaluation. Rejection of psychiatric assessment by children and parents can be intense to the extent that it seems unreasonable to others.

Psychological "Mindedness" and Related Dilemmas

The intensity is partly related to the fear that a physical illness will be missed, but probably also to a lack of psychological "mindedness," with difficulty acknowledging that psychological and physical symptoms may be closely interconnected, and a concomitant reluctance to consider that the child and family may be able to gain control over them. This reluctance is sometimes a result of frustrated efforts to manage the complaints at early stages in their presentation, and is also likely to be connected to impairment being a central feature of severe functional somatic symptoms.

Impairment often involves withdrawal and avoidance of everyday responsibilities and stresses. Many children severely affected with unexplained medical complaints and somatoform disorders are in stressful situations they find difficult to manage or seek support for on a day-to-day basis. In this context illness represents a double-edged sword; while it is an unpleasant distressing physical experience it is also an escape or way out of these stresses. The withdrawal is, however, only legitimate and acceptable if the negative experience of illness and its physical nature are acknowledged by others, thus assuming that the child is at the mercy of a "force majeure," and therefore unable to resist. A markedly affected child will often seemingly "hold on" to the illness and oppose expectations from others that he or she may have some control over the impairment. Children might challenge families and doctors when asked to contribute actively to the rehabilitation process, or simply display passive noncooperation. These children might feel too weak to resist the symptoms, or be too frightened to face the prospect of returning to everyday life and those very stressors the symptoms are helping to avoid. It is not uncommon, therefore, for some children to angrily state that the doctor or rehabilitation staff do not "believe" the symptoms because otherwise they would not be expected to do anything strenuous or demanding.

Assessment and Management

Because of the nature of these problems, assessment and treatment need to take due note of both the physical and psychosocial contributory and maintaining factors. The best approach is one using a biopsychosocial framework whereby problems are not regarded as either physical or mental, but rather whereby the relative contribution of biologic, psychological, and social factors is considered. The view that physical symptoms are wholly medically explained and therefore within the exclusive domain of the pediatrician, or alternatively are wholly medically unexplained and by implication are not within the pediatrician's domain but rather within the domain of psychiatric teams, does not correspond to clinical experience. A medical disorder may trigger or underlie medical symptoms which then become unexplained not in themselves but rather in terms of their severity or the impairment caused. For example, *excessive* lower limb weakness may follow a bone fracture and subsequent immobilization, or pseudoseizures may manifest in a child with epilepsy. In practice, pediatricians often recognize that psychosocial issues can influence pediatric problems, whether with or without an organic substrate, as demonstrated in other articles in this issue. Understanding unexplained medical problems and their management at the pediatric clinic therefore needs to take into account the triggering of physical problems or other stressors, as well as psychosocial problems that may play a part in their maintenance. A particular complicating, and not uncommon, factor in clinical practice is when the attending clinician suspects psychological issues are playing a part, as in somatization or somatoform disorders, but this is at odds with the child's and parental attitudes and views about the nature of the problem and who is the best professional to help. Engaging and working with the family to achieve a common view will thus be a requirement before effective treatment can be undertaken.

PREVIOUS REVIEWS

Several reports have reviewed the literature on unexplained physical complaints, and somatization and somatoform disorders as they manifest in children and young people. This article reviews first the main conclusions from these reviews and then considers new findings that have helped illuminate their nature and management.

The clinical picture, frequency and epidemiology, etiologic factors, and treatment of unexplained physical complaints have been reviewed comprehensively.[2–5] An early review of child psychiatric symptoms with somatic presentations[4] highlighted that the nosologic validity and boundaries of somatoform disorders, as described in DSM-IV and ICD-10 classification systems, were still comparatively untested in children. Nevertheless, there was converging evidence that functional or likely medically unexplained physical complaints were common and present in about 1 in 10 children in the general population. These symptoms often involved recurrent abdominal pains or headaches, and there was a female predominance. Concurrent psychopathology was present in excess in affected children (between one-third to one-half) and usually consisted of emotional (anxiety of depressive) disorders, disruptive problems being a considerably less common association.

Specific child personality features were noted with several affected children who were described in clinical reports as conscientious or obsessional, sensitive, insecure, and anxious; high academic expectations were also noted. An excess of stressful events commonly involving school activity but also sometimes physical illness were reported, as was illness triggering symptom onset. Family influences were thought to be important; more specifically, family health problems, preoccupation with illness, and in some cases parents appearing anxiously sensitized to the experience of physical symptoms and seeking reassurance from medical services. For a small number of families profound family disorganization and sexual abuse were relevant. Clinicians described high levels of enmeshment between family members and parental overprotection. The emerging picture was one of children with vulnerable personality features who developed functional somatic symptoms following traumatic (physical or psychosocial) events.

The review of the topic by Campo and Fritsch[2] was generally in line with these observations and conclusions. This review addressed a variety of unexplained physical symptoms, not just abdominal pains and headaches but also limb pains and aching muscles ("growing pains"), although they noted that pseudoneurologic symptoms are comparatively rare in community samples. Campo and Fritsch highlighted that presentations are often multi-symptomatic and that—in contrast with the frequency of functional symptoms—somatoform disorder presentations are rare in childhood. The excess of unnecessary and potentially dangerous and costly medical investigations and treatments to which these children are exposed, alongside the excessive use of health care services, was emphasized.

A further summary review[5] considered tentative findings about possible biologic substrates for unexplained physical complaints; for example, altered colonic motility, enhanced gastrointestinal sensitivity, and possible inflammatory changes in children with functional gastrointestinal symptoms. Evidence was starting to emerge that parental reinforcement of symptoms and discouragement of coping were likely to be factors contributing to symptom maintenance, and that the effect of external stressors on the emergence of physical symptoms might be mediated by low levels of social competence.

A recent article[3] has outlined some of the reasons for studying unexplained medical symptoms in children separately from adults, including the observation that the presenting symptoms tend to be specific to childhood and therefore questionnaires designed for adults are not appropriate, and the importance of gathering parental reports especially for preadolescents. Recent research has confirmed the presence of unexplained medical symptoms in young preschool children, and their association with anxiety symptoms in the child and distress in the parents. More unexplained somatic symptoms are reported by older than younger girls, and there is congruence generally between symptom reporting, illness attitudes conducive to somatization, and low academic attainment.

This review mentioned an unusual syndrome linked to somatization in children called "pervasive refusal" whereby children and adolescents present with profound and pervasive withdrawal, including refusal to eat, drink, talk, walk, and engage in any form of self-care. Although the nosology of this syndrome has not been established, it appears to be an extreme and serious manifestation of somatoform and other stress disorders. The review also noted factitious presentations in childhood, whereby parents fabricate childhood illness or children themselves cause damage to wounds or scratch corneas, as problems related to childhood somatization, although the active part played by young people or their parents in symptom production is at variance with the traditional assumption that in somatization and somatoform disorders unconscious mechanisms determine symptom production.

UPDATE ON MORE RECENT FINDINGS

In recent years several studies have taken these issues forward, and are reviewed here briefly. These studies address the development of instruments to assist the investigation of unexplained physical symptoms in children, the contribution of symptoms to pediatric practice, and further work on associations with psychopathology, biologic and psychological vulnerabilities, sensibility to stress in the child, and familial influences, as well as on treatment and outcome. Because much of this work has addressed recurrent abdominal pains and CFS, these conditions feature most prominently and are used as models for understanding general somatization principles.

The Use of Fit for Purpose Questionnaires and Epidemiologic Findings

An important methodological advance has been the development of questionnaires to assess physical symptoms and clusters likely to be related to somatization in children. The Children Somatization Inventory (CSI) created by Garber and colleagues[1] in 1991 is a well-standardized self-rated scale for adolescents detailing 36 common physical symptoms experienced over the previous 2-week period. The CSI has been used across different countries with results comparable to those from the original North American adolescent school sample. The most recent survey was carried out in the United Kingdom and found a median CSI symptom/severity score of 12 (5,23), with headaches, feeling low in energy, sore muscles, faintness, and nausea being the most frequent, and girls scoring higher than boys.[6] A quarter of respondents thought that their somatic symptoms were made worse by stress, and 10% reported marked impairment; a higher number of symptoms was linked to greater impairment of everyday life as well as to more emotional symptoms. This result indicates that multiple somatic symptoms in children in the general population are often likely to be an expression of somatization. The authors of the CSI have since developed a shorter 24-item version with one factor made up of multiple symptoms explaining almost 30% of the total variance.

Eminson and colleagues[7] adapted the Illness Attitudes Scales for use with young people, and demonstrated links between high symptom scores and distress about illness in a general population sample of young people. These scales have been used in young people with CFS, and have shown that these children and their parents display an enhanced general tendency to believe in the presence of a disease despite contrary medical evidence and reassurance to the contrary, a tendency that persists after the child's recovery, therefore suggesting enduring—not just illness-related—health beliefs.[8]

More recently Rask and colleagues[9] have developed, and satisfactorily validated, a parental interview to assess functional somatic symptoms in children, the Soma Assessment Interview, which may be used in clinical settings as well as in research. The instrument was used to establish rates of impairing functional symptoms in 4% of young 5- to 7-year-olds in a general population.

In contrast to unexplained physical complaints, severe somatoform disorders are rare. Kozlowska and colleagues,[10] using the Australian Pediatric Surveillance Unit, a research resource to establish rates of new rare disorders seen by pediatricians, found rates of childhood conversion disorder of 0.02 to 0.04 per 1000 total child population. The most common symptoms in this survey were loss of movement and sensation. CFS appears to be more common (0.19% in a general population survey) and partial or CFS-like syndromes even more so (about 2%).[8]

Functional Somatic Symptoms, Primary Health Care Help Seeking, and Psychiatric Comorbidity

Work by Campo and colleagues[11] has documented primary health care pediatric consultations of children with medically unexplained recurrent abdominal pain (RAP). This study found frequent complaints to be present in 2% of consulters, less frequent complaints in 11%, and a clear predominance of girls over boys (2 to 1). In about half the children parents and doctors thought there were concurrent psychosocial problems, with fears of novelty and separation and worries being the most common psychological features reported by parents. About half the children with frequent complaints were thought to be impaired in some way because of their symptoms, about a third were regarded as comparatively frequent users of medical services, and some 1 in 10 were missing substantial schooling. These data confirm that somatization expressed through RAP is a regular feature of pediatric primary care consultations.

In a further study Campo and colleagues[12] investigated psychiatric comorbidity among young people with RAP attending primary care services, and found anxiety disorders to be present in over three-quarters (depressive disorders in about half), making it highly appropriate to systematically screen for these disorders in pediatric clinics.

High levels of psychiatric comorbidity are also being recognized in other somatoform disorders. Thus, Pehlivanturk and Unal[13] identified psychiatric disorders in more than half their sample of children admitted to hospital with conversion disorders, and about three-quarters of young people with CFS have had psychiatric—mainly emotional—disorders documented in the year prior to interview.[8] Moreover, further indications of close links between anxiety and somatoform disorders are findings that anxiety disorders tend to both precede the emergence of and follow the recovery from somatoform disorders.

Biologic and Psychological Vulnerabilities

New evidence is emerging to support biologic vulnerabilities in unexplained physical complaints and somatoform disorders. Thus, in response to a water load challenge, children with RAP report significantly greater symptom increase than controls, suggesting an enhanced gastrointestinal sensitivity.[14] Campo and colleagues[15] have discussed the possibility that dysregulation of serotonergic neurotransmission is implicated in both gastrointestinal and emotional symptoms, on the basis that serotonin is an important neurotransmitter in the gastrointestinal tract and enteric nervous system, that it influences gut peristaltic activity and symptoms of nausea, and that it is also implicated in mood disorders.

The influence of biologic mechanisms on CFS is still debated; certain infections such as mononucleosis infectiosa appear particularly likely to precipitate CFS in children, and reports (most recently Lombardi and colleagues[16]; not replicated by Erlwein and colleagues[17]) continue to highlight a possible contribution of other viral agents. However, very few individuals develop CFS following viral illnesses, and the significance of viral infections needs to be clarified further.

Stress Sensitivity, Personality, and Coping

Research reports confirm psychological vulnerabilities in young people with unexplained physical symptoms and somatoform disorders, through heightened stress sensitivity, sometimes related to personality difficulty. Stressful events as illness precipitants are reported in the majority of children with conversion disorder or CFS[8,13]: mainly relationship problems and family illness in conversion, and infections and school events in CFS. Children with RAP and frequent somatic symptoms tend to report an excess of life events. Walker and colleagues[18] compared diaries on daily stressors and somatic/emotional symptoms in children with RAP and controls; more daily stressors at home and school, and strong associations between daily stressors and somatic symptoms were reported in the pain sample, especially in those reporting negative affect traits. The same research group studied stress, appraisal, and coping with pain in children with RAP,[19] also using diaries, and in line with their previous results patients with pain were less confident in their ability to change or adapt to stress, and less likely to use accommodative coping strategies.

Personality Features

These stress-management deficits might well be related to temperament or personality difficulty. Earlier evidence is being supported by findings that child temperament (eg, irregular feeding and sleeping) in the first year of life already predicts future RAP.[20] Personality anomalies (eg, prominent vulnerability, anxiousness and conscientiousness, as well as worthlessness and emotional lability) have now been documented in young people with CFS and have shown them unlikely to be merely consequences of having a chronic physical disorder.[8]

A Clinical Formulation

Kozlowska[21] has expanded David Taylor's formulation of conversion disorder reflecting children being in "intolerable predicaments." The basic concept is one of good, compliant children from families with high expectations, inarticulate family relationships, and hostility to psychological expectations. Children in intolerable situations they cannot escape or communicate about without threatening their feeling of safety will manage their fears of parental rejection, hostility, anger, or displeasure through compulsive compliance and sometimes through conversion symptoms. Compulsive compliance would minimize hostility in attachment relationships and allow for maximum physical and psychological closeness and safety. However, when compulsive compliance breaks down it leads to anxiety, fear, and anger in the child; physical illness then serves to elicit parental care and protection as well as safeguard the child from parental expectations, anger, displeasure, or rejection in the face of failure to perform.

Work on children and young people with CFS has further emphasized the crucial role of impairment as a defining feature of severe unexplained physical complaints and somatoform disorders, and as a factor contributing to its maintenance. Research has also demonstrated inefficient coping strategies, such as low use of problem solving, in children with these disorders specifically when dealing with symptoms and impairment.[8]

Parental Influences

The influence of parental and family factors is becoming increasingly documented. Mothers of children with RAP have been found to have increased histories of anxiety and depression,[22] and parental anxiety during the child's first year of life predicts RAP in the child 6 years later.[20] Parental somatization is also relevant, as children of parents with current somatization display an excess of somatic symptoms and school absence.[23]

Work on young people with CFS has demonstrated high levels of parental emotional overinvolvement with the child's illness, when compared with parents of children with other severe pediatric disorders.[8] In children with RAP detailed assessments of parental behaviors have shown that giving attention to symptoms results in doubling of symptom complaints, especially in girls, whereas distraction reduces the symptoms by half.[24] Of note, whereas children report that distraction makes the symptoms better, parents rate distraction as being more likely to have a negative impact on symptoms than attention. Understanding these attitudes is highly relevant for treatment.

Treatment and Outcome

The cornerstone of treatment is for pediatric clinicians to be interested in the child and his background, to carry out the necessary investigations, to discuss with parents tactfully that organic disease has been excluded as well as to discuss any harmful aspects in the child's environment, such as excessive academic and emotional demands (often self-imposed by the child), and to help the family modify them. More specific cognitive-behavioral techniques involve self-monitoring of the main symptoms through diaries, limiting the attention given to the symptom by others, relaxation techniques if appropriate, encouraging participation in routine activities through gradual exposure, confirming that the child is not "putting the symptom on," explaining the links between physical and psychological pain, and addressing parental anxieties and the child's reluctance to engage in a rehabilitative approach. Relaxation can be helpful for circumscribed problems such as headaches, and treatment of comorbid psychiatric disorders is also called for.

The best evidence for treatment efficacy in RAP is for family behavioral programs using techniques along the aforementioned lines (graded evidence rating A). The earlier randomized controlled trial by Sanders and colleagues[25] showed that this technique was better than treatment as usual, and has been largely replicated by Robins and colleagues.[26] Graded activity programs with cognitive-behavioral features delivered within a family treatment context have been shown to be promising and efficacious for the treatment of CFS.[27,28] For the treatment of the more severe case, the term "restrained rehabilitation" has been used to describe a coordinated multidisciplinary rehabilitation package that ensures consistency and collaboration between different professionals and families.[29] Selective serotonin reuptake inhibitors such as citaprolam have been piloted successfully for the treatment of RAP.[12]

Outcome will vary according to severity, impairment, and possibly also risk factors such as the degree of personality difficulty and family support. Mulvaney and colleagues[30] categorized children with RAP attending pediatric services into (1) low risk (70%) with low levels of symptoms and impairment expected to improve within 2 months; (2) short-term risk (16%) for those who, despite high levels of symptoms and impairment, improve greatly over several months and maintain their improvement;

and (3) long-term risk (14%) when symptoms and impairment persist and there are high initial levels of anxiety and depression, low self worth, and negative life events. The longer term adult outcome of childhood RAP has documented high levels of anxiety disorder, poor social outcome, perceived susceptibility to physical impairment, and hypochondriacal beliefs.[31] The majority (about two-thirds) of children with severe CFS have been shown to recover. Nevertheless, recovery can be slow, taking years, and one-third remain affected, with indications that poor prognosis may be linked to more disordered personalities and to maternal beliefs about psychological factors being irrelevant to the disorder.

SUMMARY

Unexplained physical complaints are frequent in the general population. These complaints are commonly associated with somatization (the tendency to express psychological distress through somatic symptoms and to request medical help) the phenomenon at the root of the somatoform disorders, of which pain and conversion in addition to CFS are seen in children. There is evidence that psychiatric comorbidity is common, particularly anxiety and to a lesser extent depressive disorders and that children with severe somatoform disorders are stress sensitive, which is probably related to personality difficulty. There are also indications of biologic vulnerability contributing to the development of physical symptoms in response to physical or other stressors. Family clustering, parental emotional overinvolvement and overattention to the child's symptoms are thought to play a part in symptom maintenance. Management needs to take into account the physical health focus of some children and their parents, alongside skepticism, and sometimes even hostility, to the possibility of a psychological contribution; this can make the initial pediatric assessment and psychiatric intervention challenging. Psychiatric pediatric liaison teams have developed techniques for dealing with these attitudes and for engaging families in the assessment and management process. Unfortunately liaison teams are not well developed.[32] Effective attention to impairing somatoform disorders is likely to require further development of specialist services of this kind. Nevertheless, for families in which a psychological contribution to symptoms is acknowledged, generic child and adolescent mental health services have much to offer in helping reduce concurrent physical symptoms and psychiatric comorbidity and possibly also help improve adult health outcomes.

REFERENCES

1. Garber J, Walker LS, Zeman J. Somatization symptoms in a community sample of children and adolescents: further validation of the Children's Somatization Inventory. Psychol Assess 1991;3:588–95.
2. Campo JV, Fritsch SL. Somatization in children and adolescents. J Am Acad Child Adolesc Psychiatry 1994;33(9):1223–35.
3. Eminson M. Medically unexplained symptoms in children and adolescents. Clin Psychol Rev 2007;27:855–71.
4. Garralda ME. A selective review of child psychiatric syndromes with a somatic presentation. Br J Psychiatry 1992;161:759–73.
5. Garralda ME. Somatization in children. J Child Psychol Psychiatry 1996;37: 13–33.
6. Vila M, Kramer T, Hickey N, et al. Assessment of somatic symptoms in British secondary school children using the Children's Somatization Inventory (CSI). J Pediatr Psychol 2009;34:989–98.

7. Eminson M, Bejamin S, Shortall A, et al. Physical symptoms and illness attitudes in adolescents: an epidemiological study. J Child Psychol Psychiatry 1996;37: 519–28.

8. Garralda ME, Chalder T. Practitioner review: chronic fatigue syndrome in childhood. J Child Psychol Psychiatry 2005;46(11):1143–51.

9. Rask CU, Christensen MF, Borg C, et al. The SOMA assessment interview: new parent interview on functional somatic symptoms in children. J Psychosom Res 2009;66(5):456–64.

10. Kozlowska K, Nunn KP, Rose D, et al. Conversion disorder in Australian pediatric practice. J Am Acad Child Adolesc Psychiatry 2007;46(1):68–75.

11. Campo JV, Jansen-McWilliams L, Comer DM, et al. Somatization in pediatric primary care: association with psychopathology, functional impairment and use of services. J Am Acad Child Adolesc Psychiatry 1999;38(9):1093–101.

12. Campo JV, Perel JM, Lucas A, et al. Citalopram treatment of pediatric recurrent abdominal pain and comorbid internalizing disorders: an exploratory study. J Am Acad Child Adolesc Psychiatry 2004;43(10):1234–42.

13. Pehlivanturk B, Unal F. Conversion disorder in children and adolescents: clinical features and comorbidity with depressive and anxiety disorders. Turk J Pediatr 2000;42:132–7.

14. Walker LS, Williams SE, Smith CA, et al. Validation of a symptom provocation test for laboratory studies of abdominal pain and discomfort in children and adolescents. J Pediatr Psychol 2006;31(7):703–13.

15. Campo JV, Dahl RE, Williamson DE, et al. Gastrointestinal distress to serotonergic challenge: a risk marker for emotional disorder? J Am Acad Child Adolesc Psychiatry 2003;42(10):1221–6.

16. Lombardi VC, Ruscetti FW, Das Gupta J, et al. Detection of an infectious retrovirus, XMRV, in blood cells of patients with chronic fatigue syndrome. Science 2009;326(5952):585–9.

17. Erlwein O, Kaye S, McClure MO, et al. Failure to detect the novel retrovirus XMRV in chronic fatigue syndrome. PLoS ONE 2010;5:e8519.

18. Walker LS, Garber J, Smith CA, et al. The relation of daily stressors to somatic and emotional symptoms in children with and without recurrent abdominal pain. J Consult Clin Psychol 2001;69(1):85–91.

19. Walker LS, Smith CA, Garber J, et al. Appraisal and coping with daily stressors by pediatric patients with chronic abdominal pain. J Pediatr Psychol 2007;32(2): 206–16.

20. Ramchandani PG, Stein A, Hotopf M, et al. Early parental and child predictors of recurrent abdominal pain at school age: results of a large population-based study. J Am Acad Child Adolesc Psychiatry 2006;45(6):729–36.

21. Kozlowska K. Good children presenting with conversion disorder. Clinical Child Psychol Psychiatry 2001;6(4):575–91.

22. Campo JV, Bridge J, Lucas A, et al. Physical and emotional health of mothers of youth with functional abdominal pain. Arch Pediatr Adolesc Med 2007;161:131–7.

23. Craig TK, Cox AD, Klein K. Intergenerational transmission of somatization behaviour: a study of chronic somatizers and their children. Psychol Med 2002;32: 805–16.

24. Walker LS, Williams SE, Smith CA, et al. Parent attention versus distraction: impact on symptom complaints by children with and without chronic functional abdominal pain. Pain 2006;122(1-2):43–52.

25. Sanders MR, Shepherd RW, Cleghorn G, et al. The treatment of recurrent abdominal pain in children: a controlled comparison of cognitive-behavioural family

intervention and standard pediatric care. J Consult Clin Psychol 1994;62(2): 306–14.

26. Robins PM, Smith SM, Glutting JJ, et al. A randomized controlled trial of a cognitive-behavioural family intervention for pediatric recurrent abdominal pain. J Pediatr Psychol 2005;30(5):397–408.

27. Stulemeijer M, de Jong LW, Fiselier TJ, et al. Cognitive behaviour therapy for adolescents with chronic fatigue syndrome: randomised controlled trial. Br Med J 2005;330(7481):14.

28. Wright B, Ashby B, Beverley DW, et al. A feasibility study comparing two treatment approaches for chronic fatigue syndrome in adolescents. Arch Dis Child 2005;90:369–72.

29. Calvert P, Jureidini J. Restrained rehabilitation: an approach to children and adolescents with unexplained signs and symptoms. Arch Dis Child 2003;88: 399–402.

30. Mulvaney S, Warren LE, Garber J, et al. Trajectories of symptoms and impairment for pediatric patients with functional abdominal pain: a 5-year longitudinal study. J Am Acad Child Adolesc Psychiatry 2006;45(6):737–44.

31. Campo JV, Di Lorenzo C, Chiappetta L, et al. Adult outcomes of pediatric recurrent abdominal pain: do they just grow out of it? Pediatrics 2001;108(1):E1.

32. Woodgate M, Garralda ME. Pediatric liaison work by child and adolescent mental health services. Child Adolesc Ment Health 2006;11:19–24.

Mental Health Concerns of the Premature Infant Through the Lifespan

Douglas Vanderbilt, MD[a,b], Mary Margaret Gleason, MD[c],*

KEYWORDS

- Preterm birth • Parent child interactions • Mental health
- Neurodevelopment

In the United States, more than 540,000 infants are born preterm each year, accounting for more than 12.8% of all births.[1] Worldwide, the World Health Organization (WHO) reports preterm birth prevalence rates of 9.6%, with a total of 12.9 million preterm births a year.[2] The cost of caring for these children in the United States is estimated to be $26 billion a year, partly because infants born with decreasing gestational age survive at increased rates and have increased needs.[3]

A recent review of the causes of prematurity from the National Academies of Science highlights the co-occurrence of numerous individual and community-level biopsychosocial risk factors that contribute to this increase in preterm births.[3] For example, a mother's history of traumatic experiences is associated with increased risk for delivering prematurely[4,5] and impoverished women are more likely than those who have financial resources to deliver a preterm infant at greater risk for morbidity and mortality.[6]

Multiple medical conditions, including maternal infections and obstetric complications, are also associated with elevated risk for preterm delivery. The interactions between biologic and social risks create vulnerability to having a child born preterm, and these biologic and social factors continue to play active roles in the life of the developing infant and family. The poorer neurodevelopmental and physical and mental health outcomes that preterm infants experience then may interact with contextual factors to perpetuate an intergenerational risk for prematurity, as seen in the elevated risk for low birth weight infants among mothers born at low birth weights.[7]

A version of this article was previously published in the *Child and Adolescent Psychiatric Clinics of North America, 19:2.*

[a] Keck School of Medicine at the University of Southern California, Los Angeles, CA, USA
[b] Developmental-Behavioral Pediatrics, Childrens Hospital Los Angeles, #76, 4650 Sunset Boulevard, Los Angeles, CA 90027, USA
[c] Departments of Psychiatry and Behavioral Sciences, and Pediatrics, Tulane Institute of Infant and Early Childhood Mental Health, 1440 Canal Street, New Orleans, LA 70112, USA
* Corresponding author.
E-mail address: mgleason@tulane.edu

Because of increased survival rates, neurodevelopmental issues, chronic medical problems, and sometimes complex family issues involved with prematurity, mental health clinicians commonly assess preterm clients and manage their behavioral and mental health problems. Understanding prematurity survival and neurodevelopmental outcomes is important for contextualizing the mental health problems seen in this high-risk population.

This article provides a brief overview of prematurity outcomes in the domains of prematurity relevant to practicing child psychiatrists. Prematurity is also examined as it relates to parental mental health challenges, infant mental health outcomes, high frequency attention problems, and psychiatric disorders. The complex interactions between prematurity and family well-being are also highlighted. Finally, evidence-based treatment modalities involved in prevention and management are explored.

INTRODUCTION TO PREMATURITY
Definitions

Table 1 presents the language used to describe degrees of prematurity and birth weight categories. Although birth weight has been the primary independent variable, degree of prematurity is now preferred because several other factors beyond prematurity, including intrauterine growth restriction, influence birth weight and are likely associated with additional risks to the infant.[8]

Outcomes Related to Prematurity

Major advances have been made in preterm survival, both at a given birth weight level and at the boundary of viability, which is currently estimated at 22 to 24 weeks gestation. In 1987, only 34% of infants born at 24 weeks survived, compared with 59% in 2000.[9]

Similarly, survival increases as gestational age progresses. In the United States, only 30% of infants born at 23 weeks survived in 2000, compared with 59% of those born at 24 weeks and 70% at 25 weeks. Variability is seen between groups, centers within networks, and internationally and could be based on research method and practice differences.[10]

The advances in preterm infant survival can be attributed to antenatal and neonatal intensive care, such as surfactant use, aggressive resuscitation, mechanical ventilators, antenatal corticosteroids, and parenteral nutritional support.[9,11] Despite these improvements in survival, corresponding improvements in developmental outcomes have not been reported.

Risk Factors for Adverse Neurodevelopmental Outcomes

Early gestational age and low birth weight are powerful determinants for the development of neurologic/behavioral problems and survival among preterm births.[12] Other

Table 1 Frequently used terms		
Term	**Abbreviation**	**Definition**
Preterm	PT	Born before 37 wk gestational age
Very preterm	VPT	Born before 32 wk gestational age
Extremely preterm	EPT	Born before 28 wk gestational age
Low birth weight	LBW	Birth weight less than 2500 g (5.5 lb)
Very low birth weight	VLBW	Birth weight less than 1500 g (3.3 lb)
Extremely low birth weight	ELBW	Birth weight less than 1000 g (2.2 lb)
Micropremie		Birth weight less than 750 g (1.7 lb)

biologic factors, such as neurologic insults of intraventricular hemorrhage (IVH), hydrocephalus, periventricular leukomalacia, bronchopulmonary dysplasia, and retinopathy of prematurity, dramatically increase the rates of severe neurodevelopmental impairments.[13] Growth and feeding problems, necrotizing enterocolitis, infections, and cardiac lesions may also result in neurologic insults and lead to worse developmental outcomes.[14,15] For example, the more severe forms of IVH (grades 3 and 4) increase the risk for neurodevelopmental disability among preterm infants from 35% to 90%.[16] Finally, multiple gestations are at risk for prematurity, death, and neurodevelopmental impairment.[17,18] Prematurity may influence neurodevelopmental outcomes through disruption of the normal brain maturation that usually occurs in the protected intrauterine environment; direct insults to the central nervous system from medical complications during delivery and the neonatal intensive care unit (NICU) course; or impacts on the family from the additional stressors of parenting a high-risk child.[19] Beyond the stresses related to concern about survival or increased care burden of a medically fragile infant, typical NICUs tend to focus on the medical optimization of the infant at the cost of prolonged separation from the parents and intrusive light and sound environmental stimuli.[20]

As has long been recognized, neurodevelopmental outcomes are also strongly associated with community, family, and caregiving environments.[21] Many risk factors, such as poverty, social support, parental discord, and parental mental health, may predate the pregnancy and may in fact increase in the perinatal period. Those who come from disadvantaged backgrounds are at a higher risk of preterm birth. The combination of a resource-deprived environment with biologic risk for prematurity creates a double jeopardy for poorer outcomes.[3] For example, parental trauma-related symptoms are also well-recognized correlates to adverse infant neurodevelopmental and cognitive outcomes.[22,23]

Research has also identified protective factors for neurodevelopmental resilience. Protective factors for extremely low birth weight (ELBW) infants include antenatal steroids, cesarean delivery, lack of social disadvantage, singleton birth, and higher gestational age.[24] A consistent pattern of improved survival is seen in girls compared with boys.[9]

General Neurodevelopmental Outcomes

Neurodevelopmental outcomes are becoming the benchmark of successful interventions.[19,25] Although a comprehensive review of neurodevelopmental outcome literature is beyond the scope of this article, important neurodevelopmental domains that may relate to child psychiatry practice are briefly reviewed. Typical domains of neurodevelopmental outcomes include neurosensory; cognitive and motor; language and social developmental; learning; and adaptive outcomes. Generally, the risk for adverse neurodevelopmental outcomes increases with earlier birth and lower birth weight.[26]

Table 2 presents common prevalence of neurodevelopmental outcomes seen in the preterm population. Beyond delays and disorders, variations of development can also be seen. For example, very low birth weight (VLBW) infants have a greater risk for having a nonverbal learning problem profile with more advanced verbal cognition, and challenges in visual spatial skills.[27–29]

PREMATURITY AND MENTAL HEALTH

The following sections review the impact of prematurity on parental mental health, infant mental health, and early parent–child relationships, and in preschool, school-aged, and adolescent/young adult survivors of prematurity.

Table 2
Neurodevelopmental outcomes of prematurity

Type of Outcome	Outcome	General Population	Low Birth Weight (<2500 g)	Very Low Birth Weight (<1500 g)	Extremely Low Birth Weight (<1000 g)
Survival		>99%	—	86%	43%–70%
Neurosensory	Vision impairment[a]	<1%	2%	4%–24%	9%–25%
	Hearing loss	<1%	—	1%–3%	1%–28%
Developmental	Cerebral Palsy	<1%	—	6%–20%	15%–23%
	Speech and language delay	6%	3%–5%	8%–45%	—
	Neurodevelopmental impairment[b]	<1%		9%–61%	22%–50%
Learning/ academic	Learning disabilities	5%–20%	17%	—	34%–45%
	Special education in school	8%	—	60%–70%	—
	Cognitive impairment	1%		7%–17%	34%–37%
Behavioral	Attention deficit hyperactivity disorder	5%–7%	7%–30%	9%–30%	15%–40%
	Autism	1%	2%–3%	—	—

Higher prevalence rates seen as birth weight declines.
  [a] Vision impairment is defined as having retinopathy of prematurity, blindness, myopia, or strabismus.
  [b] Neurodevelopmental impairment is defined as <2 standard deviations below the mean on IQ or developmental tests, cerebral palsy, blindness, or significant hearing impairment.
  Data from Refs.[12,15,19,26,81–85]

Parental Posttraumatic Stress Disorder

Preterm birth can be considered to be associated with multiple traumatic experiences. Parents can experience an initial traumatic reaction at the preterm birth based on a stressful birth experience,[30] again with the loss of the healthy imagined child, and sometimes with early separation from the infant and exposure to a highly technological, medical world that is not usually part of a birth experience. Parents may experience trauma-related symptoms, including anxiety, sleep problems, nightmares, and avoidance of medical visits in the context of caring for a seriously ill child who has been cared for in the highly technological environment of the NICU.[31] Based on semi-structured interviews, the Impact of Events Scale, or the Perinatal Posttraumatic Stress Disorder Questionnaire, posttraumatic stress disorder (PTSD) symptoms of increased arousal, re-experiencing, and avoidance can occur acutely in the few days after the birth in mothers,[32] and later in the weeks and up to 14 months post-partum in both mothers and fathers.[33–36] Research suggests that, compared with mothers of healthy newborns, mothers whose newborns are VLBW and admitted to the NICU report more symptoms of anxiety and depression that may lead to ongoing psychological distress and parenting stress.[37,38] One explanation for this pattern is the loss of control in not being able to protect their infant in the NICU. Poverty exacerbates the vulnerability for PTSD symptoms related to preterm births.[39]

In general, PTSD symptoms have been associated with poorer physical health outcomes.[40,41] Parental PTSD symptoms may jeopardize the physical health, developmental, and behavioral outcomes of high-risk infants. Early parental PTSD symptoms are associated with less sensitive and more controlling maternal behaviors.[22] Perhaps based on this interaction pattern, parental PTSD can also predict future sleep and eating problems in infants by 18 months of age.[42] Quinnell[23] reported that maternal posttraumatic stress related to prematurity accounted for almost 6% of the variance in cognitive performance at 30 months among high-risk infants. Parental symptoms of PTSD, such as dissociation, hypervigilance, and numbing, may decrease parental ability to respond sensitively to infant cues, a deficit known to interfere with parent–child interactions, cognitive functioning, and child regulatory patterns.

Maternal Depression

The prevalence of major depressive disorder (MDD) in adults peaks during childbearing years and is higher in women than men. Thus, based on typical prevalence of MDD, it may be present in 10% to 25% of pregnant women. The hormonal changes after childbirth and the major life changes associated with a new birth may make mothers especially vulnerable to postpartum depression (PPD). Given the stresses involved with preterm births, researchers have shown associations between concurrent parental distress and severity of child illness in the NICU.[43] Clinically relevant PPD symptoms after birth of a VLBW infant have been found to range from 12% to 60%,[44,45] rates that do not necessarily distinguish themselves from those for full-term births. Rates of depressive symptoms seem to be highest at the child's discharge from the hospital and decrease in most studies by 6 months of age.[46] One study reported that higher levels of maternal socioeconomic factors were associated with a slower decrease in depressive symptoms after discharge and that maternal factors seemed to be stronger predictor of this slowed decline in symptoms than the infant's medical status.[46]

Although maternal depressive symptoms directly affect the quality of the infant–maternal interaction in full-term dyads and lead to greater rates of insecure attachment, more behavioral problems, and lower cognitive scores,[47–49] their impact may be different in preterm families. For example, subclinical depressive symptoms do not increase the risk for insecure attachment relationships in term infants, but are associated with an increased risk for insecurity in preterm infants.[50] This disruption leads to lower infant social engagement, unregulated fear regulation, and increased stress reactivity.[51] Whether impacted by the challenges of parenting a preterm child, depression, or traumatic stress, negative maternal recollections of birth experience predicted greater report of internalizing and total problems at 5 years of age on the Child Behavior Checklist (CBCL) for preterm but not full-term children.[52]

Prematurity and Infant–Parent Relationships

An extensive literature highlights the importance of early parent–child relationships as providing the foundation for later development. The context of the parent–child relationship can offer a buffer against biologic and environmental risk factors, including prematurity, and suboptimal relationships can increase the risk for adverse mental health outcomes. These relationships begin before the child is born, when parents develop an internal representation of the child.[53] Infants also develop an internal representation of their parents based on the patterns of their interactions. These internal representations are shaped by ongoing interactions and experiences.

The internal representation about a preterm infant may be influenced by several external influences and fears. In an elegant experimental design, Stern and colleagues[54] recruited infants born full-term and preterm at corrected age of 6 months. They randomly labeled some infants "preterm" and others "full-term" and assigned mothers to interact and describe one of these babies. Even mothers who had preterm infants viewed preterm infants less positively than those who were term. More importantly, infants in this study randomly labelled as full-term interacted more positively with mothers than those labeled as preterm, regardless of actual birth status, highlighting the power of negative attributions on infant behaviors. Early studies of prematurity supported these stereotypes, reporting that mothers of preterm infants worked harder than term mothers to engage their infant; they initiated interactions and talked more.[55] These early reports have not been supported by more recent research, and factors in addition to prematurity have emerged. A more recent study suggested that prematurity itself has a direct influence on how dyads interact at 6 months.[56] Although most term dyads were characterized as having "sensitive maternal style and cooperative infant" interaction styles, only approximately a quarter of preterm dyads interact this way, irrespective of medical status. Preterm dyads with less optimal interaction styles were at higher risk for problems with sleeping, eating, and emotional problems at 18 months.

In the general population, a mother's state of mind regarding intimate relationships shapes interactions with her infant.[57] Negative expectations and attributions (and positive expectations) in the neonatal period explain a substantial portion of variance of the infant's behavior in interaction with the mother at 8 weeks and even at 24 months.[58,59] Similarly, maternal early caregiving experiences that shape her own internal representation of herself in intimate relationships are associated with parent–child interaction style and infant development. Mothers who had a secure view of themselves within intimate relationships were more sensitive with their 3-month-old infants than those who were insecure.[60] In fact, secure mothers who had preterm infants showed higher sensitivity to their infants than secure mothers with full-term infants. However, mothers with insecure representations of themselves showed less sensitivity with preterm infants compared with similar mothers of full-term infants.[61] Thus, maternal sense of self can be either protective or increase an infant's risk status.

Preterm infants are active participants in interactions with their parents, although their social development may be different from term infants. In a controlled study, preterm infants showed equal positive affect as their full-term counterparts in a parent–child interaction procedure; they also showed more negative affect and had a smaller latency to negative affect, and were less facially responsive than full-term infants.[62] Even after controlling for medical risks, maternal anxiety showed a moderate association with infant facial responsivity, again suggesting an important complex interaction between maternal internal experiences and infant behaviors.

In typical development, infants develop focused attachment relationships at 7 to 9 months of age and begin to show a discriminated preference for specific caregivers, whom they seek out for comfort and nurturing. The quality of the relationship is associated with the infant caregiving experiences, and a secure attachment relationship predicts a range of positive social emotional outcomes.[63] Some have theorized that preterm infants might show different patterns of attachment than full-term infants because of the medically necessary differences in the early caregiving environment.[64] However, in general, studies have not found significant differences in rates of secure attachment behaviors between preterm VLBW infants up to 20 months and term infants, and stability of the attachment classification was similar to full-term infants.[50,64–66] This pattern was not supported in a study of ELBW children, who showed higher rates of insecure attachment patterns,[67] raising the question of whether the EBLW and associated medical problems contributed to the difference. These findings suggest that prematurity alone does not have a consistent effect on security of infant attachment in VLBW and low birth weight (LBW) infants.

Only one study has examined preschool attachment in ELBW infants and found substantial deviations from usual distributions, with more children (41%) classified as atypical than expected.[68] This study raises important questions about differences in attachment in ELBW infants or the trajectory of attachment relationships beyond infancy in preterm children.

Findings from studies of infant mental health in preterm infants highlight the important contributions of parental experiences, their internal representations of their infants and the ways they interact with their infants. Medical issues and experiences may influence these internal representations. Data suggest that preterm infants may be particularly susceptible to either the protective or risk qualities in the parent–child relationship. Findings of limited differences in formal attachment quality may suggest that either the early challenges have abated by 7 to 9 months or that prematurity itself is not a direct contributor to the attachment relationship classification although further research is warranted.

Mental Health in Toddlers, Preschoolers, School-aged Children, and Adolescents Born Preterm

Mental health problems have been the focus of research on preterm infants through early adulthood. Many of the studies examining mental health issues in preterm survivors used parent report checklists to describe the mental health outcomes. Parent report measures, such as the commonly used CBCL,[69] have some logistical and psychometric strengths. Parent report measures reflect parent perceptions, which may be influenced by factors other than the child's behaviors. In fact, in a study of mothers of LBW children, mothers were twice as likely as teachers to identify their child as having behavioral problems.[70] The strongest predictors of parent CBCL responses were caregiving quality and maternal depression, not child factors. This finding provides an important reminder about caution in interpreting results of studies that measure mental health outcomes solely based on parental report.

Most studies that focus on mental health in the first few months of life have examined maternal report of temperament. Early studies suggested that infants born prematurely had more difficult temperaments than those who were full-term.[71] However, subsequent literature has yielded inconsistent results, with most studies showing little difference in the major temperamental categories of easy, difficult, and slow to warm up in preterm infants followed up as early as 6 weeks up to 4 years.[72–75] Differences between term and preterm groups are generally only reported in preterm children who have significant central nervous system insults or developmental delays.[74] Longitudinal studies suggest that any early differences in temperament decrease over time.[73,76,77]

In one of the few measures of VLBW toddler mental health, Trevaud and colleagues[78] reported that mental health scores for VLBW children were indistinguishable from reported norms on the Infant Toddler Social Emotional Assessment. Another study of preschoolers reported a 2- to 3-point difference in T-score for social and attention problems, a finding that is statistically significant but perhaps not clinically relevant. In that study of children born extremely preterm, prematurity and maternal history of adverse caregiving as a child independently predicted their social problems.[79] Degree of prematurity seems to matter in predicting early childhood mental health problems, because preschoolers born extremely preterm were rated as having substantially higher rates of hyperactivity, inattention, peer problems, and emotional problems than those born very preterm.[80–85] Early childhood literature suggests that some preterm infants may have some differences in temperamental development and early childhood mental health, but that other factors, including medical issues and parental factors, likely explain some of the differences.

Several studies have examined mental health outcomes in school-aged children born preterm, with inconsistent results. This section focuses on internalizing and externalizing symptoms. Attentional problems are discussed in the next section. In 5-year-olds, rates of total mental health and internalizing and externalizing problems are doubled in very preterm and extremely preterm children.[86] Prematurity also showed a small to moderate effect size on these outcomes, and medical problems conferred additional risks.[87,88] At 7 years of age, extremely preterm/VLBW children showed significant elevations in teacher-reported peer problems and in parent-reported hyperactivity.[89]

More studies have examined the mental health status of premature infants when they are older. In a review of controlled studies published between 1980 and 2001 focusing on very preterm children 5 to 15 years of age, Bhutta and colleagues[14] reported that 81% of the included studies showed elevated parent-reported internalizing and externalizing symptoms, with a relative risk for both domains greater than two. A more recent meta-analysis included nine well-controlled studies published between 1998 and 2008.[90] Most of these studies examined children between 10 and 14 years old and included preterm children born near 27 weeks gestational age. The meta-analysis indicated that teachers reported more internalizing symptoms compared with control children, with an effect size of 0.28. No similar pattern was seen for parent's report of child internalizing or externalizing symptoms.

Direct comparison of the two major reviews is impossible because of the different methodologies used. However, their divergent findings warrant discussion. Although the overall gestational ages were similar, the dates of the studies evaluated are different. Advances in caring for very preterm children may contribute to the more recent studies finding small to minimal effect size of prematurity on internalizing and externalizing symptoms. As with temperament and early childhood mental health, extreme prematurity (<25 weeks gestational age) confers additional risks and is associated with a sixfold risk for mental health problems and functional impairment at home and school.[91]

Other groups have also examined the mechanism of adverse mental health outcomes in school-aged children. Examining preterm-born children, Whiteside-Mansell and colleagues[92] reported that level of conflict at home and child temperament moderated the association between preterm birth and internalizing and externalizing symptoms at 8 years of age. These moderators interacted in such a way that high household conflict and difficult temperament were synergistic predictors of externalizing symptoms in preterm infants. Internalizing symptoms were affected uniquely by level of household conflict, which did not interact with temperament. Multiple studies have also reported that cognitive status may explain some externalizing symptoms in preterm children.[89,93] Internalizing symptoms are less well accounted for by other developmental domains.

Studies of preterm infants through adolescence and young adulthood show provide inconsistent results. Two large non-United States studies of very preterm children have found no difference in internalizing or externalizing symptoms according to self-report at 19 and 31 years of age.[94,95] In contrast, a large study of all children born from 1960 to 1968 in an urban hospital setting found that preterm children had twice the risk for self-reported depression and suicidal ideation compared with the more mature births.[96] However, the higher social risk status of this population may have increased susceptibility to depression in the preterm children, who experienced "two hits."

Other studies using self-report of adults born before 30 weeks gestational age also suggest an increased risk for psychopathology. More than one study reported that adult women born preterm endorse higher rates of internalizing symptoms compared with term infants.[97,98] Sociodemographic risk factors, asthma, and exposure to violence predict these symptoms.[99] Perinatal status predicted parental report of the adults' internalizing symptoms, but not the self-report.

The mechanism of the increased rate of internalizing symptoms in young adults born preterm has not been explored extensively. In one study, LBW was only associated with increased risk for adult depression if at least one parent had depression, in which case 81% met criteria for depression.[96] To the authors' knowledge, specific genetic studies of this population's psychiatric risks have not been performed. Abnormalities of hypothalamic-pituitary axis (HPA), known to be present at higher rates in preterm infants,[100] have been implicated as one possible mechanism because of the increased perinatal exposure to stress and known associations between the HPA axis and mood and anxiety disorders, especially in adversity.[101,102] However, these have not been examined in preterm children.

A decline in cerebellar volume in late adolescence in the very preterm population has been associated with a worsening of global mental health status and feelings of competence at that time.[103] Family mental health and stress may also influence the development of internalizing symptoms. Overall, however, data increasingly suggest that psychiatric outcome of preterm children and adults is influenced by complex genetic, interactional, contextual, and biologic interactions.

In young adulthood, preterm survivors also show evidence of resilience, including lower rates of alcohol use and illicit drug use and male conduct problems compared with full-term adults.[97,98] Generally, young adults born preterm, very preterm, and extremely preterm also report similar levels of overall self-esteem to their peers', and their overall measures of quality of life are indistinguishable from adults born at term.[93–95]

Despite the overall mental health resilience of young adults born preterm according to their self-report, parent reports reflect additional concerns. In two longitudinal studies that include parent's report, parents identify higher rates of mental health problems, especially internalizing symptoms, in their preterm young adults than parents of term young adults.[93,97,98] Correlations between self- and parent report in these studies are lower than in term dyads.[97] It seems plausible that parents may be highly vigilant of their child's potential vulnerability because of perinatal experiences and/or ongoing medical issue, and therefore are more sensitive to potential symptoms. Alternatively, however, surviving prematurity may confer a sense of resilience and reduce the preterm young adults' perception of symptomatology.

Overall, measures of mental health in school-aged children and adults suggest that prematurity confers some risk for mental health problems. Across reporters, internalizing symptoms in girls and young women are the most consistently reported symptoms. Because of the notable discrepancy between parent and child reports when both are available, all parent report studies must be interpreted with some caution and attention to parental factors.

ATTENTION DEFICIT HYPERACTIVITY DISORDER

Symptoms of inattention, hyperactivity, and impulsivity are common sequelae for preterm children. Rates of attention deficit hyperactivity disorder (ADHD) symptoms from various measures have increased two- to sixfold among preterm births and are related to birth weight and gestational age.[19] Using different measures, multiple reporters, and findings reported over 2 decades, high rates of attentional difficulties have been consistently reported in VLBW, very preterm, and ELBW children and adolescents, with odds ratios as high as two and medium effect sizes of prematurity on the attentional outcomes.[86,90,104]

Fewer studies actually measure ADHD diagnoses, and those that do show a wide range of prevalence. A meta-analysis used ADHD diagnoses from seven populations of preterm subjects born from the 1970s to early 1980s, Bhutta and colleagues[14] found a pooled relative risk of 2.64 compared with controls meeting diagnostic criteria from the Diagnostic and Statistical Manual IV. Rates of ADHD diagnosis in VLBW and LBW adolescents range from 7% to 23%.[105–107]

In attention symptoms seems to have some stability, because early focused attention at 7 months predicted hyperactivity and impulsivity problems at 4 to 5 years of age according to maternal report.[108] Important interactions have been seen when assessing ADHD symptoms. Among LBW children, Breslau and colleagues[39] found higher attentional problems only in urban settings, showing an interaction between biologic risk and social disadvantage. Nadeau and colleagues[89] explored identified specific working memory factors and family adversity as moderators of inattentive behaviors in EPT and VLBW children, whereas the hyperactive behaviors were explained by general intellectual delay.

Executive function is the neuropsychological processes of inhibition, strategy use, and cognitive flexibility instrumental in goal-directed behavior. Many suggest that a deficit in this processing could underlie the ADHD symptoms found in preterm samples. Shum and colleagues[109] found psychological attention measures, such as poor spatial span forward and visual attention, to be significant predictors for parent and teacher–completed rating scales among the very preterm/ELBW sample. Szatmari and colleagues[110] compared ELBW children who had higher rates of developmental delay and motor coordination problems with controls and reported a significantly elevated rate of ADHD symptoms in the ELBW group that disappeared when controlling for neurodevelopmental problems such as executive functioning. An ELBW/very preterm sample displayed significantly more executive dysfunction than normal controls.[27] These data suggest that an executive function deficit might be the key factor explaining the ADHD symptoms seen in preterm populations.

Interventions

Beyond traditional medical interventions, specific treatments and programs have been developed to optimize development, mental health, and family functioning among preterm births. Immediate interventions in the NICU include kangaroo care and the Newborn Individualized Developmental Care and Assessment Program (NIDCAP) that aim to improve preterm infant outcomes. Kangaroo care is the use of early skin-to-skin contact and breastfeeding with the mother.[111] Kangaroo care is associated with improved pain tolerance and state regulation in the NICU, enhanced breastfeeding to 18 months, and a suggestion of lessened maternal postpartum depression and anxiety.[112–115] NIDCAP is an intervention in which a trained clinician identifies individual neonate behavioral responses to enhance the NICU environment and promote more adaptive state regulation.[116] Studies have found improved short-term medical and neurophysiologic and long-term neurobehavioral outcomes compared with typical NICU care.[116] However, other studies involving less-rigorous NIDCAP training find no benefit on these outcomes.[117]

Other interventions in the NICU show promise in improving mental health outcomes associated with preterm births. For example, in a blinded, randomized, controlled trial, a self-directed educational program starting at day two of NICU stay that combined DVDs with parent assignments (eg, recognizing infant's bids for interactions) was associated with lower maternal depression after discharge and more positive interactions with the infant in the NICU.[118] Support, in the form of a single conversation with a neonatologist and psychologist, or ongoing phone support from another mother of preterm infant can be helpful in reducing maternal symptoms.[119,120] However, traditional interventions for depressive symptoms (eg, cognitive behavioral therapy) have shown limited effects in this population,[121] suggesting that traditional, effective interventions for term families may not be appropriate for parents experiencing a preterm event.

The Mother-Infant Transaction Program, which is a group treatment focused on relationship building, was shown to reduce parental stress measured by the Parenting Stress Index among a preterm intervention group.[122] A short-term individualized family-based intervention reduced maternal stress and depression in another study of preterm births.[123] Another family-based intervention that focused on educating parents about infant behavior in NICU was shown to enhance maternal knowledge and sensitivity and reduce stress.[124]

No unique interventions have been developed to target ADHD symptoms or other reported mental health symptoms in preterm children, which are admittedly inconsistently reported. Because a higher proportion of children born preterm may live in poverty, greater emphasis on the interventions among disadvantaged populations will directly benefit the preterm population.[125] Thus, attention to the post-NICU environment is crucial to maximize outcomes.[15]

SUMMARY AND IMPLICATIONS FOR CHILD PSYCHIATRISTS

Increasingly, child psychiatrists are likely to encounter children born preterm in their patient populations across several age groups. This population experiences more medical problems and higher rates of cognitive impairment than the general population. Child psychiatrists should be familiar with these outcomes, because they interact with the clinical presentation of mental health problems. In the perinatal period, parents may seek psychiatric care for their elevated rates of anxiety and depressive symptoms, which may decrease over time, but are associated with notable suffering. Infant and early childhood mental health providers must be aware that, although extreme prematurity and medical risks seem to confer an important risk for suboptimal parent–child interactions, a parent's own state of mind, attributions about the infant, and sensitivity with the infant seem to be at least as important in predicting mental health outcomes.

In school-aged children, data are difficult to interpret because nearly all are based on adult report checklists, which are likely to measure adult perceptions of child vulnerability and adult mood symptoms, in addition to child behavior patterns. In these age groups, school-aged and adolescent internalizing symptoms and ADHD seem to be the most consistently reported outcomes. The high consistency of problems with attention and executive functioning suggests that these have a direct link to prematurity itself and must be carefully considered in every patient who has a history of preterm birth. As with all psychiatric patients, differences between self- and parent report provide important information about family interactions and a rich clinical picture. The degree of inconsistency across studies for other psychiatric disorders suggests that clinicians must be vigilant in reviewing symptoms of depression and anxiety, especially in adolescents, but that a biopsychosocial formulation that includes parent mental health will be most useful in guiding treatment.

Finally, longitudinal studies report that global measures of competence and self-worth are equivalent in preterm patients and their term peers. Across all age groups, data suggest that premature status is associated with increased risk for adverse mental health outcomes, especially when accompanied by additional financial, medical, or psychiatric risk factors. Some specific mechanisms explaining particular mental health outcomes likely will be identified in the future. However, the current literature confirms that, for prematurely born and full-term children, the number of risk factors rather than the specific risk factors predict early mental health outcomes.[126]

The study of psychiatric outcomes in preterm children is still in its infancy. Much of the literature has used parent reports, and observational measures, biologic correlates, or data related to parent's internal experiences and symptoms have received limited attention. The early childhood literature suggests that when these are included, the direct effects of prematurity decrease, except in the most extreme medical problems. Clinicians and prematurely born children and their families will benefit from further research that integrates the biologic, child and parent psychological, and environmental factors that may influence mental health resilience in this population.

REFERENCES

1. March of Dimes. PeriStats. Available at: http://www.marchofdimes.com/prematurity/. Accessed February 21, 2010.
2. March of Dimes. White paper on preterm birth: the global and regional toll. Available at: http://www.marchofdimes.com/files/66423_MOD-Complete.pdf. Accessed February 21, 2010.
3. Behrman RE, Butler AS. Institute of Medicine. Committee on understanding premature birth and assuring healthy Outcomes: preterm birth: causes, consequences, and prevention. Washington, DC: National Academies Press; 2007.
4. Lederman SA, Rauh V, Weiss L, et al. The effects of the World Trade Center event on birth outcomes among term deliveries at three lower Manhattan hospitals. Environ Health Perspect 2004;112:1772.
5. Misra DP, O'Campo P, Strobino D. Testing a sociomedical model for preterm delivery. Paediatr Perinat Epidemiol 2001;15:110.
6. Roberts EM. Neighborhood social environments and the distribution of low birthweight in Chicago. Am J Public Health 1997;87:597.
7. Sanderson M, Emanuel I, Holt VL. The intergenerational relationship between mother's birthweight, infant birthweight and infant mortality in black and white mothers. Paediatr Perinat Epidemiol 1995;9:391.
8. Tyson JE, Parikh NA, Langer J, et al. Intensive care for extreme prematurity—moving beyond gestational age. N Engl J Med 2008;358:1672.
9. Fanaroff AA, Hack M, Walsh MC. The NICHD neonatal research network: changes in practice and outcomes during the first 15 years. Semin Perinatol 2003;27:281.
10. Hack M, Taylor HG, Klein N, et al. Functional limitations and special health care needs of 10- to 14-year-old children weighing less than 750 grams at birth. Pediatrics 2000;106:554.
11. Hack M, Fanaroff AA. Outcomes of children of extremely low birthweight and gestational age in the 1990s. Semin Neonatol 2000;5:89.
12. Stephens BE, Vohr BR. Neurodevelopmental outcome of the premature infant. Pediatr Clin North Am 2009;56:631.
13. Schmidt B, Asztalos EV, Roberts RS, et al. Impact of bronchopulmonary dysplasia, brain injury, and severe retinopathy on the outcome of extremely

low-birth-weight infants at 18 months: results from the trial of indomethacin prophylaxis in preterms. JAMA 2003;289:1124.

14. Bhutta AT, Cleves MA, Casey PH, et al. Cognitive and behavioral outcomes of school-aged children who were born preterm: a meta-analysis. JAMA 2002; 288:728.

15. Perlman JM. Neurobehavioral deficits in premature graduates of intensive care—potential medical and neonatal environmental risk factors. Pediatrics 2001;108:1339.

16. Volpe JJ. Neurology of the newborn. 4th edition. Philadelphia: WB Saunders; 2001. p. 501–3.

17. Laptook AR, O'Shea TM, Shankaran S, et al. Adverse neurodevelopmental outcomes among extremely low birth weight infants with a normal head ultrasound: prevalence and antecedents. Pediatrics 2005;115:673.

18. Pharoah PO. Neurological outcome in twins. Semin Neonatol 2002;7:223.

19. Aylward GP. Neurodevelopmental outcomes of infants born prematurely. J Dev Behav Pediatr 2005;26:427.

20. Mayes LC. The assessment and treatment of the psychiatric needs of medically compromised infants: consultation with preterm infants and their families. Child Adolesc Psychiatr Clin N Am 1995;4:555.

21. Wilson RS. Risk and resilience in early mental development. Dev Psychol 1985; 21:795.

22. Muller-Nix C, Forcada-Guex M, Pierrehumbert B, et al. Prematurity, maternal stress and mother-child interactions. Early Hum Dev 2004;79:145.

23. Quinnell FA. Postpartum posttraumatic stress as a risk factor for atypical cognitive development in high-risk infants. Milwaukee, Wisconsin: University of Wisconsin-Milwaukee Editor; 2001. p. 113.

24. Gargus RA, Vohr BR, Tyson JE, et al. Unimpaired outcomes for extremely low birth weight infants at 18 to 22 months. Pediatrics 2009;124:112.

25. Stephens BE, Bann CM, Poole WK, et al. Neurodevelopmental impairment: predictors of its impact on the families of extremely low birth weight infants at 18 months. Infant Ment Health J 2008;29:570.

26. Vanderbilt D, Wang JC, Parker S. The do's in preemie neurodevelopment. Contemp Pediatr 2007;254:84.

27. Anderson PJ, Doyle LW, Victorian Infant Collaborative Study Group. Executive functioning in school-aged children who were born very preterm or with extremely low birth weight in the 1990s. Pediatrics 2004;114:50.

28. Fletcher JM, Landry SH, Bohan TP, et al. Effects of intraventricular hemorrhage and hydrocephalus on the long-term neurobehavioral development of preterm very-low-birthweight infants. Dev Med Child Neurol 1997;39:596.

29. Gabrielson J, Hard AL, Ek U, et al. Large variability in performance IQ associated with postnatal morbidity, and reduced verbal IQ among school-aged children born preterm. Acta Paediatr 2002;91:1371.

30. Alcorn KL, O'Donovan A, Patrick JC, et al. A prospective longitudinal study of the prevalence of post-traumatic stress disorder resulting from childbirth events. Psychol Med 2010;1:1.

31. Peebles-Kleiger MJ. Pediatric and neonatal intensive care hospitalization as traumatic stressor: implications for intervention. Bull Menninger Clin 2000; 64:257.

32. Vanderbilt D, Bushley T, Young R, et al. Acute posttraumatic stress symptoms among urban mothers with newborns in the neonatal intensive care unit: a preliminary study. J Dev Behav Pediatr 2009;30:50.

33. DeMier RL, Hynan MT, Harris HB, et al. Perinatal stressors as predictors of symptoms of posttraumatic stress in mothers of infants at high risk. J Perinatol 1996;16:276.
34. Holditch-Davis D, Bartlett TR, Blickman AL, et al. Posttraumatic stress symptoms in mothers of premature infants. J Obstet Gynecol Neonatal Nurs 2003; 32:161.
35. Kersting A, Dorsch M, Wesselmann U, et al. Maternal posttraumatic stress response after the birth of a very low-birth-weight infant. J Psychosom Res 2004;57:473.
36. Shaw RJ, Bernard RS, Deblois T, et al. The relationship between acute stress disorder and posttraumatic stress disorder in the neonatal intensive care unit. Psychosomatics 2009;50:131.
37. Carter JD, Mulder RT, Bartram AF, et al. Infants in a neonatal intensive care unit: parental response. Arch Dis Child Fetal Neonatal Ed 2005;90:F109.
38. Doering LV, Moser DK, Dracup K. Correlates of anxiety, hostility, depression, and psychosocial adjustment in parents of NICU infants. Neonatal Netw 2000;19:15.
39. Breslau J, Miller E, Breslau N, et al. The impact of early behavior disturbances on academic achievement in high school. Pediatrics 2009;123:1472.
40. Saxe GN, Vanderbilt D, Zuckerman B. Traumatic stress in injured and ill children. PTSD Res Q 2003;14:1.
41. Schnurr PP, Jankowski MK. Physical health and post-traumatic stress disorder: review and synthesis. Semin Clin Neuropsychiatry 1999;4:295.
42. Pierrehumbert B, Nicole A, Muller-Nix C, et al. Parental post-traumatic reactions after premature birth: implications for sleeping and eating problems in the infant. Arch Dis Child Fetal Neonatal Ed 2003;88:F400.
43. Klebanov PK, Brooks-Gunn J, McCormick MC. Classroom behavior of very low birth weight elementary school children. Pediatrics 1994;94:700.
44. Davis L, Edwards H, Mohay H, et al. The impact of very premature birth on the psychological health of mothers. Early Hum Dev 2003;73:61.
45. Singer LT, Salvator A, Guo S, et al. Maternal psychological distress and parenting stress after the birth of a very low-birth-weight infant. JAMA 1999; 281:799.
46. Poehlmann J, Schwichtenberg MAJ, Bolt D, et al. Predictors of depressive symptom trajectories in mothers of infants born preterm or low birthweight. J Fam Psychol 2009;23:690.
47. Korja R, Savonlahti E, Ahlqvist-Bjorkroth S, et al. Maternal depression is associated with mother-infant interaction in preterm infants. Acta Paediatr 2008; 97:724.
48. Murray L, Fiori-Cowley A, Hooper R, et al. The impact of postnatal depression and associated adversity on early mother-infant interactions and later infant outcome. Child Dev 1996;67:2512.
49. Sharp D, Hay DF, Pawlby S, et al. The impact of postnatal depression on boys' intellectual development. J Child Psychol Psychiatry 1995;36:1315.
50. Poehlmann J, Fiese BH. The interaction of maternal and infant vulnerabilities on developing attachment relationships. Dev Psychopathol 2001;13:1.
51. Feldman R, Granat A, Pariente C, et al. Maternal depression and anxiety across the postpartum year and infant social engagement, fear regulation, and stress reactivity. J Am Acad Child Adolesc Psychiatry 2009;48:919.
52. Latva R, Korja R, Salmelin RK, et al. How is maternal recollection of the birth experience related to the behavioral and emotional outcome of preterm infants? Early Hum Dev 2008;84:587.

53. Benoit D, Parker KC, Zeanah CH. Mothers' representations of their infants assessed prenatally: stability and association with infants' attachment classifications. J Child Psychol Psychiatry 1997;38:307.

54. Stern M, Karraker KH, Sopko AM, et al. The prematurity stereotype revisited: Impact on mothers' interactions with premature and full-term infants. Infant Ment Health J 2000;21:495.

55. Macey TJ, Harmon RJ, Easterbrooks MA. Impact of premature birth on the development of the infant in the family. J Consult Clin Psychol 1987;55:846.

56. Forcada-Guex M, Pierrehumbert B, Borghini A, et al. Early dyadic patterns of mother-infant interactions and outcomes of prematurity at 18 months. Pediatrics 2006;118:e107.

57. Madigan S, Bakermans-Kranenburg MJ, Van Ijzendoorn MH, et al. Unresolved states of mind, anomalous parental behavior, and disorganized attachment: a review and meta-analysis of a transmission gap. Attach Hum Dev 2006;8:89.

58. Greenberg MT, Crnic KA. Longitudinal predictors of developmental status and social interaction in premature and full-term infants at age two. Child Dev 1988;59:554.

59. Keren M, Feldman R, Eidelman AI, et al. Clinical interview for high-risk parents of premature infants (CLIP) as a predictor of early disruptions in the mother-infant relationship at the nursery. Infant Ment Health J 2003;24:93.

60. Coppola G, Cassibba R, Costantini A. What can make the difference? Premature birth and maternal sensitivity at 3 months of age: the role of attachment organization, traumatic reaction and baby's medical risk. Infant Behav Dev 2007;30:679.

61. Korja R, Savonlahti E, Haataja L, et al. Attachment representations in mothers of preterm infants. Infant Behav Dev 2009;32:305.

62. Hsu H-C, Jeng SF. Two-month-olds' attention and affective response to maternal still face: a comparison between term and preterm infants in Taiwan. Infant Behav Dev 2008;31:194.

63. Moss E, Bureau JF, Cyr C, et al. Correlates of attachment at age 3: construct validity of the preschool attachment classification system. Dev Psychol 2004;40:323.

64. Easterbrooks MA. Quality of attachment to mother and to father: effects of perinatal risk status. Child Dev 1989;60:825.

65. Frodi A, Thompson R. Infants' affective responses in the strange situation: effects of pre-maturity and of quality of attachment. Child Dev 1985;56:1280.

66. Goldberg S, Perrotta M, Minde K, et al. Maternal behavior and attachment in low–birth–weight twins and singletons. Child Dev 1986;57:34.

67. Mangelsdorf SC, Plunkett JW, Dedrick CF, et al. Attachment security in very low birth weight infants. Dev Psychol 1996;32:914.

68. Sajaniemi N, Mäkelä J, Saolkorpi T, et al. Cognitive performance and attachment patterns at four years of age in extremely low birth weight infants after early intervention. Eur Child Adolesc Psychiatry 2001;10:122.

69. Achenbach T, Rescorla L. Manual for the ASEBA Preschool form. Burlington (VT): University of Vermont; 2000.

70. Spiker D, Kraemer HC, Constantine NA, et al. Reliability and validity of behavior problem checklists as measures of stable traits in low birth weight, premature preschoolers. Child Dev 1992;63:1481.

71. Field TM, Hallock NF, Dempsey JR, et al. Mothers' assessments of term and preterm infants with respiratory distress syndrome: reliability and predictive validity. Child Psychiatry Hum Dev 1978;9:75.

72. Chapieski ML, Evankovich KD. Behavioral effects of prematurity. Semin Perinatol 1997;21:221.
73. Hughes MB, Shults J, McGrath J, et al. Temperament characteristics of premature infants in the first year of life. J Dev Behav Pediatr 2002;23:430.
74. Larroque B, N'Guyen S, Guadeney A, et al. Temperament at 9 months of very preterm infants born at less than 29 weeks' gestation: the EPIPAGE study. J Dev Behav Pediatr 2005;26:48.
75. Olafsen KS, Kaaresen PI, Handegård BH, et al. Maternal ratings of infant regulatory competence from 6 to 12 months: influence of perceived stress, birth-weight, and intervention: a randomized controlled trial. Infant Behav Dev 2008;31:408.
76. Riese ML. Longitudinal assessment of temperament from birth to 2 years: a comparison of full-term and preterm infants. Infant Behav Dev 1987;10:347.
77. Washington J, Minde K, Goldberg S. Temperament in preterm infants: style and stability. J Am Acad Child Adolesc Psychiatry 1986;26:493.
78. Treyvaud K, Anderson VA, Howard K, et al. Parenting behavior is associated with the early neurobehavioral development of very preterm children. Pediatrics 2009;123:555.
79. Assel MA, Landry SH, Swank PR, et al. How do mothers' childrearing histories, stress and parenting affect children's behavioural outcomes? Child Care Health Dev 2002;28:359.
80. Woodward LJ, Moor S, Hood KM, et al. Very preterm children show impairments across multiple neurodevelopmental domains by age 4 years. Arch Dis Child Fetal Neonatal Ed 2009;94:339.
81. Behrman RE, Butler AS, editors. Preterm birth: causes, consequences, and prevention. Washington, DC: The Institute of Medicine, The National Academies Press; 2006.
82. Cole C, Hagadorn J, Kim C, et al. Criteria for determining disability in infants and children: low birth weight. Agency for Healthcare Research and Quality (AHRQ), 2003; Evidence Report/Technology Assessment 70. Available at: www.ahrq.gov/clinic/epcsums/lbwdissum.htm. Accessed January 24, 2010.
83. Developmental Disabilities. Topic home. The Centers for Disease Control and Prevention. Available at: http://www.cdc.gov/ncbddd/dd/default.htm. Accessed January 25, 2010.
84. Law J, Boyle J, Harris F, et al. Prevalence and natural history of primary speech and language delay: findings from a systematic review of the literature. Int J Lang Commun Disord 2000;35:165.
85. U.S. Department of Education. 26th Annual Report to Congress on the Implementation of the Individuals with Disabilities Education Act. Available at: http://www.2.ed.gov/about/reports/annual/osep/2004/index.html. Accessed February 21, 2010.
86. Delobel-Ayoub M, Arnaud C, White-Koning M, et al. Behavioral problems and cognitive performance at 5 years of age after very preterm birth: the EPIPAGE study. Pediatrics 2009;123:1485.
87. Reijneveld SA, de Kleine MJ, van Baar AL, et al. Behavioural and emotional problems in very preterm and very low birthweight infants at age 5 years. Arch Dis Child Fetal Neonatal Ed 2006;91:423.
88. Schiariti VM, Hoube JS, Lisonkova SM, et al. Caregiver-reported health outcomes of preschool children born at 28 to 32 weeks' gestation. J Dev Behav Pediatr 2007;28:9.
89. Nadeau L, Boivin M, Tessier R, et al. Mediators of behavioral problems in 7-year-old children born after 24 to 28 weeks of gestation. J Dev Behav Pediatr 2001;22:1.

90. Aarnoudse-Moens CS, Weisglas-Kuperus N, van Goudoever JB, et al. Meta-analysis of neurobehavioral outcomes in very preterm and/or very low birth weight children. Pediatrics 2009;124:717.

91. Samara M, Marlow N, Wolke D, et al. Pervasive behavior problems at 6 years of age in a total-population sample of children born at <=25 weeks of gestation. Pediatrics 2008;122:562.

92. Whiteside-Mansell L, Bradley RH, Casey PH, et al. Triple risk: do difficult temperament and family conflict increase the likelihood of behavioral malad-justment in children born low birth weight and preterm? J Pediatr Psychol 2009;34:396.

93. Grunau RE, Whitfield MF, Fay TB. Psychosocial and academic characteristics of extremely low birth weight (<=800 g) adolescents who are free of major impair-ment compared with term-born control subjects. Pediatrics 2004;114:e725.

94. Dalziel SR, Lim VK, Lambert A, et al. Psychological functioning and health-related quality of life in adulthood after preterm birth. Dev Med Child Neurol 2007;49:597.

95. Tideman E, Ley D, Bjerre I, et al. Longitudinal follow-up of children born preterm: somatic and mental health, self-esteem and quality of life at age 19. Early Hum Dev 2001;61:97.

96. Nomura Y, Brooks-Gunn J, Davey C, et al. The role of perinatal problems in risk of co-morbid psychiatric and medical disorders in adulthood. Psychol Med 2007;37:1323.

97. Hack M, Youngstrom EA, Cartar L, et al. Behavioral outcomes and evidence of psychopathology among very low birth weight infants at age 20 years. Pediatrics 2004;114:932.

98. Lindstrom K, Lindblad F, Hjern A. Psychiatric morbidity in adolescents and young adults born pre-term: a Swedish national cohort study. Pediatrics 2009;123:e47.

99. Hack MM, Youngstrom EA, Cartar L, et al. Predictors of internalizing symptoms among very low birth weight young women. J Dev Behav Pediatr 2005;93.

100. Haley DW, Weinberg J, Grunau RE. Cortisol, contingency learning, and memory in preterm and full-term infants. Psychoneuroendocrinology 2006;31:108.

101. Arborelius L, Owens MJ, Plotsky PM, et al. The role of corticotropin-releasing factor in depression and anxiety disorders. J Endocrinol 1999;160:1.

102. Hein C, Nemeroff CB. The role of childhood trauma in the neurobiology of mood and anxiety disorders: preclinical and clinical studies. Biol Psychiatry 2001;49:1023.

103. Parker J, Mitchell A, Kalpakidou A, et al. Cerebellar growth and behavioural & neuropsychological outcome in preterm adolescents. Brain 2008;131:1344.

104. Anderson P, Doyle LW. Neurobehavioral outcomes of school-age children born extremely low birth weight or very preterm in the 1990s. JAMA 2003;289(24):3264.

105. Botting N, Powls A, Cooke RW, et al. Attention deficit hyperactivity disorders and other psychiatric outcomes in very low birthweight children at 12 years. J Child Psychol Psychiatry 1997;38:931.

106. Indredavik MS, Vik T, Heyerdahl S, et al. Psychiatric symptoms and disorders in adolescents with low birth weight. Archives of disease in childhood. Fetal Neonatal Ed 2004;89:F445.

107. Whitaker AH, Van Rossem R, Feldman JF, et al. Psychiatric outcomes in low-birth-weight children at age 6 years: relation to neonatal cranial ultrasound abnormalities. Arch Gen Psychiatry 1997;54:847.

108. Lawson KR, Ruff HA. Early focused attention predicts outcome for children born prematurely. J Dev Behav Pediatr 2004;25:399.

109. Shum D, Neulinger K, O'Callaghan M, et al. Attentional problems in children born very preterm or with extremely low birth weight at 7–9 years. Arch Clin Neuropsychol 2008;23:103.

110. Szatmari P, Saigal S, Rosenbaum P, et al. Psychiatric disorders at five years among children with birthweights less than 1000g: a regional perspective. Dev Med Child Neurol 1990;32:954.

111. Whitelaw A, Sleath K. Myth of the marsupial mother: home care of very low birth weight babies in Bogota, Colombia. Lancet 1985;1:1206.

112. de Alencar AE, Arraes LC, de Albuquerque EC, et al. Effect of kangaroo mother care on postpartum depression. J Trop Pediatr 2009;55:36.

113. Hake-Brooks SJ, Anderson GC. Kangaroo care and breastfeeding of mother-preterm infant dyads 0–18 months: a randomized, controlled trial. Neonatal Netw 2008;27:151.

114. Lee SB, Shin HS. Effects of kangaroo care on anxiety, maternal role confidence, and maternal infant attachment of mothers who delivered preterm infants. Taehan Kanho Hakhoe Chi 2007;37:949.

115. Warnock FF, Castral TC, Brant R, et al. Brief report: maternal kangaroo care for neonatal pain relief: a systematic narrative review. J Pediatr Psychol 2009. Available at: http://www.jpepsy.oxfordjournals.org/cgi/content/abstract/jsp123v1?ct=ct. Accessed February 25, 2010.

116. Als H, Duffy FH, McAnulty GB, et al. Early experience alters brain function and structure. Pediatrics 2004;113:846.

117. Maguire CM, Walther FJ, Sprij AJ, et al. Effects of individualized developmental care in a randomized trial of preterm infants <32 weeks. Pediatrics 2009;124:1021.

118. Melnyk BM, Feinstein NF, Alpert-Gillis L, et al. Reducing premature infants' length of stay and improving parents' mental health outcomes with the creating opportunities for parent empowerment (cope) neonatal intensive care unit program: a randomized, controlled trial. Pediatrics 2006;118:e1414.

119. Naoyuki K, Teruyo N, Yuko I, et al. Effects of interview on mood status of pregnant women with high-risk delivery. Pediatr Int 2009;51:498.

120. Preyde M, Ardal F. Effectiveness of a parent "buddy" program for mothers of very preterm infants in a neonatal intensive care unit. Can Med Assoc J 2003; 186:169.

121. Hagan R, Evans SF, Pope S. Preventing postnatal depression in mothers of very preterm infants: a randomised controlled trial. BJOG 2004;111:641.

122. Kaaresen PI, Ronning JA, Ulvund SE, et al. A randomized, controlled trial of the effectiveness of an early-intervention program in reducing parenting stress after preterm birth. Pediatrics 2006;118:e9.

123. Meyer EC, Coll CT, Lester BM, et al. Family-based intervention improves maternal psychological well-being and feeding interaction of preterm infants. Pediatrics 1994;93:241.

124. Browne JV, Talmi A. Family-based intervention to enhance infant-parent relationships in the neonatal intensive care unit. J Pediatr Psychol 2005;30:667.

125. Heckman JJ. Skill formation and the economics of investing in disadvantaged children. Science 1900;312:2006.

126. Sameroff AJ, Fiese BH. Models of development and developmental risk. In: Zeanah CH, editor. Handbook of infant mental health. 2nd edition. New York: Guilford Press; 2000. p. 3.

Psychiatric Features in Children with Genetic Syndromes: Toward Functional Phenotypes

Matthew S. Siegel, MD[a,b,c,*], Wendy E. Smith, MD[d,e]

KEYWORDS

- Children • Phenotype • Behavioral • Genetic
- Neuropsychiatric

In the past decade, rapid advances in genetics have increased diagnostic precision and allowed for further characterization of phenotypes of many genetic syndromes, including behavioral phenotypes. An excellent example is the identification of *MECP2* as the causative gene for Rett syndrome; molecular testing has refined the diagnostic process for a previously mysterious phenomenologically defined disorder and will likely result in *Diagnostic and Statistical Manual of Mental Disorders*, Fifth Edition (DSM-V) nosologic reclassification. With wide availability of molecular diagnostic testing and more precise diagnostic options, increasing attention is being paid by specialists involved in the care of children with genetic conditions, including developmental psychology, child psychiatry, pediatric neurology, genetics, pediatrics, and speech language pathology (though often from singular perspectives), to define the characteristic behavioral phenotypes of genetic disorders (**Table 1**).[1]

A version of this article was previously published in the *Child and Adolescent Psychiatric Clinics of North America, 19:2*.

[a] Department of Psychiatry, Tufts University School of Medicine, 136 Harrison Avenue, Boston, MA 02110, USA

[b] Developmental Disorders Program, Spring Harbor Hospital, 123 Andover Road, Westbrook, ME 04092, USA

[c] Department of Psychiatry, Division of Child Psychiatry, Maine Medical Center, 66 Bramhall Street, Portland, ME 04092, USA

[d] Division of Genetics, Department of Pediatrics, The Barbara Bush Children's Hospital, Maine Medical Center, 22 Bramhall Street, Portland, ME 04102, USA

[e] Maine Medical Partners, Pediatric Specialty Care, 1577 Congress Street, Portland, ME 04102, USA

* Corresponding author. Department of Psychiatry, Division of Child Psychiatry, Maine Medical Center, 66 Bramhall Street, Portland, ME 04092.

E-mail address: siegem@springharbor.org

Pediatr Clin N Am 58 (2011) 833–864
doi:10.1016/j.pcl.2011.06.010
0031-3955/11/$ – see front matter © 2011 Elsevier Inc. All rights reserved.

Table 1
Role of cognitive and psychiatric features in diagnosis

Diagnosis (Mutation)	Cognitive Features	Psychiatric Features	Role in Diagnosis
Down syndrome (Trisomy 21)	Moderate to severe intellectual disability Strengths: grammar Weaknesses: expressive language Visual processing better than auditory	>50%: Hyperactivity, impulsiveness, inattention, and stubbornness 30% Anxiety, depression 10% Autism	Minimal, diagnosis made on physical or medical features *Diagnostic Testing:* Karyotype
Fragile X syndrome (*FMR1*; triplet repeat expansion)	Mild to severe intellectual disability Difficulty with abstract thinking, sequential cognitive processing, short-term memory, math, and visual-motor processing	Attention dysfunction, hyperarousal, social anxiety, social cognition and communication challenges 25%–50% Autism	Significant, often the presenting symptoms *Diagnostic Testing:* FMR1 PCR and Southern blot for CGG repeat length
Rett syndrome (*MECP2*)	Severe to profound intellectual disability Limited language acquisition and use	Stage I: Decreased interactions Stage II: Social withdrawal, irritability, autistic-like behaviors, sleep disturbance Stage III: Improvement in alertness, interactions, ongoing sleep disturbance Stage IV: Persistence of poor communication, irritability	Moderate, presents simultaneously with neurologic features *Diagnostic Testing:* MECP2 sequencing; del/dup testing
Prader-Willi syndrome (15q11-q13; imprinting—loss of paternal contribution)	Mild to borderline intellectual disability Strengths: visuospatial performance, reading and decoding, and long-term memory. Weaknesses: short-term memory, auditory processing, socialization, mathematical skills, and sequential processing	Extreme hyperphagia, self-injurious behaviors (skin picking), OCD Social cognition deficits Cognitive inflexibility, explosiveness, poor affect regulation Depression/mood disorder/psychosis	Minimal, obesity related to hyperphagia may be a major clinical diagnostic clue *Diagnostic Testing:* Methylation PCR followed by FISH

Angelman syndrome (15q11-q13; imprinting—loss of maternal contribution)	Severe to profound intellectual disability Minimal expressive speech, better receptive language	Social and happy; frequent, inappropriate, and unexpected laughter Positive interpersonal bias, social disinhibition with a diminished fear of strangers Fear of crowds and noise, hyperactivity/inattention, sleep disturbance	Significant *Diagnostic Testing:* Methylation PCR followed by FISH; *UBE3A* sequencing
Williams syndrome (deletion 7q11.23)	Mild intellectual disability (75%) Strengths: auditory rote memory and language Weaknesses: severe visuospatial construction deficits and language	Adaptive behavior less than expected for IQ Superficial sociability Externalizing: inattention, impulsivity, attention seeking, hyperactivity, and temper tantrums Internalizing: obsessions/preoccupations, fears, anxiety, sadness/depression ADHD (>50%) Sleep disturbance	Minimal, physical and medical issues often prompt diagnosis *Diagnostic Testing:* Locus-specific FISH or CGH microarray
Deletion 22q11.2	Borderline to mild intellectual disability Verbal IQ is higher than performance Strengths: language abilities Weaknesses: receptive and high-order language skills, abstract reasoning, and visuospatial deficits	Emotional dysregulation ADHD Anxiety and phobias Poor social adaptation with withdrawal Autism 30%: Psychotic symptoms	Moderate, particularly when there are few medical issues *Diagnostic Testing:* Locus-specific FISH or CGH microarray
Smith-Magenis syndrome (deletion 17p11.2)	Moderate intellectual disability (range from mild to severe) Weaknesses: short-term memory, visuomotor coordination, sequencing, and response speed Speech delay is common, with receptive language better than expressive	Sleep disturbance (inverted melatonin circadian rhythms) Self-injurious behaviors Stereotypy: self-hug, lick-and-flip, mouthing objects, teeth grinding, body rocking, spinning Socially adult-oriented, demanding of adult attention, egocentric, delayed empathic skills	Significant, often predominate overall phenotype *Diagnostic Testing:* Locus-specific FISH or CGH microarray

(continued on next page)

Table 1
(continued)

Diagnosis (Mutation)	Cognitive Features	Psychiatric Features	Role in Diagnosis
Turner syndrome (45, X and variants)	Infrequent intellectual disability (5%) Performance IQ lower than verbal Learning disabilities in math common Significantly impaired nonverbal abilities Impaired executive functioning skills: attention and concentration, problem-solving ability, organization and working memory, impulsivity and processing speed	ADHD 18 times higher than general population Social immaturity, anxiety Younger girls: immature, hyperactive and anxious Older girls: anxiety, depression, and social relationship challenges	Minimal, generally diagnosed on physical or medical features *Diagnostic Testing:* Karyotype
Lesch-Nyhan syndrome (HPRT deficiency)	Mild to moderate intellectual disability	Chronic, compulsive, self-injurious behaviors resulting in self-mutilation: biting, eye poking, fingernail pulling, psychogenic vomiting, arching, head snapping, head banging Language pattern: repeated ambivalent statements with anxiety and vulgarity Frequent compulsive aggression toward others (grabbing and pinching)	Significant *Diagnostic Testing:* Urine urate/creatinine ratio (>2.0 suggestive) followed by HPRT enzyme activity determination; sequencing is available

Abbreviations: ADHD, attention-deficit/hyperactivity disorder; CGH, comparative genomic hybridization; FISH, fluorescent in situ hybridization; HPRT, hypoxanthine-guanine phosphoribosyltransferase; OCD, obsessive compulsive disorder.

Although children with genetic diagnoses represent a small proportion of referrals to general child psychiatry practitioners, information about these conditions has a role beyond direct applicability to the diagnosed child. Given that rates of mental illness are higher in all individuals with developmental delay, children with a neurodevelopmental disorder are more likely to present to a practitioner, and awareness of phenotypic features allows for the identification of previously undiagnosed individuals, as well as for more complete evaluation of individuals with known diagnoses. From a population perspective, examining psychopathology in individuals with known genetic diagnoses leads to an increased understanding of gene-brain-behavior pathways[2] that may have far-reaching implications in the general population.

In genetics, a clinical diagnosis is often suspected on the basis of specific physical, developmental, medical, and behavioral features; all of these features comprise the overall phenotype of the individual. The behavioral phenotype of genetic conditions encompasses specific cognitive, language, and social aspects as well as behavioral deviance and psychopathology. It is important to remember that despite a common diagnosis, a "classic" behavioral phenotype may not occur in all affected individuals and may be affected by genotype, environmental factors, and intellectual disability.[2]

The mental health field historically has struggled with the concept of distinct psychiatric or neurobehavioral illness in a person with developmental delay, sometimes termed dual diagnosis. Reiss and colleagues[3] have eloquently described the troublesome issue of diagnostic overshadowing, whereby all features of an individual's presentation are ascribed to developmental delay. Such an error of attribution leads to the underdiagnosis of distinct and treatable disorders or impairments, and increases illness burden. Social traits, in particular, have been difficult for clinicians to evaluate, specifically whether deficits are due to a particular genetic diagnosis, a common downstream effect of psychosocial disadvantage and stigmatization, or secondary to developmental delay and intellectual disability.[4] In contrast, clinicians must be alert to the possibility of overpathologizing developmentally appropriate behavior in a delayed child.

A common conundrum for the child psychiatrist is that neither psychiatric nor behavioral models fully capture the individual presenting phenotype. The field has evolved from detailed narrative descriptions of characteristic behavioral traits for a specific disorder to a second generation of research that uses validated instruments applying DSM criteria to define prevalence rates of psychopathology. Concerns have been raised that creating a behavioral or psychiatric phenotype solely from studies measuring psychopathology based on DSM criteria is reductionistic,[5] as many individuals with genetic syndromes have behaviors or features that do not appear in the DSM, and if a particular diagnostic category is not assessed in the research, it is then omitted from the evidence base. The neurodevelopmental disorders with well-described genetic bases have far more specificity than DSM disorders, and social phenotypes or traits, in particular, are not well characterized in the DSM Fourth Edition, Text Revised.

Behavioral phenotypes themselves, however, do not fully capture what a child psychiatrist is evaluating, which should be particularly focused on what may contribute to impairment in functioning. Such an evaluation requires the integration of cognitive, social, psychiatric, and behavioral features that contribute to impairment, leading to description and possible understanding of an individual functioning phenotype. With this context in mind, here the authors review several readily identified genetic syndromes, with a particular focus on psychiatric features that affect the functional phenotype.

GENETIC TESTING

Significant advances have been made in methods and availability of genetic testing in the past decade, allowing for increased precision in establishing a diagnosis for many individuals. In fact, the long-honored chromosome analysis (or karyotype), once the mainstay of genetic testing, is now often replaced as a first-line test with molecular methods, including fluorescent in situ hybridization (FISH), comparative genomic hybridization (CGH) microarray, and gene sequencing. A good analogy for genetic testing is a set of encyclopedias on a shelf. A karyotype can determine how many volumes are present or if large sections are rearranged onto other volumes. FISH testing can indicate whether a specific section or chapter is missing; CGH can determine if *any* chapter is missing. DNA sequencing can tell if there is a typo in a specific sentence.

A karyotype remains the primary means of documenting chromosome number and structure; this is the only testing method able to diagnose chromosome translocations. A karyotype is obtained by inducing living cells to replicate in the laboratory but halting the process in metaphase when the chromatin is condensed into the characteristic chromosomes; these chromosomes are then stained and the banding patterns are compared to identify and sort the individual chromosome pairs.

FISH is a method used to detect the presence or absence of a specific portion of DNA as determined by the probe used. Patient DNA is collected and denatured to a single-stranded form; a locus-specific DNA probe with an attached fluorescent marker is then hybridized to the patient DNA. If the probe target is present in patient DNA, the probe binds and its presence is detected using a fluorescent microscope. Absence of the locus-specific DNA probe indicates that the target area is deleted from the patient DNA.

CGH, or microarray, uses a multiplex platform to compare numerous (tens of thousands) segments of patient DNA to control DNA using a computerized reading method. Patient DNA and control DNA are allowed to hybridize and bind to a computer chip where specific chromosome loci are represented by specific locations on the chip. A computer then assesses whether the patient DNA and control DNA are present in equal amounts at each test locus. If excess control DNA is detected at a particular location, the inference is that this area was deleted in the patient sample; if excess patient DNA is detected, a duplication of patient DNA is implied. CGH is being used increasingly as a first-line diagnostic tool.

For disorders in which a specific gene is identified to be causative, targeted DNA testing is often used to establish a diagnosis. The specific type of DNA testing method used depends on the molecular cause of the condition. For diagnoses in which point mutations (single nucleotide alterations, insertions, or deletions) are the main etiology, gene sequencing is often used. For well-characterized conditions, sequencing may be simplified into common mutation testing or exon-specific sequencing if there are particular "hot spots" within the known gene. It is important to remember that gene sequencing only tests for alterations in the specific gene targeted and will not provide any other genetic information.

An excellent resource for information about genetic testing, including available testing options for many genetic diagnoses, is www.genetests.org, a National Institutes of Health supported Web site designed to provide current genetic diagnostic information via a searchable laboratory directory.

Pre- and posttest genetic counseling is a necessary component of all genetic testing. Families must be informed of the advantages and limitations of various tests, particularly the sensitivity and specificity of testing and implications of test results for other family members. This counseling is often complex and should be provided by a someone who is very familiar with all of the potential issues; genetic counselors are Masters degree trained individuals with board certification from the American Board of Genetic Counseling.

TRISOMY 21 (DOWN SYNDROME)
Genetics, Etiology, and Epidemiology

Initially described by John Langdon Down in 1866, the condition known eponymously as Down syndrome (DS) was determined to be caused by trisomy of chromosome 21 in the 1950s. Whereas the vast majority of individuals (more than 95%) with trisomy 21 have an entire additional chromosome 21 secondary to nondisjunction during gametogenesis, a smaller percentage of individuals will have trisomy 21 related to a chromosome translocation. An even smaller percentage of affected individuals will have variable physical features related to somatic mosaicism or partial duplication of chromosome 21q22 involved in other chromosome rearrangements. A diagnosis of trisomy 21 can be confirmed with chromosome analysis, although determining low-level mosaicism may require additional testing.

The incidence of trisomy 21 varies during gestation, but is thought to be approximately 1 in 800 live births.[6] There is no identified ethnic, population, or socioeconomic predilection. The risk of trisomy 21 increases with increasing maternal age, related to maternal nondisjunction; however, the vast majority of babies with trisomy 21 are born into families without advanced parental age.

Advances in medical and surgical care of individuals with chromosome abnormalities has had a tremendous impact on the life expectancy of individuals with trisomy 21. Although mortality within the first several years of life is increased over the general population, related in part to higher neonatal mortality and congenital structural cardiac disease, current life expectancy is estimated to be greater than 50 to 60 years.[7]

Physical Features and Medical Issues

The overwhelming majority of individuals with trisomy 21 will be diagnosed in the neonatal period based on characteristic facial features and concomitant medical issues. An increasing proportion of infants are also diagnosed prenatally through widely available screening tests offered to all pregnant women.[8]

The characteristic facial features of individuals with trisomy 21 vary slightly over time, but the overall facial gestalt is always present. Microcephaly with occipital flattening is common, and midface hypoplasia tends to center the facial features. Notably, the palpebral fissures are up-slanting and there is often an exaggerated inner-canthal or epicanthal fold that accentuates a flat and broad nasal bridge. The nose and mouth are small. The ears tend to be small and round, and are often low set (the peak of the pinna is not intersected by an imaginary line drawn through the inner and outer canthal folds) and posteriorly rotated. The neck is short and there is frequently thickening or redundant skin posteriorly. Individuals with trisomy 21 are shorter than their family prediction, and this is most apparent in the proximal arms and legs as well as the hands and feet.

Congenital malformations of multiple organ systems may be seen in trisomy 21.[9] Cardiac malformations are seen in 40% to 50% of individuals and include most commonly ventricular septal defects, endocardial cushion defects, and persistent patent ductus arteriosus as well as a variety of other malformations. Gastrointestinal malformations, including duodenal atresia, and Hirschsprung disease are seen at rate higher than in the general population. Other common medical issues include an increased risk for seizures,[10] thyroid disease (autoimmune hypothyroidism),[11] celiac disease,[12] refractive errors, strabismus, hearing loss, eustachian tube dysfunction, occipito-atlanto-axial instability, and acute leukemia as well as an increased susceptibility to infections. Appropriate growth charts and Health Care Supervision recommendations are available from the American Academy of Pediatrics[13] as well as the major DS awareness and support organizations.

Cognitive and Psychiatric Features

Developmental delay is universally present in individuals with DS, most commonly moderate to severe intellectual disability, with a wide range in severity. Language delay is common, with greater impairment in expressive skills as compared with receptive skills.[14] Language pragmatics are spared, while there are challenges for grammar. Visual processing is more developed than auditory processing.[15]

Individuals with DS historically were described as placid and good tempered, but this generalization has not been supported. Several investigators have characterized a pattern of hyperactivity, impulsivity, inattention, and stubbornness/disobedience, with Pueschel and colleagues[16] describing this pattern in more than half of the 40 school-age children with DS studied. Some children demonstrate a stubborn persistence, need for sameness, and repetitive or perseverative qualities.[17]

Rates of comorbid psychiatric disorders are higher than in the general population, although lower than rates in the total population with intellectual disability.[18] Up to one-third of children with DS meet criteria for at least one psychiatric disorder[19] including attention-deficit/hyperactivity disorder (ADHD), conduct disorder, and anxiety disorder.[20]

Psychiatric features change with developmental level. Preschool- to school-age children with DS commonly display hyperactivity and impulsivity, noncompliance and tantruming, agitation, anxiety or disruptiveness, repetitive movements, and sensory dysregulation, but are rarely disinterested in social interaction.[19] Postpubertal individuals show a significant decrease in hyperactivity but increased internalizing symptoms, including social withdrawal.[21] Depression has been described in children and adolescents with DS. Symptoms observed are those typical of depressive disorders (ie, depressed mood, crying, decreased interests, and so forth),[22] and self-care may deteriorate. The differential diagnosis of a mood disorder in DS individuals should include hypothyroidism, B-12 deficiency, bereavement, and obstructive sleep apnea.[23] Increased anxiety and extreme social withdrawal may be present in DS children with major depressive disorder. In addition, 7% to 10% of individuals with DS meet criteria for autism, and when it occurs there is a high probability of one or more family members displaying a broader autism phenotype.[24]

Accurate psychiatric diagnosis can be a challenge, and experts in the treatment of individuals with DS encourage a focus "beyond overt behaviors in search of diagnostic clues, such as alterations in mood, arousal or activity level, physiologic disturbance, atypical development or neurocognitive function."[19]

The evidence base for DS-specific psychopharmacologic treatment is limited. At this time treatment borrows from conventional intervention pathways for psychiatric illness in the general population. In one group of children with DS, a small open-label trial of rivistigamine showed positive effects on several aspects of cognitive functioning.[25]

FRAGILE X SYNDROME
Genetics, Etiology, and Epidemiology

Fragile X syndrome (FXS) is recognized as the most common inherited form of mental retardation, with an incidence of approximately 1 in 3000, including affected males and females. The premutation/intermediate length mutation carrier frequency is much higher, approximately 1% in females[26] and 1 in 800 males.

FXS is one of several "triplet repeat" neurologic disorders caused by expansion of a disease-specific trinucleotide repeat within a disease-specific gene. In FXS this trinucleotide repeat, CGG, expands within the promoter of the *FMR1* gene located at Xq27.3. Expansion of the number of CGG repeats leads to decreased or absent formation of FMRP, a protein critical to the translation of molecular messages within the developing brain.

In the general population, the number of CGG repeats in *FMR1* is typically 20 to 50. CGG repeats within this range can be stable over generations and carry no risk of expansion to a full mutation in the next generation. When the number of CGG repeats expands to greater than 50, the risk of expansion to a full mutation, more than 200 CGG repeats, increases. CGG repeats between 50 and 200 are termed premutations; premutation carriers may have mild features, but are often indistinguishable from non-premutation carriers. When a premutation in *FMR1* is passed from a carrier mother to a child, there is a substantial risk of expansion to produce a full mutation in the child; full mutations of *FMR1* are methylated and FMRP is not expressed. This situation results in FXS in males (who have only one copy of *FMR1*) and variable features, ranging from mild to complete FXS, in females, because of X-inactivation and the contribution of the normal *FMR1* gene to cellular functioning.

Molecular testing for FXS in affected individuals and individuals at risk for being carriers is readily available.[27] More than 99% of patients can be diagnosed using the polymerase chain reaction (PCR) to determine CGG repeat size (most accurate for CGG repeat lengths within the normal or low permutation range) and Southern blotting to determine the size of large mutations as well as methylation status. Determining methylation status in males with a full mutation can provide some prognostic information. Determination of premutation size in at risk family members is essential for accurate genetic counseling. Methylation PCR is frequently used to rapidly identify individuals who require more in-depth testing. Point mutations in *FMR1* have been identified in a very small percentage of affected individuals. Cytogenetic studies cannot be used reliably for detection of a fragile site in either affected individuals or carriers; this is important as cytogenetics was the primary means of diagnosis until well into the 1990s.

Physical Features and Medical Issues

The classic physical and facial features associated with FXS in males may not be evident until later childhood, if at all. These features include macrocephaly, large and prominent ears, a long face, postpubertal macroorchidism, and a subtle connective tissue disorder characterized by a highly arched palate, small joint hyperextensibility, flat feet, and mitral valve prolapse.[28] In early childhood clinical suspicion is most often raised by the developmental and behavioral phenotype, as physical examination features are not as clear.[29,30]

In infancy, boys with FXS may have feeding difficulties related to hypotonia, gastroesophageal reflux, or oral motor/sensory issues.[31] Medical problems in childhood can include seizures in approximately one-third of affected individuals, recurrent sinus or middle ear infections in up to 25%, mild scoliosis in 20%, and problems with small joint hyperextensibility, particularly in the hands in the vast majority of boys.[32] Older adolescents and adults may develop mitral valve prolapse (50%) and hypertension. The hyperextensibility generally improves. The American Academy of Pediatrics has published Health Care Supervision guidelines for individuals with FXS.[33]

Cognitive and Psychiatric Features

Affected males typically show mild to severe intellectual disability and difficulty with abstract thinking, sequential cognitive processing, short-term memory, math, and visual-motor processing.[34] IQ correlates inversely with the number of trinucleotide repeats, and executive functioning, visual-spatial skills, and attention are more impaired than would be expected for IQ level.[35] Language skills plateau at approximately 48 months, and speech is typically rapid with tangentiality and perseveration. One-third of patients have a significant decline in IQ in middle to late childhood due to peaking in the rate of development relative to chronologic age. Large prospective longitudinal studies have shown that children with FXS do not lose skills, but do not maintain the same developmental trajectory as same-age peers.[36]

Individuals with FXS struggle with attentional dysfunction, hyperarousal, social anxiety, and communication challenges. Females with the full mutation may show social anxiety, social awkwardness, and schizotypal features.[37] Female premutation carriers have an elevated rate of emotional problems; 30% show anxiety, social phobia or depression, but no cognitive deficits.[38] This statistic suggests that the behavioral features of social avoidance and anxiety are independent of the effects of cognitive deficits. Adult male premutation carriers have attention-switching problems including a preference for fixed routines and a tendency to focus on details.[39]

Anxiety has been widely recognized as a major focus of impairment.[40] Avoidance of social interactions may be due to hyperarousal, as children with FXS have enhanced autonomic reactivity to sensory stimuli and a decrease in prepulse inhibition.[41,42] Gaze aversion is a prominent feature, particularly over the age of 8 to 9 years, and may disrupt social interactions. Of note, the gaze aversion is accompanied by an appropriate recognition of the other person. Studies have shown neuronal dysfunction involving the fusiform gyrus, plus evidence that direct gaze is processed abnormally.[43] Direct gaze, eye contact, and socialization are associated with hyperarousal and a high level of stress.[44]

There are high rates of autistic-like symptoms, such as gaze aversion, hand flapping, language impairment and perseveration, and social cognition deficits,[45] and one-quarter to one-half of children with FXS meet criteria for autism, although individuals with FXS account for only 1% of those diagnosed with autism. In one study, autistic and psychiatric symptoms were found to be stable over time in 18 males with FXS through adulthood.[46]

Treatment of emotional and behavioral problems in children with FXS is best approached from a multimodal perspective. Speech and language therapy, behavioral interventions, special education, and psychopharmacology all have a role.

Treatment of emotional dysregulation and behavioral outbursts has been investigated from behavioral and pharmacologic perspectives. In controlled studies, most problem behaviors in FXS children were maintained by social escape, suggesting that an exposure protocol treatment for social interaction paired with social skills training may be an effective intervention. A pilot study of behavioral shaping to increase eye contact was recently published by Hall[47] and suggests the ability to use cognitive behavioral techniques to improve core behavioral deficits in FXS. Treatment with a selective serotonin reuptake inhibitor (SSRI) targeting social anxiety may be helpful, and a survey of fluoxetine usage in FXS suggested that it may be effective for depression and mood lability in females and aggression in males.[48]

Aggression, agitation, and mood dysregulation may respond to an atypical antipsychotic—anecdotal reports from topic experts indicate low doses of aripiprazole, 2.5 to 5 mg at night, may be beneficial.[49] Lithium has also been anecdotally reported to be helpful with aggression and mood stabilization in adolescents; opinion on the use of propranolol, a β-blocking agent, is mixed, although one case report suggested improvement.[50]

There have been 3 controlled studies of treatment of ADHD in FXS: 15 children with FXS, 3 to 11 years old, received methylphenidate (MPH), 0.3 mg/kg twice a day or dextroamphetamine, 0.2 mg/kg daily for 1 week. Ten of the 15 were judged to be responders to MPH; however, improvements could not be demonstrated on most outcome measures.[51,52] A double-blind randomized controlled trial using L-acetylcar-nitine, 50 mg/kg twice a day, reported improvement in hyperactivity at the 1-year mark in boys with FXS.[53] A survey of parents whose children were taking clonidine sug-gested beneficial effects in a majority,[54] and the same author has suggested clonidine or tenex as an intervention of choice for children with sensory hypersensitivity and hyperarousal.

Sporadic case reports have looked at other agents including imipramine.[55] Several attempts have also been made to use compounds targeting neurobiologic deficits produced by the absence of FMRP.[56]

RETT SYNDROME
Genetics, Etiology, and Epidemiology

Classic Rett syndrome has a prevalence of approximately 1 in 10,000 females,[57] although emerging information regarding the range of phenotypes associated with *MECP2* alterations in both males and females will expand the clinical impact of this gene over time. *MECP2* is located at Xq28 and encodes the MeCP2 protein respon-sible for decreasing transcription, and thus expression, of other genes. Loss of this inhibition in the brain probably results in overexpression of normally tightly regulated genes in brain development.[58]

Molecular testing is available to confirm a clinical diagnosis of Rett syndrome; however, mutations are found by sequencing the *MECP2* gene in only approximately 80% of girls with classic features and 40% with variant phenotypes.[59,60] Reliable genotype-phenotype correlations cannot be made for most identified mutations.[61] Other methods are used to detect deletions and duplications; the latter are more common in severe *MECP2*-related phenotypes.[62] Most *MECP2* mutations associated with classic Rett syndrome are not inherited, although asymptomatic mothers have been identified.

Physical Features and Medical Issues

Clinical diagnostic criteria are available for establishing a diagnosis of Rett syndrome along with variant phenotypes.[63] These criteria highlight the more specific features of the syndrome and place less emphasis on the nonspecific features to reduce erro-neous diagnosis and exclude other potential causes of similar generalized features.

Rett syndrome is most often diagnosed in childhood once the developmental trajec-tory of affected girls is recognized. Classic Rett syndrome typically progresses through recognizable clinical stages throughout the lifetime.[64,65] Stage I is the "early-onset stagnation" phase marked by mildly delayed development, although continued progress, and reduced interactions with others. This stage typically begins in toddlerhood and lasts weeks or months, only to be followed by a similarly brief State II. Stage II is the "rapid developmental regression" phase during which there is true loss of acquired motor, language, and social skills, which may happen quite dramat-ically or over time. This phase is accompanied by a more pronounced decrease in interaction with others and objects, and development of atypical behaviors or actions such as hair pulling. Growth failure develops during this time, with slowing of linear growth and head circumference. By early childhood, length and head circumference are usually at least 2 standard deviations below the mean, and the head circumference may continue to decrease to more than 3 standard deviations below the mean by late childhood.

Following State II is Stage III, the "pseudostationary phase," when the stereotypical, repetitive hand motions (wringing, washing motions, or clapping) are most obvious. Breathing patterns can change, and sleep/wake cycles are often disturbed. Interaction skills and elements of personality reappear, leading to an apparent "wake-up." Seizures are seen in some affected girls, and dystonia is not infrequent leading to orthopedic complications. This phase can last for many years. Stage IV, "late motor deterioration," commences when the ability to walk is lost. During this phase there is progressive neurologic deterioration leading to rigidity, although purposeful eye movements and intense visual awareness are often preserved. Autonomic dysfunction is also common.

Medical complications are related to the developmental and neurologic issues. Feeding problems due to neurologic impairment can be compounded by gastro-esophageal reflux. Seizures are common, and are diagnosed in 80% of affected individuals, although they can resolve with time. Orthopedic complications secondary to neurologic manifestations are typical. Cardiac rhythm disturbances due to prolonged QTc interval are seen and have been associated with sudden death.

Cognitive and Psychiatric Features

Most affected girls experience severe to profound intellectual disability, but there is little evidence for deterioration over time.[66] There is severe impairment in the development of expressive and receptive language, and most girls lose all speech by 40 months, although use of some words may be preserved.[67]

Behavioral and emotional features vary by stage of progression. In Stage I subtle symptoms include decreased eye contact and reduced interest in toys. During Stage II the emergence of stereotypic hand movements is paired with social withdrawal, and autistic-like behaviors with irritability, sleep disturbance, and screaming and crying episodes.

In Stage III there is generally an improvement in behavior, less irritability and fewer autistic-like features, better social and communication skills, and better alertness and attention span. Stereotypical, midline, asymmetric hand movements are almost constant but can be voluntarily controlled for short periods of time.[68] Stage III is also characterized by sleep disturbance with initial insomnia, frequent arousals, and daytime napping. Stage IV (late motor deterioration) heralds reduced mobility and increased rigidity, spasticity, and dystonic posturing, but no decline in cognition, communication, or hand skills.[69] Eye gaze becomes the most important interactional mode.

There are no proven pharmacologic treatments for the syndrome. Topic experts have suggested that agitation can be treated with low-dose neuroleptics or SSRIs, and sleep disturbance can be ameliorated with melatonin or antihistamines.[70]

PRADER-WILLI SYNDROME
Genetics, Etiology, and Epidemiology

The genes within the proximal region of the long arm of chromosome 15 demonstrate tightly regulated, specific parent-of-origin expression. This differential expression is controlled by imprinting, by which methylation of the DNA causes the selective silencing of genes from either the paternal or the maternal homolog. The genes within this region are variably expressed, with some genes expressed only when inherited paternally and others only when inherited maternally.

Loss of the paternally expressed genetic information at 15q11-q13 results in the medical and physical features recognized as Prader-Willi syndrome (PWS). PWS has an estimated incidence of 1 in 10,000 to 1 in 15,000, and has no racial or ethnic predilection. There are several different molecular etiologies for PWS including a common 4-Mb deletion of the paternally inherited chromosome 15 (75%), maternal uniparental disomy (UPD; inheritance of both copies of chromosome 15 from the mother), or an imprinting defect (<5%).

Molecular testing for PWS is readily available. Most testing algorithms begin with methylation-sensitive PCR, which can diagnose PWS independent of molecular etiology by determining whether both a methylated (maternal) and unmethylated (paternal) signal are detected.[71] The absence of the unmethylated (paternal) contribution confirms the diagnosis. Additional testing, including FISH and UPD studies, are required to distinguish the underlying cause and provide appropriate genetic counseling.

Physical Features and Medical Issues

The medical and physical features of PWS change dramatically within the first few years of life. Infancy is universally marked by profound central hypotonia and feeding difficulties, often leading to failure to thrive. With time the hypotonia improves, but global developmental delays become more prominent. In childhood, central obesity results from extreme hyperphagia, usually beginning between 1 and 6 years of age.

Physical features include short stature, small and narrow hands and feet, hypogonadism, and fair pigmentation as compared with family members. The facial features are notable for bitemporal narrowing, almond-shaped eyes, and a narrow nasal bridge. Medical issues are often related to obesity, with a high proportion of fat mass to lean body mass. Decreased vomiting and a high pain threshold may predispose affected individuals to acute injuries.

Clinical criteria have been developed and validated to allow for prompt diagnosis in suggestive clinical situations.[72,73] Treatment with recombinant human growth hormone has been shown to improve linear growth and, possibly, body composition.[74,75]

Cognitive and Psychiatric Features

Mild (33%) to borderline (60%) intellectual disability is common; however, up to 5% of those with PWS have an IQ in the normal range.[76] Individuals with PWS show challenges with short-term memory, auditory processing, socialization, mathematical skills, and sequential processing. Relative strengths are present in visuospatial performance, reading and decoding, and long-term memory. There is a particular aptitude for jigsaw puzzles.

Individuals with PWS have very high rates of maladaptive behaviors, the most striking of which is compulsive hyperphagia, characterized by compulsive food seeking, food hoarding,[77] and gorging. Management is primarily behavioral, by restricting access to food, which can be a major challenge.

Obsessive-compulsive features are widely recognized, including ritualistic behaviors, hoarding nonfood items, hair pulling, skin picking, ordering, and "just right" behaviors.[78] Compulsive behaviors cause significant impairment in almost half of affected individuals, but frank obsessional thinking is rare.[79] Cognitive inflexibility, with a drive for sameness, usually comes to clinical attention around 5 years of age with perseveration in speech, becoming "stuck" on issues, and need for a consistent daily schedule. There is a high incidence of responding to minor frustrations with explosive tantrums. Individuals with PWS tend to be egocentric and will argue, lie, manipulate, and confabulate to change rules, obtain their wishes, or justify behavior. These characteristics may produce a picture of oppositionality and stubbornness which, when paired with typically solitary behavior and social withdrawal, leads to poor peer relations.[80] Specific social cognition deficits have been identified, including difficulty recognizing social cues and processing social information.[81]

In adolescence, explosiveness and poor affect regulation may evolve into prolonged periods of clinical depression, and in some cases into a hypomanic state with confusion, restlessness, and increased goal-directed behavior lasting days to weeks; 15% to 17% of individuals with PWS meet criteria for a mood disorder.[82] In one study, 28% of individuals with PWS developed severe affective disturbance with psychotic features in late adolescence to adulthood; there are emerging genotype-phenotype correlations.[83,84]

Self-injury rates are high throughout life; in one series 81% of PWS individuals engaged in self-injurious behavior (SIB).[85] Skin picking is the most common form of self-injury[79] followed by nose picking, nail and lip biting, nail pulling, and hair pulling.

The primary treatment for most of the functionally impairing features is behavioral and has been reviewed elsewhere.[86] All individuals require long-term behavioral treatment, and interventions have included placing food under restricted access, token economies, video modeling, and others.

Pharmacologic management experience is anecdotal. A tendency toward effects greater than expected for dose, both therapeutic and undesired, has been noted, and dosages one-quarter to one-half of typical are often sufficient[87] for effect. Reduced metabolism by components of cytochrome P450 complex has been documented in one-third of PWS individuals and may provide a clue to this finding.[88] SSRIs may improve compulsive behaviors and skin picking, but careful monitoring of mood is necessary.[89] Additional small studies and case reports have demonstrated success in improving mood and skin-picking behaviors with topiramate,[90,91] reduction of violent outbursts with carbamazepine[92] and lithium,[93] and improvement in maladaptive behaviors without weight gain using low-dose risperidone (average of 1.6 mg/d).[94] Methylphenidate has been noted to be helpful for ADHD symptomatology.[95] Medications have not been effective in curbing the drive for food or decreasing appetite.

ANGELMAN SYNDROME
Genetics, Etiology, and Epidemiology

Within the 15q11-q13 region are genes with specific parent of origin expression; some genes are exclusively expressed from the paternal allele and others are expressed only from the maternal allele. When there is loss of the normal expression of maternal alleles, Angelman syndrome (AS) results.[96] This loss of expression can result from several molecular mechanisms including a deletion within the maternal chromosome homolog (70%–75%), paternal UPD of chromosome 15 (2%–5%), and imprinting defects (2%–5%). Mutations within one gene located within this region, UBE3A, have been shown to cause AS in 20% to 25% of affected individuals.

Molecular testing to diagnose AS is available.[97] Testing begins with methylation-sensitive PCR, which can confirm a diagnosis in most affected individuals. If an abnormal methylation pattern is detected, additional FISH or UPD studies will determine the etiology. In individuals with classic features and normal methylation studies, UBE3A mutation analysis is indicated.

AS is seen in all ethnic groups, and has an overall incidence of approximately 1 in 12,000 to 1 in 20,000.[98]

Physical Features and Medical Issues

Most individuals with AS are diagnosed in childhood as the physical examination features, developmental profile and medical issues become apparent.[99] Seizures, often difficult to control, dominate the medical issues, and usually emerge at 18 to 24 months. Microcephaly develops over time as well. Some individuals have hypopigmentation, strabismus or oral motor coordination difficulties.

Cognitive and Psychiatric Features

Global developmental delays in very early childhood evolve into severe to profound intellectual disability. Marked expressive speech delay is common, with many children using few, if any words; receptive language skills are often more advanced.

The behavioral phenotype of individuals with AS is characteristic and part of available clinical diagnostic criteria.[100] Individuals appear social and happy but laugh frequently, inappropriately and unexpectedly with minimal stimulation. Laughter is not uncontrollable; laughing and smiling behavior increases in the presence of adult speech, touch, eye contact, smiling or laughing.[101] Although individuals with AS have a markedly positive interpersonal bias, social disinhibition, a diminished fear of strangers, fear of crowds and noise are commonly problematic.[102]

Hyperactivity/inattention is commonly reported, particularly in childhood, and improvement is noted with age.[103] Sleep disturbance, seen in approximately 25% of individuals includes reduced total sleep time, increased sleep onset latency, disrupted sleep architecture with frequent nocturnal awakenings, reduced rapid-eye-movement sleep and periodic leg movements.[104] Other less frequent but problematic behaviors include excessive mouthing/chewing, hand flapping, aggression and an attraction to water; food related behaviors include pica, gorging food and food fads.[105] No controlled psychopharmacologic data exist.

WILLIAMS SYNDROME

Genetics, Etiology, and Epidemiology

The co-occurrence of idiopathic hypercalcemia and supravalvar aortic stenosis was initially described in the 1960s[106–108] and the full syndrome was eponymously named after cardiologists Williams and Buren. WS is primarily a sporadic condition with an approximate incidence of 1 in 10,000. A common chromosome microdeletion of 1.5 Mb at 7q11.23 is responsible for the full phenotype[109]; absence of the *ELN* gene is associated with the cardiac and connective tissue features, and loss of the *LIMK1* and *GTF2I* genes appear to be critical for the WS cognitive and developmental phenotype, respectively.[110,111] Molecular testing, via FISH or CGH microarray, is able to document the microdeletion in 99% of individuals with WS.

Physical Features and Medical Issues

Most diagnoses of WS are made early in childhood based on the classic cardiac malformations, supravalvar aortic stenosis and, less commonly, pulmonic stenosis, accompanied by short stature, typical facial features, and characteristic developmental and behavioral features. The facial features of individuals with WS change over time but are notable for bitemporal narrowing, a long philtrum, a wide mouth with full lips, a "stellate" appearance of the iris, an infraorbital crease, and full cheeks. Because of the defect in elastin, the face ages more than expected based on chronologic age, resulting in narrowing of the face and furrowing along the nasolabial folds.

Individuals with WS tend to have a deep or hoarse voice, hypotonia, ligamentous laxity, soft skin, and a predisposition to viscous organ diverticulae and rectal prolapse.

Fifteen percent of individuals have variable hypercalcemia. A history of failure to thrive in infancy is common. Health care supervision guidelines are available from the American Academy of Pediatrics.[112]

Cognitive and Psychiatric Features

Seventy-five percent of individuals with WS have intellectual disability, usually in the mild range. Adaptive behavior, however, is less than expected for IQ. Strengths in auditory rote memory and language are seen, but severe visuospatial construction deficits[113] and language disorder are problematic.

Externalizing maladaptive behaviors are common and include inattention (>90%), impulsivity, attention seeking, hyperactivity, and temper tantrums. Internalizing features are also frequent, including obsessions/preoccupations, fears, anxiety, sadness/depression, and irritability. Fights and aggressive behavior are less common than the frequency seen in the general intellectual disability (ID) population.

Individuals with WS display a superficial sociability, comprising a keen interest in people and increased empathy, appearing most clearly pathologic in their guileless approach to strangers.[114] Affected children show increased social interest from infancy onward,[114] and display a positive interpersonal bias when categorizing others[115]; face-seeking and positive face stimuli are overvalued.[116] Individuals with WS rely on superficial signals but fail to recognize more subtle cues in the interactions with others,[117] resulting in excessive empathy and lack of social inhibition.[118] Along with this capacity to empathize with others, affected individuals perform poorly on theory of mind tasks that require inferring mental states as a basis for others' behavior,[119] and in particular show deficits in the social cognition component.

The most striking psychopathologic features are on the anxiety axis, which are more prevalent than in the general ID population.[120] Individuals show high levels of anxiety, and many develop depression as adults, which may relate to the accumulation of unsuccessful social experiences. Use of the DICA-R (Diagnostic Interview for Children and Adolescents—Revised) in WS individuals revealed minimal separation anxiety or obsessive compulsive disorder, but high rates of worry about future events. Eighteen percent met criteria for generalized anxiety disorder, and 35% met full criteria for a specific phobia, commonly with associated avoidance behavior. Unlike neurotypical children, individuals with WS show maintenance of concrete fears, out of proportion to their developmental delay.[121] Common phobias involve natural environment fears (storms, high places), fears of being alone, and fears involving animals. Cognitive behavioral therapy using exposure and response prevention is recommended for treatment of these phobias.

More than half of affected children have ADHD, primarily inattentive and combined types.[122] Hyperactivity and aggression, if present, may decrease with age. There have been 2 small placebo-controlled pharmacologic treatment studies, in which MPH was shown to be effective at a dose of 0.5 mg/kg or 10 mg twice a day in a majority of those studied.[123,124]

An increased rate of sleep disturbance, particularly initiating and maintaining sleep, has been seen in up to half of affected individuals; polysomnography showed no increased sleep apnea but increased wake time, decreased stage 1 and 2 sleep, increased stage 3 and 4 sleep, and fivefold higher periodic limb movements. Clonazepam has been reported to be helpful.[125]

DELETION 22Q11.2 (VELO-CARDIO-FACIAL SYNDROME; DIGEORGE SYNDROME)
Genetics, Etiology, and Epidemiology

Encompassing a wide range of physical phenotypes, including several eponymous syndromes, this microdeletion is thought to be the most common contiguous gene deletion, with general population estimates ranging from 1 in 3800 to 1 in 6000.[126] The deletion is found in much higher frequency within populations selected for cardinal physical features including cleft lip/palate/bifid uvula and conotruncal cardiac malformations.

The classic 3-Mb deletion includes 30 genes, several of which appear to play a role in the phenotype. *TBX1* has been shown to be associated with the cardiovascular malformations,[127] *COMT* may have a role in the behavioral and psychological issues,[128] and *CTLD* appears to be associated with hypotonia.[129]

Deletions of 22q11.2 can be detected via specific FISH. Recently, CGH microarray has been used as first-line molecular testing for individuals with developmental delays.[130] This technology is able to detect the classic deletion as well as smaller, variant deletions that would not be detected via FISH, as the probe target is not deleted. The clinical information emerging as a result of the variant deletions will likely contribute to more specific genotype-phenotype correlations, particularly with regard to the congenital anomalies and psychiatric issues.[131,132]

In contrast to most other microdeletion syndromes, approximately 10% of 22q11.2 deletions are inherited from variably affected parents.[133,134] As with all chromosome deletions, there is a 50% risk of passing the deletion from parent to child.

Physical Features and Medical Issues

Deletion 22q11.2 is known for wide phenotypic variability, and long lists of possible features have been compiled.[135] Multisystem involvement is apparent in most individuals.

Velo-cardio-facial syndrome (VCFS) classically involves abnormalities of the palate, ranging from velopharyngeal insufficiency to overt clefting; structural cardiac defects involving the aorta, ventricular septum, conotruncal structures and proximal vasculature, and subtle facial features including a long face, long nose with a full tip, retrognathia, hooded eyes, and atypical ear morphology. Short stature is common, as are long, tapered fingers and hypotonia.

Several clinical diagnoses have been associated with deletions of 22q11.2, including DiGeorge syndrome, conotruncal anomaly face syndrome, Cayler syndrome, and some families with Opitz G/BBB syndrome.[136–138]

Cognitive and Psychiatric Features

Individuals with deletion 22q11.2 commonly have IQ scores in the borderline range, with a mean of 70, although some may have mild intellectual disability. Verbal IQ is higher than performance,[139] and the most common learning disability area is math. There is a relative strength in language abilities, despite frequent and dramatic early language delay. Investigators have documented receptive and high-order language deficits, abstract reasoning deficits, and visuospatial deficits.

Executive functioning challenges include distractibility, attention deficits, and abstract thinking problems.[140] Individuals can be impulsive, disinhibited, and prone to temper tantrums. What is often characterized as mood swings (emotional dysregulation) has been attributed by one expert author to better represent a feature of ADHD or oppositional behavior, rather than a bipolar diathesis, as they occur in the absence of other symptoms of a manic disorder, such as grandiosity, increased energy, decreased need for sleep, or racing thoughts.[141]

Younger children with VCFS show attention problems, anxiety and phobia symptoms, and poor social adaptation with withdrawal, shyness, and awkwardness.[142] The development of anxiety may be related to gene/environment interaction whereby hypernasal speech, decreased facial expression, and poor social interaction skills are met with negative reinforcement from peers.[143,144] With age, anxiety persists rather than diminishes, and 8 times as many individuals develop psychotic disorders when compared with age- and IQ-matched controls.[142]

While rates of anxiety are generally high, Gothelf and colleagues[143] have particularly noted obsessive compulsive disorder (OCD), the most prevalent symptoms being excessive washing and cleaning, hoarding, and somatic worries.

Two-thirds of school-aged children and adolescents will meet criteria for a psychiatric disorder; there is no correlation with IQ.[144] Fifty percent of affected individuals meet criteria for autism spectrum diagnoses by the Autism Diagnostic Interview–Revised (primarily Pervasive Developmental Disorder–Not Otherwise Specified), 27% have psychotic symptoms, and 12% schizophrenia.[145]

The emergence of psychotic symptoms in adolescence to early adulthood is of great concern to families. Approximately 30% of individuals develop psychotic symptoms that tend to have a chronic course and are less responsive to neuroleptic treatment than other psychoses.[146] Paranoid schizophrenia has also been reported in up to 30% of adults.[140] Increased rates of psychotic illnesses among relatives have also been documented.[147] The presence of subthreshold psychotic symptoms, anxiety, and depression, and lower verbal IQ during childhood significantly predicted the onset of a psychotic disorder at 17.5 years, but ADHD did not put the subjects at increased risk.[148] Overall, approximately 2% of all cases of schizophrenia and 6% of those with onset in childhood were found to have deletion 22q11.2[148]; all deletion-positive individuals had physical features or medical history indicating this diagnosis.

Genotype/phenotype correlations are emerging regarding the remaining *COMT* gene in affected individuals, the gene product involved in dopamine degradation. Two polymorphisms have been identified within this gene, a high-activity VAL allele and a lower activity MET allele. Individuals with the 22q11.2 deletion and a remaining MET allele may be at risk for more severe psychotic symptoms, and have higher rates of OCD and ADHD in childhood.[149]

Treatment should be multimodal and includes behavioral treatment for anxiety disorders, social skills training, and psychopharmacology. An annual psychiatric examination by a child psychiatrist with particular attention to subthreshold psychotic symptoms, and consideration of treatment with atypical antipsychotics, is recommended. Given the high rates of cardiac involvement in individuals with this deletion, an electrocardiogram should be obtained, and QTc monitored[149] particularly during treatment of ADHD. One open-label study of low-dose MPH (0.3 mg/kg) reduced ADHD symptoms in 75% of treated individuals.[150] Significant improvement in OCD symptoms has been noted with fluoxetine, 30 to 60 mg/d. Metyrosine, a tyrosine hydroxylase inhibitor, has been associated with a decrease in psychiatric symptoms.[151]

SMITH-MAGENIS SYNDROME
Genetics, Etiology, and Epidemiology

Smith-Magenis syndrome (SMS) has been recognized since the 1980s[152–154] and is caused by a deletion of chromosome 17p11.2.[155,156] The phenotype changes significantly over the life span, and diagnosis is largely dependent on the presence of structural malformations or recognition of the behavioral phenotype.

The critical region for SMS is a 1-Mb region[157,158] within the classic deletion of approximately 4 Mb.[159,160] Several genes within this region have been implicated in the features of SMS syndrome, including *RAI1*. A standard karyotype will identify the deletion in at least 90% of affected individuals. Deletion-specific FISH is available and can increase diagnostic yield to more than 95%. Smaller deletions may be detected using CGH microarray. A small number of affected individuals have been found to have mutations within *RAI1*.[161]

Physical Features and Medical Issues

In contrast to many microdeletion syndromes, the behavioral and developmental features of SMS predominate the phenotype and may be the presenting symptoms prompting diagnostic testing in childhood.

The facial features of children and adults with SMS are described as "coarse" with a prominent brow ridge, deeply set eyes, and a prominent mandible. Ophthalmalogic abnormalities, cardiac anomalies, hearing loss, short stature, and small hands and feet are frequent. Neurologic abnormalities, including seizures, hypotonia, diminished reflexes, and high pain tolerance are common. Hypercholesterolemia is also common.

Infants with SMS have a particular phenotype, quite different from that seen in older children. The facial features of babies are more subtle, with midface hypoplasia and up-slanting palpebral fissures. Affected infants are hypotonic, quiet, and "complacent," often with feeding difficulties.[162,163]

Cognitive and Psychiatric Features

Most individuals have moderate intellectual disability, with a range from mild to severe, with no verbal/performance difference,[164] and the level of cognitive and adaptive functioning has been shown to depend on deletion size.[165] Short-term memory, visuomotor coordination, sequencing, and response speed are weaknesses.[166] Speech delay is common, with receptive language better than expressive, and there is usually limited adaptive functioning. Sleep disturbance, stereotypy, and SIB are the primary psychiatric features and are not usually recognized until the age of 18 months, and evolve with time.

A lifelong sleep disturbance can cause significant impairment. This problem begins as long naps as an infant, but evolves to become an inverted melatonin circadian rhythm problem, including difficulty falling asleep, shortened sleep cycles, frequent and prolonged awakenings at night, and daytime sleepiness.[167] Treatment of the sleep disturbance with a β1-adrenergic antagonist (acebutolol, 10 mg/kg) during the day, and exogenous administration of melatonin in the evening have been shown in case series to lead to improved sleep and reduced behavioral problems.[168,169]

SIB is seen in over 95% of affected individuals; typical topography includes wrist biting, head banging, skin picking, nail removal, and foreign body insertion. These behaviors can be severe and persistent, and the frequency and range of topography increase with age.[170] There is also a characteristic "self-hug"—a spasmodic squeezing of the upper body, of which there are 2 subtypes: (1) self-hugging and spasmodically tensing the upper body, and (2) hand clasping at chest level and squeezing arms against body. This behavior has been interpreted as a ticlike pattern of involuntary expression of excitement.[171] Other odd or stereotypic behaviors include lick-and-flip, mouthing objects, teeth grinding, body rocking, and spinning objects.

Children with SMS are socially adult-oriented and demanding of adult attention. These children are egocentric and have delayed empathic skills out of proportion to their cognitive level. In fact, withdrawal of adult attention is often the primary antecedent to SIB and aggressive/disruptive behavior.[172] While most children are affectionate and have a primarily positive affect, affective lability, property destruction, impulsivity, nervousness, physical aggression, and argumentative behavior are also seen.[173] There is a single case report of use of risperidone to target aggression in a 13-year-old with SMS.[174]

TURNER SYNDROME

Genetics, Etiology, and Epidemiology

By definition, Turner syndrome (TS) occurs only in females and has an incidence of approximately 1 in 3000 live-born infant girls. At the most basic level, TS results when there is a single functioning X chromosome as a result of loss of the second sex chromosome in its entirety or more specifically, portions of the short arm of either the second X chromosome or the Y. Half of affected individuals will have a 45,X karyotype; a wide range of other structural X-chromosome malformations and mosaic chromosome constitutions make up the remaining karyotypes.[175] A standard peripheral blood karyotype will confirm a diagnosis as well as detect X-chromosome variations and mosaicism.

Physical Features and Medical Issues

Cardinal features of TS include lymphedema, cardiac malformations, short stature, and primary ovarian failure. The age at which a diagnosis of TS is made is highly dependent on the physical features that are present: in infancy, lymphedema of the hands and feet or characteristic cardiac malformations may prompt diagnostic testing, whereas in childhood short stature is the common diagnostic feature, as is delayed puberty or primary ovarian failure in adolescents and adults. Prenatal diagnosis, based on the presence of an increased nuchal translucency or cystic hygroma, is also possible.

Left-sided congenital structural malformations, such as aortic valve abnormalities and aortic coarctation, are seen in less than half of affected individuals.[176,177] Renal malformations are also fairly common in TS, as are recurrent otitis media, strabismus, hypothyroidism, inflammatory bowel disease, overweight, and benign nevi.[178,179] Subtle facial features, including down-slanting palpebral fissures and low-set ears, or physical examination findings (wide neck, low posterior hairline, broad chest) are present in some affected individuals. Appropriate growth charts and Health Care Supervision recommendations are available from the American Academy of Pediatrics.[180]

Cognitive and Psychiatric Features

In general, affected girls have an IQ in the normal range; only 5% have intellectual disability. Performance IQ is usually lower than verbal, and learning disabilities in math are common. Nonverbal abilities are often significantly impaired, including visual-spatial, visual-perceptual, and visual-constructional abilities.[181] Impaired executive functioning skills may include attention and concentration, problem-solving ability, organization and working memory, impulsivity, and processing speed. Russell and colleagues[182] found an 18-fold increased prevalence for ADHD among those with TS versus controls.

Psychiatric features include social immaturity, anxiety, hyperactivity, and social challenges. Younger girls are generally immature, hyperactive, and anxious. Older girls tend to have anxiety, depression, and social relationship challenges. Girls with TS have been shown to have more difficulty maintaining relationships, and tend to have fewer friends and be more socially isolated than controls.[183]

There is debate as to whether the shyness, anxiety, low self esteem, and depression noted with increased prevalence in TS are due to neurodevelopmental deficits, or due to self-consciousness over physical appearance and infertility. When compared with their unaffected sisters, in an effort to neutralize environmental effects, girls with TS had more social thought and attention problems.[184]

Rigorous neuropsychological investigation into the social interaction difficulties and anxiety seen in TS has demonstrated weakness with discriminating facial affect,[185] and affective prosody[186] and specific significant deficits with mental rotation, object assembly, and face recognition.[187] There is a specific partial deficit in social gaze processing, involving recognition of emotional cues expressed in the upper face, particular for expression of "fear" in the eye region.[188] Impaired appraisal of facial affect and decreased ability to habituate to fearful stimuli may stem from impaired functional connectivity between the amygdala and fusiform gyrus, suggesting that standard cognitive behavioral therapy exposure protocols for treatment of anxiety may have to be modified for these individuals.[189]

Although there are few treatment data psychotherapy is generally recommended, focusing on coping and adaptive skills, social skills training, stress management, improving self esteem, and using internal and external strategies to compensate for cognitive weaknesses.[190]

LESCH-NYHAN SYNDROME
Genetics, Etiology, Epidemiology, Physical Features, and Medical Issues

Lesch-Nyhan syndrome is an X-linked disorder of purine metabolism resulting from decreased activity of hypoxanthine-guanine phosphoribosyltransferase. This diagnosis is often suspected because of the specific physical and behavioral phenotype seen in childhood; choreoathetosis, seizures, dystonia, and dysarthria are also frequently present. The diagnosis is established by measuring plasma or urine uric acid levels, which are markedly elevated. Medical treatment is primarily symptomatic, and allopurinol is used to prevent complications related to hyperuricemia/uricosuria.

Cognitive and Psychiatric Features

IQ is typically in the mild to moderate range of intellectual disability. The psychiatric presentation is dominated by chronic SIB, resulting in self-mutilation.

Self-injury consists most frequently of biting, followed by eye poking, fingernail pulling, and psychogenic vomiting. Biting behavior tends to target the lips and fingers, followed by the arms and tongue, and the biting pattern is often asymmetric. Other movements that can produce self-injury, such as arching, head snapping, and head banging, are also seen.[191] The SIB appears to be a compulsive behavior that the child tries to control but generally is unable to resist.[192] As with other compulsive behaviors, control improves with age but affected individuals may enlist others to assist in controlling these impulses, or may self-restrain. A characteristic language pattern involving repeated ambivalent statements with anxiety and vulgarity is seen along with frequent compulsive aggression toward others, grabbing, and pinching—with resultant apologies.

Based on a theory that many of the neuropsychiatric features are related to abnormalities in dopamine function, treatments with the dopamine precursor levodopa have been tried, but were unsuccessful. A case report of deep brain stimulation in the globus pallidus pars interna in a single 19-year-old describes cessation of self-mutilation.[193] Other effective treatment avenues include behavioral therapy with an extinction protocol based on active withdrawal of attention. Benzodiazepines can reduce anxiety, but may exacerbate extrapyramidal side effects and behavioral features. Stress and anxiety increase self-injury, so reduction in these factors is important. Use of restraints and protective equipment is common. SSRIs can be used to treat anxiety, Risperidone at low dose has been suggested by topic experts for SIB and aggression. No controlled pharmacologic treatment data are available.

COMMON INBORN ERRORS OF METABOLISM

Several other inborn errors of metabolism are associated with marked behavioral or psychiatric manifestations. Not all of these diagnoses are established in infancy through newborn screening, and many may not be diagnosed until the behavioral phenotype is well established. Although in general these diagnoses are rare, consideration should be given to a metabolic evaluation in individuals with suggestive medical and psychological features.

Phenylketonuria (PKU), resulting from a deficiency of phenylalanine hydroxylase, is part of newborn screening programs in all 50 US states. Early diagnosis and medical management to maintain phenylalanine levels within the recommended therapeutic range of 2 to 6 mg/dL (120–360 μmol/L) in childhood reduces the risk of mental retardation, behavioral problems, and learning difficulties.[194,195] Liberalization of the phenylalanine restricted diet, with subsequent elevations of blood phenylalanine levels to greater than 10 to 20 mg/dL are often accompanied by difficulty with attention, reduced executive functioning, and anxiety/depression.[196–199] Many of these symptoms can be reduced by decreasing the blood phenylalanine concentration through diet modification or medications, although there does remain an increased risk for psychiatric disorders.[200]

Most individuals with the mucopolysaccharidoses (MPS) are diagnosed based on specific physical or medical issues related to the intracellular storage of nonmetabolized mucopolysaccharides. The MPS disorders are also often associated with behavioral problems, including abnormal levels of activity (either lethargy or hyperactivity), aggression, oppositional behavior, sleep disturbance, and difficulties in interpersonal skills. The SanFillipo syndromes (MPS III) are particularly notable for the degree of behavioral involvement, which often dominates the overall phenotype. A variable period of normal development is followed by delays in language acquisition, severe temper tantrums, inattention, explosive reactions to change, sleep disturbance and, ultimately, dementia. A limited number of diagnosis-specific therapies are available, primarily targeting the medical complications.

The recurrent hyperammonemia associated with the urea cycle disorders (UCDs) has been implicated in residual developmental delays and mental retardation seen in many patients. However, neurocognitive disabilities and decreased IQ are seen in individuals without episodic hyperammonemia and in asymptomatic carriers of the most common form, X-linked ornithine transcarbamylase deficiency. There is increasing recognition of a characteristic nonverbal learning disability and difficulties with attention and executive functioning in individuals of all ages, regardless of the degree of hyperammonemic symptomatology.[201,202]

SUMMARY

The identification of specific genetic diagnoses, including genotype-specific variations, presents the unique opportunity to study genotype/phenotype connections in child psychiatry. Multiple investigators have spent the last 2 decades characterizing the psychopathologic features associated with specific diagnoses, and the latest research seeks to connect specific facets of behavioral functioning, such as social gaze processing in TS, with genetic variance. These advances have implications for understanding functional deficits in the broader population, and support a dimensional approach to psychopathologic characterization. Each disorder, as it is more fully characterized, presents a microcosm whereby particular facets of functional impairment, such as direct gaze aversion in FXS, or components of theory of mind in Williams syndrome, can be mapped and linked at a genomic level to inform highly specific treatments with potential broader application.

REFERENCES

1. Reiss AL. Childhood developmental disorders: an academic and clinical convergence point for psychiatry, neurology, psychology and pediatrics. J Child Psychol Psychiatry 2009;50(1–2):87–98.
2. Skuse DH. Behavioural phenotypes: what do they teach us? Arch Dis Child 2000;82:222–5.
3. Reiss S, Levitan GW, Szysko J. Emotional disturbance and mental retardation: diagnostic overshadowing. Am J Ment Defic 1982;86(6):567–74.
4. Dykens EM, Rosner BA. Psychopathology in persons with Williams-Beuren syndrome. In: Morris CA, Lenhoff HM, Wang PP, editors. Williams-Beuren syndrome: research, evaluation and treatment. 1st edition. Baltimore (MD): The Johns Hopkins University press; 2006. p. 274–93.
5. Feinstein C, Singh S. Social phenotypes in neurogenetic syndromes. Child Adolesc Psychiatr Clin N Am 2007;16(3):631–48.
6. Besser LM, Shin M, Kucik JE, et al. Prevalence of Down syndrome among children and adolescents in metropolitan Atlanta. Birth Defects Res A Clin Mol Teratol 2007;79:765–74.
7. Bittles AH, Glasson EJ. Clinical, social, and ethical implications of changing life expectancy in Down syndrome. Dev Med Child Neurol 2004;(46):282–6.
8. Driscoll DA, Gross SJ. On behalf of the professional practice guidelines committee. Screening for fetal aneuploidy and neural tube defects. Genet Med 2009;11(11):818–21.
9. Torfs CP, Christianson RE. Anomalies in Down syndrome individuals in a large population based registry. Am J Med Genet 1998;77:431–8.
10. Goldberg-Stern H, Strawsburg RH, Patterson B, et al. Seizure frequency and characteristics in children with Down syndrome. Brain Dev 2001;23:375–8.
11. Prasher VP. Down syndrome and thyroid disorders: a review. Downs Syndr Res Pract 1999;6:25–42.
12. Hill I, Dirks M, Liptak G, et al. Guidelines for the diagnosis and treatment of celiac disease in children: recommendations of the North American Society for Pediatric Gastroenterology, Hepatology and Nutrition. J Pediatr Gastroenterol 2004;40(1):1–19.
13. American Academy of Pediatrics Committee on Genetics. Health supervision for children with Down syndrome. Pediatrics 2001;107:442–9.
14. Miller JF. Individual differences in vocabulary acquisition in children with Down syndrome. Prog Clin Biol Res 1995;393:93–103.
15. Myers BA, Pueschel SM. Psychiatric disorders in persons with Down syndrome. J Nerv Ment Dis 1991;179(10):609–13.
16. Pueschel SM, Myers BA. Environmental and temperament assessments of children with Down's syndrome. J Intellect Disabil Res 1994;38(pt2):195–202.
17. Pueschel SM, Gallagher PL, Zartler AS, et al. Cognitive and learning processes in children with Down syndrome. Res Dev Disabil 1987;8(1):21–37.
18. State MW, King BH, Dykens E. Mental retardation: a review of the past 10 years. Part II. J Am Acad Child Adolesc Psychiatry 1997;36(12):1664–9.
19. Capone G, Goyal P, Ares W, et al. Neurobehavioral disorders in children, adolescents, and young adults with Down syndrome. Am J Med Genet 2006;142C(3):158–72.

20. Dykens EM, Shah B, Sagun J, et al. Maladaptive behavior in children and adolescents with Down's syndrome. J Intellect Disabil Res 2002;46:484–92.
21. Evans DW, Gray FL. Compulsive-like behavior in individuals with Down syndrome: its relation to mental age level, adaptive, and maladaptive behavior. Child Dev 2000;71(2):288–300.
22. Cooper SA, Collacott RA. Clinical features and diagnostic criteria of depression in Down's syndrome. Br J Psychiatry 1994;165(3):399–403.
23. Pary RJ, Loschen EL, Tomkowiak SB. Mood disorders and down syndrome. Semin Clin Neuropsychiatry 1996;1(2):148–53.
24. Ghaziuddin M. Autism in Down's syndrome: a family history study. J Intellect Disabil Res 2000;44(Pt 5):562–6.
25. Heller JH, Spiridigliozzi GA, Crissman BG, et al. Safety and efficacy of rivastigmine in adolescents with Down syndrome: a preliminary 20-week, open-label study. J Child Adolesc Psychopharmacol 2006;16(6):755–65.
26. Strom CM, Crossley B, Redman JB, et al. Molecular testing for Fragile X syndrome: lessons learned from 119,232 tests performed in a clinical laboratory. Genet Med 2007;9:46–51.
27. Sherman S, Pletcher BA, Driscoll DA. Fragile X syndrome: diagnostic and carrier testing. Genet Med 2005;7:584–7.
28. American Academy of Pediatrics Committee on Genetics. Health supervision for children with Fragile X syndrome. Pediatrics 1996;98:297–300.
29. Jacquemont S, Hagerman RJ, Leehey MA, et al. Penetrance of the fragile X-associated tremor/ataxia syndrome in a premutation carrier population. J Am Med Assoc 2004;291:460–9.
30. Tarleton JC, Saul RA. Molecular genetic advances in fragile X syndrome. J Pediatr 1993;122:169–85.
31. Lachiewicz AM, Dawson DV, Spiridiglioaai GA. Physical characteristics of young boys with Fragile X syndrome: reasons for difficulties in making a diagnosis in young males. Am J Med Genet 2000;92:229–36.
32. Hagerman RJ, Hagerman PJ. The fragile X premutation: into the phenotypic fold. Curr Opin Genet Dev 2002;12:278–83.
33. Grigsby J, Bennett R, Brega A, et al. Fragile X-associated tremor-ataxia syndrome (FXTAS): An X-linked neurodegenerative phenotype. Presented at the American College of Medical Genetics Meeting. Dallas (TX), 2005 [Abstract #280].
34. Dykens EM, Hodapp RM, Evnas DW. Profiles and development of adaptive behavior in children with Down syndrome. Am J Ment Retard 1994;98(5):580–7.
35. Mazzocco MM. Advances in research on the Fragile X syndrome. Ment Retard Dev Disabil Res Rev 2000;6(2):96–106.
36. Skinner M, Hooper S, Hatton DD, et al. Mapping nonverbal IQ in young boys with Fragile X syndrome. Am J Med Genet Am 2005;132(1):25–32.
37. Hagerman RJ, Hills J, Scharfenaker S, et al. Fragile X syndrome and selective mutism. Am J Med Genet 1999;83(4):313–7.
38. Franke P, Leboyer M, Gansicke M, et al. Genotype-phenotype relationship in female carriers of the permutation and full mutation of FMR-1. Psychiatry Res 1998;80(2):113–27.
39. Cornish K, Kogan C, Turk J, et al. The emerging Fragile X permutation phenotype: evidence from the domain of social cognition. Brain Cogn 2005;57(1):53–60.
40. Hatton DD, Bailey DB Jr, Hargett-Beck MQ, et al. Behavioral style of young boys with Fragile X syndrome. Dev Med Child Neurol 1999;41(9):625–32.

41. Miller LJ, Mcintosh DN, McGrath J, et al. Electrodermal responses to sensory stimuli in individuals with Fragile X syndrome: a preliminary report. Am J Med Genet 1999;83(4):26–79.

42. Roberts JE, Boccia ML, Bailey DB Jr, et al. Cardiovascular indices of physiological arousal in boys with Fragile X syndrome. Dev Psychobiol 2001;39(2): 107–23.

43. Garrett AS, Menon V, MacKenzie K. Here's looking at you, kid: neural systems underlying face and gaze processing in Fragile X syndrome. Arch Gen Psychiatry 2004;61(3):281–8.

44. Hall SS, Lightbody AA, Huffman LC. Physiologic correlates of social avoidance behavior in children and adolescents with Fragile X syndrome. J Am Acad Child Adolesc Psychiatry 2009;48(3):320–9.

45. Hall S, DeBernardis M, Reiss A. Social escape behaviors in children with Fragile X syndrome. J Autism Dev Disord 2006;36(7):935–47.

46. Sabaratnam M, Murthy NV, Wijeratne A, et al. Autistic-like behaviour profile and psychiatric morbidity in Fragile X syndrome: a prospective ten-year follow-up study. Eur Child Adolesc Psychiatry 2003;12(4):172–7.

47. Hall SS, Maynes NP, Reiss AL. Using percentile schedules to increase eye contact in children with Fragile X syndrome. J Appl Behav Anal 2009;42(1): 171–6.

48. Hagerman RJ, Fulton MJ, Leaman A, et al. A survey of fluoxetine therapy in Fragile X syndrome. Dev Brain Dysfunct 1994;7:155–64.

49. Hagerman RJ. Lessons from Fragile X regarding neurobiology, autism, and neurodegeneration. J Dev Behav Pediatr 2006;27(1):63–74.

50. Cohen IL, Tsiouris JA, Pfadt A. Effects of long acting propranolol on agonistic and stereotyped behaviors in a man with pervasive developmental disorder and Fragile X syndrome:a double blind, placebo controlled study. J Clin Psychopharmacol 1991;11(6):398–9.

51. Hagerman RJ, Murphy MA, Wittenberger MD. A controlled trial of stimulant medication in children with Fragile X syndrome. Am J Med Genet 1988; 30(1–2):377–92.

52. Hagerman RJ. Influence of stimulants on electrodermal studies in Fragile X syndrome. Microsc Res Tech 2002;57:168–73.

53. Torrioli MG, Nernacotola S, Mariotti P, et al. Double-blind, placebo-controlled study of L-acetylcarnitine for the treatment of hyperactive behavior in Fragile X syndrome. Am J Med Genet 1999;87(4):366–8.

54. Hagerman RJ, Riddle JE, Roberts LS, et al. A survey of the efficacy of clonidine in Fragile X syndrome. Dev Brain Dysfunction 1995;8:336–44.

55. Hilton DK, Martin CA, Heffron WM, et al. Imipramine treatment of ADHD in a Fragile X child. J Am Acad Child Adolesc Psychiatry 1991;30(5):831–4.

56. Reiss AL, Hall SS. Fragile X syndrome: assessment and treatment implications. Child Adolesc Psychiatr Clin N Am 2007;16(3):668.

57. Laurvick CL, de Klerk N, Bower C, et al. Rett syndrome in Australia: a review of the epidemiology. J Pediatr 2006;148:347–52.

58. Ellaway C, Christodoulou J. Rett syndrome: clinical characteristics and recent genetic advances. Disabil Rehabil 2001;23:98–106.

59. Kammoun F, de Roux N, Boespflug-Tanguy O, et al. Screening of MECP2 coding sequence in patients with phenotypes of decreasing likelihood for Rett syndrome: a cohort of 171 cases. J Med Genet 2004;41:e85.

60. Li MR, Pan H, Bao XH, et al. MECP2 and CDKL5 gene mutation analysis in Chinese patients with Rett syndrome. J Hum Genet 2007;52:38–47.

61. Weaving LS, Williamson SL, Bennetts B, et al. Effects of MECP2 mutation type, location and X-inactivation in modulating Rett syndrome phenotype. Am J Med Genet Am 2003;118:103–14.
62. Archer HL, Whatley SD, Evans JC, et al. Gross rearrangements of the MECP2 gene are found in both classical and atypical Rett syndrome patients. J Med Genet 2006;43:451–6.
63. Hagberg B, Hanefeld F, Percy A, et al. An update on clinically applicable diagnostic criteria in Rett syndrome: comments to Rett Syndrome Clinical Criteria Consensus Panel Satellite to European Paediatric Neurology Society Meeting, Baden Baden, Germany, 11 September 2001. Europ J Paediatr Neurol 2002; 6:293–7.
64. Hagberg B, Gilberg C. Rett syndrome, clinical and biological aspects, Rett Variants-Rettoid types, Clinics in Developmental Medicine, vol. 127. Cambridge (UK): MacKeith Cambridge University Press; 1993. p. 40–60.
65. Witt-Engerström I. Rett syndrome in Sweden. Acta Paediatr Scand 1990; 369(Suppl):1–60.
66. Cass H, Reilly S, Owen L, et al. Findings from a multidisciplinary clinical case series of females with Rett syndrome. Dev Med Child Neurol 2003;45(5):325–37.
67. Lavas J, Slotte A, Jochym-Nygren M, et al. Communication and eating proficiency in 125 females with Rett syndrome: the Swedish Rett Center Survey. Disabil Rehabil 2006;28(20):1267–79.
68. Lotan M, Ben-Zeev B. Rett syndrome. A review with emphasis on clinical characteristics and intervention. Scientific World Journal 2006;6(6):1517–41.
69. Ben-Zeev B. Rett syndrome. Child Adolesc Psychiatr Clin N Am 2007;16(3): 723–4.
70. Monaghan KG, Wiktor A, Van Dyke DL. Diagnostic testing for Prader-Willi syndrome and Angelman syndrome: a cost comparison. Genet Med 2002;4: 448–50.
71. Holm VA, Cassidy SB, Butler MG, et al. Prader-Willi syndrome: consensus diagnostic criteria. Pediatrics 1993;91:398–402.
72. Gunay-Aygun M, Schwartz S, Heeger S, et al. The changing purpose of Prader-Willi syndrome clinical diagnostic criteria and proposed revised criteria. Pediatrics 2001;108:E92.
73. Eiholzer U, l'Allemand D, van der Sluis I, et al. Body composition abnormalities in children with Prader-Willi syndrome and long-term effects of growth hormone therapy. Horm Res 2000;53:200–6.
74. Hoybye C. Endocrine and metabolic aspects of adult Prader-Willi syndrome with special emphasis on the effect of growth hormone treatment. Growth Horm IGF Res 2004;14:1–15.
75. Curfs LM, Fryns JP. Prader-Willi syndrome: a review with special attention to the cognitive and behavioral profile. Birth Defects Orig Artic Ser 1992;28(1):99–104.
76. Benarroch F, Hirsch HJ, Gentsil L. Prader-Willi syndrome: medical prevention and behavioral challenges. Child Adolesc Psychiatr Clin N Am 2007;16(3): 695–708.
77. Stein DJ, Keating J, Zar HJ, et al. A survey of the phenomenology and pharmacotherapy of compulsive and impulsive-aggressive symptoms in Prader Willi syndrome. J Neuropsychiatry Clin Neurosci 1994;6(1):23–9.
78. Dykens EM, Leckman JF, Cassidy SB. Obsessions and compulsions in Prader-Willi syndrome. J Child Psychol Psychiatry 1996;37:995–1002.
79. Dykens EM, Cassidy SB. Correlates of maladaptive behavior in children and adults with Prader-Willi syndrome. Am J Med Genet 1995;60(6):546–9.

80. Koenig K, Klin A, Schultz R. Deficits in social attribution ability in Prader-Willi syndrome. J Autism Dev Disord 2004;34(5):573–82.
81. Vogels A, De Hert M, Descheemaeker MJ, et al. Psychotic disorders in Prader-Willi syndrome. Am J Med Genet 2004;127A(3):238–43.
82. Boer H, Holland A, Whittington J, et al. Psychotic illness in people with Prader Willi syndrome due to chromosome 15 maternal uniparental disomy. Lancet 2002;359(9301):135–6.
83. Soni S, Whittington J, Holland AJ. The course and outcome of psychiatric illness in people with Prader-Willi syndrome: implications for management and treatment. J Intellect Disabil Res 2007;51:32–42.
84. Symons FJ, Butler MG, Sanders MD, et al. Self-injurious behavior and Prader-Willi syndrome: behavioral forms and body locations. Am J Ment Retard 1999; 104(3):260–9.
85. Whitman BY. Tools for psychological and behavioral management. In: Butler MG, editor. Management of Prader-Willi syndrome. 3rd edition. New York: Springer; 2006. p. 317–43.
86. Roof E, The use of psychotropic medications in Prader-Willi syndrome. Presented at the 20th Annual PWSA (USA) National Conference. Orlando (FL), July 27, 2005.
87. Dykens E, Shah B. Psychiatric disorders in Prader-Willi syndrome: epidemiology and management. CNS Drugs 2003;17:167–78.
88. Hellings JA, Warnock JK. Self-injurious behavior and serotonin in Prader-Willi syndrome. Psychopharmacol Bull 1994;30(2):245–50.
89. Shapira NA, Lessig MC, Lewis MH. Effects of topiramate in adults with Prader-Willi syndrome. Am J Ment Retard 2004;109(4):301–9.
90. Smathers SA, Wilson JG, Nigro MA. Topiramate effectiveness in Prader-Willi syndrome. Pediatr Neurol 2003;28(2):130–3.
91. Gupta BK, Fish DN, Yerevanian BI. Carbamazepine for intermittent explosive disorder in a Prader-Willi syndrome patient. J Clin Psychiatry 1987;48(10):423.
92. Jerome L. Prader-Willi and bipolar illness. J Am Acad Child Adolesc Psychiatry 1993;32(4):876–7.
93. Durst R, Rubin-Jabotinksy K, Raskin S. Risperidone in treating behavioural disturbances of Prader-Willi syndrome. Acta Psychiatr Scand 2000;102(6):461–5.
94. Wigren M, Hansen S. ADHD symptoms and insistence on sameness in Prader-Willi syndrome. J Intellect Disabil Res 2005;49(6):449–56.
95. Knoll JH, Nicholls RD, Magenis RE, et al. Angelman and Prader Willi syndromes share a common chromosome 15 deletion but differ in parental origin of the deletion. Am J Med Genet 1989;32:285–90.
96. ASHG/ACMG. Diagnostic testing for Prader-Willi and Angelman syndromes: Report of the ASHG/ACMG test and technology transfer committee. Am J Hum Genet 1996;58:1085–8.
97. Clayton-Smith J, Pembrey ME. Angelman syndrome. J Med Genet 1992;29: 412–5.
98. Steffenburg S, Gillberg CL, Steffenburg U, et al. Autism in Angelman syndrome: a population-based study. Pediatr Neurol 1996;14:131–6.
99. Williams CA, Beaudet AL, Clayton-Smith J, et al. Angelman syndrome 2005: updated consensus for diagnostic criteria. Am J Med Genet Am 2006;140:413–8.
100. Horsler K, Oliver C. Environmental influences on the behavioral phenotype of Angelman syndrome. Am J Ment Retard 2006;111(5):311–21.
101. Artigas-Pallares J, Brun-Gasca C, Gabau-Vila E, et al. Aspectos medicos y conductuales del syndrome Angelman. Rev Neurol (Madrid) 2005;41:649–56.

102. Barry RJ, Leitner RP, Clarke AR. Behavioral aspects of Angelman syndrome: a case control study. Am J Med Genet Am 2005;132(1):8–12.
103. Pelc K, Cheron G, Boyd SG, et al. Are there distinctive sleep problems in Angelman syndrome? Sleep Med 2008;9(4):434–41.
104. Clarke D, Marston G. Problem behaviours associated with 15q- Angelman syndrome. Am J Ment Retard 2000;105:25–31.
105. Williams JCP, Barrett-Boyes BG, Lowe JB. Supravalvar aortic stenosis. Circulation 1961;24:1311–8.
106. Buren AJ, Apitz J, Harmjanz D. Supravalvar aortic stenosis in association with mental retardation and a certain facial appearance. Circulation 1962;27:1235–40.
107. Garcia RE, Friedman WF, Kaback MM, et al. Idiopathic hypercalcemia and supravalvar aortic stenosis. N Engl J Med 1964;27:117–20.
108. Ewart AK, Morris CA, Atkinson D, et al. Hemizygosity at the elastin locus in a developmental disorder, Williams syndrome. Nat Genet 1993;5:11–6.
109. Frangiskakis JM, Ewart AK, Morris CA, et al. LIM-kinase 1 hemizygosity implicated in impaired visuospatial constructive cognition. Cell 1996;86:59–69.
110. Morris CA, Mervis CB, Hobart HH, et al. GTF2I hemizygosity implicated in mental retardation in Williams syndrome: genotype-phenotype analysis of five families with deletions in the Williams syndrome region. Am J Med Genet Am 2003;123(1):45–59.
111. American Academy of Pediatrics Committee on Genetics. Health supervision for children with Wiliams syndrome. Pediatrics 2001;107:1192–204.
112. Mervis CB, Klein-Tasman BP. Williams syndrome: cognition, personality and adaptive behavior. Ment Retard Dev Disabil Res Rev 2000;6(2):148–58.
113. Jones W, Bellugi U, Lai Z, et al. Hypersociability in Williams syndrome. J Cogn Neurosci 2000;12(Suppl 1):30–46.
114. Bellugi U, Adolphs R, Cassidy C. Towards the neural basis for hypersociability in a genetic syndrome. Neuroreport 1999;22(5):197–207.
115. Frigerio E, Burt DM, Gagliardi C. Is everybody always my friend? Perception of approachability in Williams syndrome. Neuropsychologia 2006;44(2):254–9.
116. Gagliardi C, Frigerio E, Burt DM, et al. Facial expression recognition in Williams syndrome. Neuropsychologia 2003;41(6):733–8.
117. Gosch A, Pankau R. Personality characteristics and behavior problems in individuals of different ages with Williams syndrome. Dev Med Child Neurol 1997;39(8):527–33.
118. Plesa-Skwerer D, Tager-Flusberg H. Social cognition in Williams-Seuren syndrome. In: Morris CA, Lenhoff HM, Wang PP, editors. Williams-Beuren syndrome. Baltimore (MD): Johns Hopkins University Press; 2006. p. 237–53.
119. Dykens EM. Anxiety, fears and phobias in persons with Williams syndrome. Dev Neuropsychol 2003;23(1–2):291–316.
120. Spence SH, McCathie H. The stability of fears in children: a two-year prospective study: a research note. J Child Psychol Psychiatry 1993;34(4):579–85.
121. Leyfer OT, Woodruff-Borden J, Klein-Tasman BP, et al. Prevalence of psychiatric disorders in 4 to 16-year-olds with Williams syndrome. Am J Med Genet Br 2006;141(6):615–22.
122. Power TJ, Blum NJ, Jones SM, et al. Brief report: response to methylphenidate in two children with Williams syndrome. J Autism Dev Disord 1997;27(1):79–87.
123. Bawden HN, MacDonald GW, Shea S. Treatment of children with Williams syndrome with methylphenidate. J Child Neurol 1997;12(4):248–52.
124. Arens R, Wright B, Elliott J, et al. Periodic limb movement in sleep in children with Williams syndrome. J Pediatr 1998;133(5):670–4.

125. Botto LD, May K, Fernhoff PM, et al. A population-based study of the 22q11.2 deletion: phenotype, incidence, and contribution to major birth defects in the population. Pediatrics 2003;112:101–7.

126. Merscher S, Funke B, Epstein JA, et al. TBX1 is responsible for cardiovascular defects in velo-cardio-facial/DiGeorge syndrome. Cell 2001;104:619–29.

127. Lachman HM, Morrow B, Shprintzen RJ, et al. Association of codon 108/158 catechol-o-methyl transferase gene polymorphism with the psychiatric manifestations of velo-cardio-facial syndrome. Am J Med Genet 1996;67:468–72.

128. Sirotkin H, Morrow B, DasGupta, et al. Isolation of a new clathrin heavy chain gene with muscle-specific expression from the region commonly deleted in velo-cardio-facial syndrome. Hum Mol Genet 1996;5:617–24.

129. Sagoo GS, Butterwort AS, Sanderson S, et al. Array CGH in patients with learning disability (mental retardation) and congenital anomalies: updated systematic review and meta-analysis of 19 studies and 13,926 subjects. Genet Med 2009;11(3):139–46.

130. Carlson C, Sirotkin H, Pandita R, et al. Molecular definition of 22q11 deletions in 151 velo-cardio-facial syndrome patients. Am J Hum Genet 1997;61:620–9.

131. Rauch A, Zink S, Zweier, et al. Systematic assessment of atypical deletions reveals genotype-phenotype correlation in 22q11.2. J Med Genet 2005;42:871–6.

132. Swillen A, Devriendt K, Vantrappen G, et al. Familial deletions of 22q11.2: the Leuven experience. An J Med Genet 1998;80:531–2.

133. Kates WR, Antshel K, Roizen N, et al. Velo-cardio-facial syndrome. In: Butler MG, Meaney FJ, editors. Genetics of developmental disabilities. New York: Marcel Dekker; 2004. p. 383–418.

134. Shprintzen RJ, Morrow B, Kucherlapati R. Vascular anomalies may explain many of the features of velo-cardio-facial syndrome. Am J Hum Genet 1997;61:34A.

135. Matsuoka R, Takao A, Kimura M, et al. Confirmation that the conotruncal anomaly face syndrome is associated with a deletion within 22q11.2. Am J Med Genet 1994;53:285–9.

136. McDonald-McGinn DM, Driscoll DA, Bason L, et al. Autosomal dominant "Opitz" GBBB syndrome due to a 22q11.2 deletion. Am J Med Genet 1995;59:103–13.

137. Giannotti A, Digilio MC, Marino B, et al. Cayler cardiofacial syndrome and del 22q11: part of the CATCH22 phenotype. Am J Med Genet 1994;53:303–4.

138. Wang PP, Woodlin MF, Kreps-Falk R, et al. Research on behavioral phenotypes: velocardiofacial syndrome. Dev Med Child Neurol 2000;42(6):422–7.

139. Shprintzen RJ, Goldberg RB, Young D, et al. The velo-cardio-facial syndrome: a clinical and genetic analysis. Pediatrics 1981;67(2):167–72.

140. Gothelf D. Velocardiofacial syndrome. Child Adolesc Psychiatr Clin N Am 2007;16(3):677–94.

141. Feinstein C, Eliez S, Blasey C, et al. Psychiatric disorders and behavioral problems in children with velocardiofacial syndrome: usefulness as phenotypic indicators of schizophrenia risk. Biol Psychol 2002;51(4):312–8.

142. Gothelf D, Feinstein C, Thompson T, et al. Risk factors for the emergence of psychotic disorders in adolescents with 22q11.2 deletion syndrome. Am J Psychiatry 2007;164(4):663–9.

143. Gothelf D, Presburger G, Zohar AH, et al. Obsessive-compulsive disorder in patients with velocardiofacial (22q11 deletion) syndrome. Am J Med Genet 2004;126B(1):99–105.

144. Woodlin M, Wang PP, Aleman D, et al. Neuropsychological profile of children and adolescents with the 22q11.2 microdeletion. Genet Med 2001;3(1):34–9.

145. Vorstman JA, Morcus ME, Duijff SN, et al. The 22q11.2 deletion in children: high rate of autistic disorders and early onset of psychotic symptoms. J Am Acad Child Adolesc Psychiatry 2006;45(9):1104–13.

146. Gothelf D, Frisch A, Munitz H, et al. Clinical characteristics of schizophrenia associated with velo-cardio-facial syndrome. Schizophr Res 1999;35(2):105–12.

147. Pulver AE, Nestadt G, Goldberg R. Psychotic illness in patients diagnosed with velo-cardio-facial syndrome and their relatives. J Nerv Ment Dis 1994;182(8):476–8.

148. Sporn A, Addington A, Reiss AL, et al. 22q11 deletion syndrome in childhood onset schizophrenia: an update. Mol Psychiatry 2004;9(3):225–6.

149. Gothelf D, Michaelovsky E, Frisch A, et al. Association of the low-activity COMT 158Met allele with ADHD and OCD in subjects with velocardiofacial syndrome. Int J Neuropsychopharmacol 2007;10(3):301–8.

150. Gothelf D, Gruber R, Presburger G, et al. Methylphenidate treatment for attention-deficit/hyperactivity disorder in children and adolescents with velocardiofacial syndrome: an open-label study. J Clin Psychiatry 2003;64(10):1163–9.

151. Graf WD, As Unis, Yates CM, et al. Catecholamines in patients with 22q11.2 deletion syndrome and the low-activity COMT polymorphism. Neurology 2001; 57(3):410–6.

152. Smith ACM, McGavran L, Waldstein G. Deletion of the 17 short arm in two patients with facial clefts. Am J Med Genet 1982;34(Suppl):A410.

153. Smith ACM, McGavran L, Robinson J, et al. Interstitial deletion of (17) (p11.2p11.2) in nine patients. Am J Med Genet 1986;24:393–414.

154. Stratton RF, Dobns WB, Greenberg F, et al. Interstitial deletion of (17) (p11.2p11.2): report of six additional patients with a new chromosome deletion syndrome. Am J Med Genet 1986;24:421–32.

155. Behjati F, Mullarkey M, Bergbaum A, et al. Chromosome deletion 17p11.2 (Smith-Magenis syndrome) in seven new patients, four of whom had been referred for fragile X investigation. Clin Genet 1997;51:71–4.

156. Elsea SH, Purandare SM, Adell RA, et al. Definition of the critical interval for Smith-Magenis syndrome. Cytogenet Cell Genet 1977;79:276–81.

157. Lucas RE, Vlangos CN, Das P, et al. Genomic organization of the approximately 1.5 Mb Smith-Magenis syndrome critical interval: transcription map, genomic contig, and candidate gene analysis. Eur J Hum Genet 2001;9:892–902.

158. Bi W, Yan J, Stankiewicz P, et al. Genes in a refined Smith-Magenis syndrome critical deletion interval on chromosome 17p11.2 and the syntenic region of the mouse. Genome Res 2002;12:713–28.

159. Vlangos CN, Yim DKC, Elsea SH. Refinement of the Smith-Magenis syndrome critical region to ~950kb and assessment of 17p11.2 deletions. Are all deletions created equally? Mol Genet Metab 2003;79(2):134–41.

160. Potocki L, Shaw CJ, Stankiewicz P, et al. Variability in clinical phenotype despite common chromosomal deletion in Smith-Magenis syndrome [del(17)(p11.2p11.2)]. Genet Med 2003;5(6):430–4.

161. Slager RE, Newton TL, Vlangos CN, et al. Mutations in RAI1 associated with Smith-Magenis syndrome. Nat Genet 2003;33:466–8.

162. Gropman A, Smith ACM, Allanson J, et al. Smith Magenis syndrome: aspects of the infant phenotype. Am J Hum Genet 1998;63(Suppl):A19.

163. Gropman A, Wolters P, Smith ACM. Neurodevelopmental assessment and functioning in five young children with Smith-Magenis syndrome. Am J Hum Genet 1999;65(Suppl):A141.

164. Udwin O, Webber C, Horn I. Abilities and attainment in Smith-Magenis syndrome. Dev Med Child Neurol 2001;43(12):823–8.

165. Madduri N, Peters SU, Voigt RG, et al. Cognitive and adaptive behavior profiles in Smith-Magenis syndrome. J Dev Behav Pediatr 2006;27(3):188–92.

166. Dykens EM, Finucane BM, Gayley C. Brief report: cognitive and behavioral profiles in persons with Smith-Magenis syndrome. J Autism Dev Disord 1997; 27(2):203–11.

167. Smith AC, Dykens E, Greenberg F. Behavioral phenotype of Smith-Magenis syndrome (del 17p11.2). Am J Med Genet 1998;81(2):179–85.

168. De Leersnyder H, de Blois MC, Vekemans M, et al. Beta(1)-adrenergic antagonists improve sleep and behavioural disturbances in a circadian disorder, Smith-Magenis syndrome. J Med Genet 2001;38(9):586–90.

169. De Leersnyder H. Inverted rhythm of melatonin secretion in Smith-Magenis syndrome: from symptoms to treatment. Trends Endocrinol Metab 2006;17(7):291–8.

170. Finucane B, Dirrigi KH, Simon EW. Characterization of self-injurious behaviors in children and adults with Smith-Magenis syndrome. Am J Ment Retard 2001; 106(1):52–8.

171. Finucane BM, Konar D, Haas-Givler B. The spasmodic upper-body squeeze: a characteristic behavior in Smith-Magenis syndrome. Dev Med Child Neurol 1994;36(1):78–83.

172. Taylor L, Oliver C. The behavioural phenotype of Smith-Magenis syndrome: evidence for a gene-environment interaction. J Intellect Disabil Res 2008; 52(10):830–41.

173. Dykens EM, Smith AC. Distinctiveness and correlates of maladaptive behavior in children and adolescents with Smith-Magenis syndrome. J Intellect Disabil Res 1998;42(Pt 6):481–9.

174. Niederhofer H. Efficacy of risperidone treatment in Smith-Magenis syndrome. Psychiatr Danub 2007;19(3):189–92.

175. Sybert VP. The adult patient with Turner syndrome. In: Albertson-Wikland K, Ranke MB, editors. Turner syndrome in a life span perspective: research and clinical aspects. New York: Elsevier; 1995. p. 205–18.

176. Gotzsche CO, Krag-Olsen B, Nielsen J, et al. Prevalence of cardiovascular malformations and association with karyotypes in Turner's syndrome. Arch Dis Child 1994;71:433–6.

177. Arulanantham K, Kramer MS, Gryboski JD. The association of inflammatory bowel disease and X chromosome abnormality. Pediatrics 1980;66:63–7.

178. Germain EL, Plotnick LP. Age-related anti-thyroid antibodies and thyroid abnormalities in Turner syndrome. Acta Paediatr Scand 1986;75:750–5.

179. Lippe B, Geffner ME, Dietrich RB, et al. Renal malformations in patients with Turner syndrome: Imaging in 141 patients. Pediatrics 1988;82:852–6.

180. American Academy of Pediatrics Committee on Genetics. Health supervision for children with Turner syndrome. Pediatrics 1995;96:1166–73.

181. Ross JL, Stefanatos GA, Kushner H, et al. Persistent cognitive deficits in adult women with Turner syndrome. Neurology 2002;58(2):218–25.

182. Russell HF, Wallis D, Mazzocco MM, et al. Increased Prevalence of ADHD in Turner syndrome with no evidence of imprinting effects. J Pediatr Psychol 2006;31(9):945–55.

183. Siegel PT, Clopper R, Stabler B. The psychological consequences of Turner syndrome and review of the National Cooperative Growth Study psychological substudy. Pediatrics 1998;102(2 Pt 3):488–91.

184. Mazzocco MM, Baumgardner T, Freund LS, et al. Social functioning among girls with Fragile X or Turner syndrome and their sisters. J Autism Dev Disord 1998; 28(6):509–17.

185. McCauley E, Kay T, Ito J, et al. The Turner syndrome: cognitive deficits, affective discrimination, and behavior problems. Child Dev 1987;58(2):464–73.
186. Ross JL, Stefanatos G, Roeltgen D, et al. Ullrich-Turner syndrome: neurodevelopmental changes from childhood through adolescence. Am J Med Genet 1995;58(1):74–82.
187. Rae C, Joy P, Harasty J, et al. Enlarged temporal lobes in Turner syndrome: an X-chromosome effect? Cereb Cortex 2004;14(2):156–64.
188. Lawrence K, Campbell R, Swettenham J. Interpreting gaze in Turner syndrome: impaired sensitivity to intention and emotion, but preservation of social cueing. Neuropsychologia 2003;41(8):894–905.
189. Skuse DH, Morris JS, Dolan RJ. Functional dissociation of amygdale-modulated arousal and cognitive appraisal in Turner syndrome. Brain 2005;128(pt 9): 2084–96.
190. Kesler SR. Turner syndrome. Child Adolesc Psychiatr Clin N Am 2007;16(3): 709–22.
191. Anderson LT, Ernst M. Self-injury in Lesch-Nyhan disease. J Autism Dev Disord 1994;24(1):67–81.
192. Harris JC. Developmental neuropsychiatry, vol II. New York: Oxford University Press; 1995. p. 307.
193. Taira T, Kobayashi T, Hori T. Disappearance of self-mutilating behavior in a patient with Lesch-Nyhan syndrome after bilateral chronic stimulation of the globus pallidus interna. J Neurosurg 2003;98(2):414–6.
194. Lesch M, Nyhan WL. A familial disorder of uric acid metabolism and central nervous system dysfunction. Am J Med 1964;36:561–70.
195. Arnold GL, Kramer BM, Kirby RS, et al. Factors affecting cognitive, motor, behavioral and executive functioning in children with phenylketonuria. Acta Paediatr 1998;87:565–70.
196. Griffiths P, Tarrini M, Robinson P. Executive function and psychosocial adjustment in children with early treated phenylketonuria; correlation with historical and concurrent phenylalanine levels. J Intellect Disabil Res 1997;41:317–23.
197. Pietz J, Fatkenheur B, Burgard P, et al. Psychiatric disorders in adult patients with early-treated phenylketonuria. Pediatrics 1997;99:345–50.
198. Realmuto G, Garfinkle BD, Tuchman M, et al. Psychiatric diagnosis and behavioral characteristics of phenylketonuric children. J Nerv Ment Dis 1986;174: 536–40.
199. Seashore MR, Freidman E, Novelly RA, et al. Loss of intellectual function in children with phenylketonuria after relaxation of dietary phenylalanine restriction. Pediatrics 1985;75:226–32.
200. Williams K. Benefits of normalizing plasma phenylalanine: impact on behavior and health. J Inherit Metab Dis 1998;21:785–90.
201. Enns GM. Neurologic damage and neurocognitive dysfunction in urea cycle disorders. Semin Pediatr Neurol 2008;15(3):132–9.
202. Gropman AL, Batshaw ML. Cognitive outcome in urea cycle disorders. Mol Genet Metab 2004;81:S58–62.

Developmental and Psychosocial Issues in Cystic Fibrosis

Michelle M. Ernst, PhD[a,c,*], Mark C. Johnson, MD[b,c], Lori J. Stark, PhD[a,c]

KEYWORDS

- Cystic fibrosis • Chronic illness • Adherence • Quality of life
- Coping

Cystic fibrosis (CF) is the most common life-limiting genetic disorder of Whites, affecting approximately 30,000 individuals in the United States.[1] It is an autosomal recessive disorder resulting from aberrations in the gene that encodes the cystic fibrosis transmembrane conductance regulator (CFTR) protein, thereby causing abnormal ion transport throughout the body. In the lungs, this leads to problems with mucous clearance, which subsequently sets the stage for chronic lung infection and inflammation. Respiratory symptoms are experienced by nearly every patient. Gastrointestinal consequences include exocrine pancreatic insufficiency (in an estimated 90% of individuals), which sets the stage for CF-related diabetes (CFRD) in an estimated 50% of adults older than 30 years of age. Other gastrointestinal effects include poor nutrient absorption (especially for fat), biliary cirrhosis, bile duct proliferation, and excessive absorption of fluid, increasing the risk for intestine obstruction. In fact, 20% of patients with CF have meconium ileus within the first 24 hours of life. More early symptoms that indicate CF include respiratory infections (most often cough or pulmonary infiltrates) and failure to thrive. Additional symptoms that occur across

A version of this article was previously published in the *Child and Adolescent Psychiatric Clinics of North America, 19:2*.

This study was supported by grant D24 DK 059492 from the National Institutes of Health (L.J.S.).

[a] Division of Behavioral Medicine and Clinical Psychology, Cincinnati Children's Hospital Medical Center, University of Cincinnati College of Medicine, 3333 Burnet Avenue, Cincinnati, OH 45229-3039, USA

[b] Division of Child and Adolescent Psychiatry, Cincinnati Children's Hospital Medical Center, University of Cincinnati College of Medicine, 3333 Burnet Avenue, Cincinnati, OH 45229-3039, USA

[c] Department of Pediatrics, Cincinnati Children's Hospital Medical Center, University of Cincinnati College of Medicine, 3333 Burnet Avenue, Cincinnati, OH 45229-3039, USA

* Corresponding author. Division of Behavioral Medicine and Clinical Psychology, Cincinnati Children's Hospital Medical Center, University of Cincinnati College of Medicine, 3333 Burnet Avenue, Cincinnati, OH 45229-3039.

E-mail address: Michelle.Ernst@cchmc.org

the life span include chronic sinusitis, nasal polyps (present in 25% of patients), and late onset puberty. Infertility is present in nearly 95% of men as a result of absence of the vas deferens and for 20% of women as a result of ion transport issues in the genitourinary system, such as abnormal cervical mucus.[2] Pain is common throughout the disease course.[3] Whereas 50 years ago most children with CF died before 6 years of age, in 2007 the median predicted survival age was 37.4 years. A total of 95% of patients die from complications related to pulmonary infection, with females more at risk for mortality than males.[1]

Children suspected to have CF are diagnosed by identification of clinical symptoms and analysis of sweat chloride values (ie, the sweat test). Testing sometimes has to be delayed until the infant produces sufficient sweat for the procedure. Currently, more than 70% of patients with CF are diagnosed by 2 years of age, with some children diagnosed prenatally. As a result of newborn screening programs (NBS), more children with CF are being diagnosed during the newborn phase. Evidence suggests that newborn screening programs are effective in promoting early health care for affected infants, corresponding with improved outcomes in nutritional status and decreased hospitalization.[4]

Given the chronic, progressive, and disabling nature of CF, multiple treatments are prescribed, most on a daily basis. Maintenance of lung health is of primary concern and pulmonary treatments include airway clearance techniques (ACT) (eg, coughing, breathing exercises, and chest percussion) and acute and chronic antibiotic treatment. Gastrointestinal treatments include pancreatic enzyme replacement and vitamins. High-caloric dietary intake and vitamin supplements are often necessary to offset the poor gastrointestinal absorption of fats and nutrients. Patients with CF are recommended to consume between 110% and 200% of the dietary reference intakes for energy (DRI) for healthy individuals to enhance nutrition and growth.[5] Thus, this illness requires children, with the aid of their families, to adopt multiple health-related behaviors in addition to managing more typical developmental demands. The comprehensive nature of CF experience and treatment makes CF a family diagnosis.

Despite the enormous treatment burden and shortened mortality, individuals with CF and their families have been shown to be tremendously resilient, with most patients and parents reporting a high quality of life and normative levels of psychopathology.[6] Nonetheless, the morbidity and mortality factors are understandably challenging for many children and their families, and there is a subset of patients and families for whom more significant psychological distress is noted. This article applies a developmental perspective to describing the psychosocial factors affecting psychological adjustment and health-related behaviors relevant to infants, preschool, and school-age children, and adolescents with CF. Topics particularly pertinent to each developmental period are noted. In addition, psychological factors related to noteworthy medical milestones are also examined in respect to their interface with and effect on psychosocial functioning. Clinical implications and recommendations are presented throughout.

PERINATAL

Attachment, the reciprocal bonding relationship between the infant and the parent that evolves based on the mutual connection of their dyad, is a primary task of this developmental stage. The parent's and the infant's mental representations and behaviors are involved in the attachment process. The parent-child relationship is a critical context for the developing infant, and the quality of attachment predicts important child psychosocial factors such as emotional and behavioral regulation, social skills, and the ability to cope with stress. Parental distress can have negative implications for attachment, particularly when coupled with parental depression and anxiety.[7]

The attachment period often coincides with the time of CF diagnosis. The diagnostic process is emotionally challenging. Even before a definitive CF diagnosis, parents of infants with positive CF screens during NBS report high levels of depressive and anxious symptoms, frequently accompanied by hypervigilence such that parents misinterpret common newborn behaviors as evidence of CF. Negative emotions such as worry, sadness, and guilt caused by the hereditary component of CF are common.[8] Worse coping with a positive screen has been found when parents were not knowledgeable about the NBS process, had little knowledge about CF, and were experiencing more general adjustment issues related to the newborn period (significant sleep deprivation, adjusting to role of new parent). In addition, parents' distress was reported to be amplified when the medical team communicated the results of the screen in an impersonal fashion and before the infant was old enough to undergo a sweat test (thus extending the waiting period).[8] Once a CF diagnosis is confirmed, parents typically continue to experience fluctuating states of psychological distress and normalcy as they take on the role of medical parent,[4] and may be particularly vulnerable to depressive symptoms when their infants are still only a few months old. Glasscoe and colleagues[9] studied the mental health of parents of infants with CF and reported that mothers and fathers of infants less than 9 months old had higher relative risk of scoring at or more than the clinical cut-off for mild depression (on the Beck Depression Inventory) compared with parents of age-matched healthy controls (relative risk 2.6 and 2.26, for mothers and fathers, respectively). No increased risk was found in parents of older infants.

Despite this risk of heightened distress in parents during the initial attachment period, there do not seem to be higher rates of maladaptive attachments between infants with CF and their parents, again highlighting the resiliency of families with CF.[4,10] However, when maladaptive attachment does occur, it has been found to have a negative effect on the health status of infants with CF. Infants with CF who have problematic attachment styles have been found to have significantly poorer nutritional status and lower body mass index (BMI, calculated as weight in kilograms divided by the square of height in meters).[10] Apart from the positive findings related to general attachment patterns, other research has found differences between families with CF and healthy controls in specific parent and child behaviors. For example, one study using direct observation to explore differences in interpersonal behaviors of children with CF between the ages of 12 and 24 months and their parents versus healthy dyads found parents of children with CF showed more controlling, serious, and less encouraging behaviors, whereas their children displayed more whining and less responsivity to parent behaviors.[11] Thus, even in the earliest stages of development, the toll of CF may begin to influence family interactions.

Clinical Implications

Screening for parent mental health concerns is critical during early infancy to provide appropriate intervention and maximize parental ability to engage meaningfully and positively with their child. Paying close attention to parents' emotional responses to the CF diagnosis such as guilt or worry is important because persistent negative emotions may have significant effects on child and parent mental health. For example, a study of parents of children with CF in ages ranging from 5 to 12 years found that more than 40% of the parents in their sample blamed themselves for their child's illness as a coping strategy. Use of self-blame was significantly associated with worse emotional adjustment for the children with CF and their parents.[12] Providing education and support during the early diagnostic period may ameliorate some of these unhelpful reactions, thereby preventing long-term negative correlates.[13]

In addition, early signs of problematic interactions between child and parent should be a cue to closely track important physiologic outcomes and to look more closely at how health behavior patterns are unfolding. Helping parents implement developmentally appropriate effective routines around general daily activities as well as CF-specific treatment tasks can promote positive reciprocal relationships and increase enjoyment of time spent together. These types of interventions may be particularly important for treatment-related activities that are shown to have poor adherence later in development. For example, Grasso and colleagues[14] reported that using music during ACT in infants and toddlers led to parents rating their own and their child's enjoyment of the time better and made the time go more quickly.

EARLY CHILDHOOD: PRESCHOOL

During the preschool period, developmental issues related to expanding language skills, cognitive development in areas such as understanding causality and assessment of ability to control environment, and emotional/behavioral regulation development may be of particular relevance to the experience of CF. Developing language skills helps the child process and express their experiences so that parents and health care providers can have a better understanding of the child's cognitive and emotional events. Although much research has tied children's causal attribution to Piagetian stages, with young children attributing illness to magical or superstitious factors, recent research suggests that preschool children may have a more sophisticated understanding of illness which also incorporates biologic factors.[15] In the one study that looked directly at causal attributions in a CF sample, more than half of the 4- to 6-year-old children with CF knew that they had been born with the illness and only 1 of the 17 preschool children studied stated they were being punished with their CF.[16] However, few knew what the various treatments were for.[16] The preschool child is also still developing accuracy in understanding which events can or cannot be controlled, which has significant implications for the young child with CF who may be in a myriad of stressful environmental situations beyond their control such as medical procedures and treatments.[17] The young child with CF may exhibit extreme behavioral reactions to attempt to escape these procedures, and may develop heightened aversion for future medical events.

The interface of behavioral self-regulation and CF-related tasks is particularly noteworthy in this age range, when preschool children are already contending with increasing awareness of behavioral limits, whereas parents are developing strategies to enhance compliance. Even when children have mild disease and low levels of symptoms, treatment burden is significant: daily nutrition goals, enzyme supplementation, and ACT are recommended to preserve growth and lung health. The increased opportunities for parent/child conflict may alter parenting strategies such that parents may become either more authoritative or harsh (particularly for health-related behaviors deemed essential for survival) or more permissive as a result of parenting resources stretched thin by the chronic illness, a choose-your-battles approach, or overprotection. These additive behavioral demands associated with CF treatment can challenge the emotional resources of children and parents and can have negative implications for child and parent mental health, general family functioning, and health-related outcomes. There is little research exploring general psychosocial functioning in young children with CF. However, Ward and colleagues[18] recently published the results of a study comparing parent-reported behavioral functioning of preschool children with CF with normative data. Although increases in child internalizing or externalizing mental health issues were not found, nearly half of the children with CF were found to have moderate to large sleep and/or eating problems, and 40% of the children had poor compliance with ACT. Thus, although not appearing to have significant psychological impairment, these preschool children with CF did struggle with health-related processes and behaviors.

Problematic mealtime behaviors are a particularly salient health-related concern for children with CF because they are at high risk for poor growth as a result of chronic lung infection and dietary fat malabsorption. Nutritional status, in turn, is related to lung functioning, health complications, and morbidity in CF. Although nutritional guidelines for children with CF recommend eating between 110% and 200% of the DRI, studies of infants, toddlers, and preschool children report typical consumption of only 100% of DRI, with fewer than one-quarter of the children achieving the minimum recommendation for children with CF.[19,20] As might be expected given the sense of urgency parents feel and the higher demands placed on the children, mealtimes with preschool children with CF have been shown to be more problematic than in healthy families. Children with CF show a higher frequency of behaviors that interfere with eating such as crying and whining, delaying meals by talking, spitting out food, and leaving the table.[20–22] At the same time, parents of children with CF engage in behaviors such as increased coercion, commands, physical prompts, and actual feeding of preschool children compared with a healthy sample.[22] Parents often cite mealtime as a particular concern, and report thinking that they have little control over their children's eating patterns.[23]

Although CF-related eating concerns persist throughout development, assessment and intervention during early childhood may change the trajectory of maladaptive behaviors and interactions. In general, behavioral problems in children in this age range are best treated through behavior modification. A recent randomized clinical trial of behavioral modification involving toddlers and preschool children with CF found an increase in average daily caloric intake of approximately 850 kcal, corresponding to 120% of DRI. This finding was significantly better than a treatment-as-usual control condition in which the children's caloric intake declined during the same period. The gains found in the behavioral treatment group were maintained at 3- and 12-month follow-up. The intervention consisted of 6 weekly individual sessions during which parents received nutrition counseling and training in behavioral modification principles. Specific behavioral techniques highlighted included active praising of desired eating behaviors, ignoring noneating behaviors, setting time limits for meals, using successive approximation to determine weekly goals, and providing tangible reinforcement for goal achievement.[24]

The management of developmental and treatment-related concerns for the preschool child may have negative implications for broader family interaction patterns as well as the adjustment of other family members. For example, Spieth and colleagues[22] compared mealtimes of families of a preschool child with CF with those of families of children without CF. Relative to the healthy control families, the families with a child with CF had greater deficits in family functioning in areas such as communication, emotional expression, interpersonal involvement, and appropriate behavioral expectations and enforcement. Greater marital role strain and decreased home recreation time have also been reported in families caring for a preschool child with CF.[25] There is also evidence that parents of preschool children with CF are at risk for problematic psychosocial functioning. For example, in the study by Ward and colleagues,[18] parents of preschool children with CF reported increased levels of depression (33%), anxiety (16%), and stress (34%).

Siblings in the household may also be affected. Research across chronic illnesses has shown that the presence of a child with chronic illness in the family has a negative effect on siblings, particularly in the areas of peer activities and psychological functioning.[26] Although sibling psychosocial functioning has not been studied in CF, research has examined differences in how parents treat the child with CF compared with a healthy sibling. A study comparing parenting practices toward sibling dyads in which the younger sibling had CF versus sibling dyads of 2 healthy children found greater discrepancy in patterns of differential treatment in the families with CF. Mothers spent more time with the younger sibling who had CF in mealtimes and play-times. In addition, mothers rated the quality of their time with their ill child as extremely positive, but reported as much negative time as positive time during interactions with their well child despite no evidence that these children had worse behaviors.[27] The strong emotional reactions of having a child with a life-limiting illness may promote more positive feelings toward that child and more negative parenting relationships with well children. Beyond the effects this differential treatment may have on the sibling's adjustment, the quality of the sibling relationship may be negatively affected, which may have long-term social implications for both children.[28]

Clinical Implications

Given that the young child's experience with medical issues affects longer-term psychosocial and biologic outcomes, it is imperative that children be given developmentally appropriate but accurate information about their illness even during these early ages. The findings that children may be able to understand illness causality at a more sophisticated level than previously believed is encouraging, and should be capitalized on in helping children understand the relationship between their illness and the resulting daily treatments and medical procedures. Interventions to maximize coping with early distressing CF-related experiences is also important for current and future interactions with health care provision, and research suggests that adequate pain management and nonpharmacologic interventions such as distraction can be helpful in decreasing aversive responses to procedural anxiety and pain.[17]

Helping families maintain healthy family dynamics despite treatment burden is a priority with children at this age. Although most research has applied behavioral therapy to dietary recommendations in this age group, behavioral strategies can be applied more broadly to improve adherence across CF tasks.[29] Ensuring that parents are knowledgeable in behavioral management strategies is critical to positively affect their young child's health behaviors in ways that promote prosocial behaviors and increase parental self-efficacy. Inquiring about the functioning of specific family members as well as overall family interaction patterns can also identify areas for clinical intervention. One positive effect of CF on family relationships is that parents of a child with CF have been shown to spend more time with that child in play and less time in chores compared with parents who have healthy children, perhaps reflecting prioritizing the resource of time when confronted with a life-limiting disease.[25] Validating the importance of prioritization with parents in conjunction with more effective parenting strategies may help them redistribute some of their limited resources of time and energy to self-care, marital health, and maximizing the quality of time spent with all children in the home.

SCHOOL AGE

The school-age period is characterized by evolving cognitive skills and an increased emphasis on peer relationships. As children's cognitive and language skills expand, they are able to communicate better about their own beliefs and expectations related to their illness. This development may facilitate effective psychoeducation that targets misinformation and addresses unfounded fears or concerns. It is essential that children's sense of ownership and control of their chronic illness be encouraged during this period to develop skills and self-efficacy related to self-management and collaboration throughout the life span. The opportunity to develop child self-care skills seems to be missed frequently. Savage and Callery[30] observed family-provider interactions during CF clinic visits, and found that most school-age children were marginalized by staff, felt bored, and perceived the interaction to be only between their parent and the provider. In addition, children's own health priorities were not addressed. For example, diet consultations were focused toward the parent and emphasized weight gain, whereas children reported that their primary desired outcome for increased nutrition was more energy.[30] Children are more interested in adopting healthier behaviors if these behaviors are framed toward outcomes personally desired and meaningful to school-age children.

Although cognitive changes can affect children's relationships with health providers, peer relationships are a core catalyst for the psychosocial development of the school-age child. Children's identity and sense of competence begin to be developed largely through a process of comparison with their peers.[31] For the child with CF, this peer comparison process may highlight their CF-related differences (eg, frequent coughing, taking enzymes with meals, more fatigue, school absences). Children who were diagnosed at birth or in early childhood may, in effect, undergo a second diagnostic period during which they realize at a deeper level the effect of CF on multiple aspects of their life. School-age children with CF describe significant concerns related to being different than their peers, with a high premium on appearing normal.[32] Coping with negative peer reactions such as teasing or overprotection in response to the visible manifestations of CF is reported to be one of the most stressful daily events for children with CF.[32] Even with supportive peers, children seek to diminish the emphasis placed on their illness. Children are often unsuccessful at hiding the more visible aspects of the disease, and may be setting themselves up for worse peer issues because providing the CF context for atypical behaviors may minimize negative peer perceptions.[33] Keeping illness status a secret can also negatively affect the ability to develop and maintain intimate friendships.[31,32]

Support from peers who share the same medical illness has often been promoted to circumvent the potential for stigmatization, decrease the sense of alienation, and increase sharing of adaptive strategies to maintain quality of life. Before the mid-1990s, children with CF were encouraged to attend CF-related summer camps and other venues for peer support, and although empirical evidence is lacking, research with other chronic illnesses suggests that these experiences were beneficial for increasing adjustment.[34] However, in the mid-1980s CF medical communities became cognizant of *Burkholderia cepacia*, a particularly treatment-resistant constellation of bacteria that can be contracted from environmental sources and person-to-person transmission, and that often corresponds with rapid decline in lung functioning for patients with CF. It was soon determined that CF summer camps were the setting for epidemic spread of this bacteria, and these programs were closed.[35] Other treatment-resistant bacteria have since been identified, and evidence of epidemic spread has been found within outpatient CF clinics as well as on inpatient hospital wards.[35] In reaction, CF centers have implemented strict segregation policies (eg, isolating children with CF from each other during clinics), and have strongly recommended that patients with CF should not interact with each other.[36] There is little research into the emotional consequence of the stricter infection-control policies. However, some studies suggest that parents and children are in agreement with the policies because of the health benefits incurred by segregation but also identify costs such as decreased social support, feeling alienated, and missing friends with CF.[37,38] Thus, children and adolescents with CF, although having similar challenges with healthy peers as do other children with chronic illnesses, are not afforded the benefits of support from those peers with CF who would most closely understand their experiences.

The additive psychosocial challenges incurred by CF during this age period seem to increase the risk of psychological distress in these children, although there is some disagreement in the literature.[10,39] In a study using semistructured diagnostic interviews,[40] 60% of children with CF met criteria for a psychological diagnosis, with an anxiety diagnosis present in 35%. Externalizing diagnoses were also present, with a prevalence of 22.5% for oppositional defiant disorder and 12.5% for conduct disorder. Depression rates have been found to range from 2% to 9% in some studies to 33% in more recent studies.[39] Poorer adjustment in this age group has been related to higher levels of stress, lower self-efficacy, increased monitoring for CF-related cues, and less internal health locus of control.[40,41] Other cognitive factors from the general chronic illness literature that may be relevant are illness uncertainty (the degree to which children experience confusion related to illness status and course)[42] and parental perception of child vulnerability.[43] The life-limiting nature of CF, growth problems, and significant respiratory symptoms may render parents of children with CF particularly susceptible to viewing their child as fragile. The communication of this perception (either overtly or subtly) coupled with the unpredictable course of CF may negatively affect children's developing self-concept because they may learn to perceive themselves as lacking the skills needed to manage disease-related factors.

Behavioral and cognitive-behavioral interventions are generally considered to be first-line treatments for depression and anxiety in the general population of school-age children.[44,45] There is a dearth of literature applying these evidence-based treatment protocols to enhance adjustment in the CF population. However, 2 recent studies did integrate cognitive-behavioral features such as problem-solving, anticipatory guidance, behavioral modeling, and relaxation training into their interventions. In one study, children 8 to 12 years old with CF were randomly assigned to either a control group or to a Building CF Life Skills intervention that targeted problem-solving and social skills.[46] The intervention was delivered in 1 home visit and 1 small-group intervention. Loneliness and perceived effect of CF were improved relative to control immediately after intervention as well as at the 9-month follow-up. The use of a group intervention was particularly noteworthy in this study given the usual strategy of isolating children with CF from each other for infection-control purposes. Here, any children with drug-resistant infections were in separate clinic rooms connected by a real-time video camera link, which gave the children a rare opportunity to form a live CF peer group.[46] Another study used a CD-ROM program to increase CF-related knowledge and expand the coping repertoire of 10- to 17-year-old children. Results showed that children randomly assigned to the CD-ROM condition had greater disease-related knowledge and generated more coping strategies to hypothetical challenging situations when compared with a wait-list control.[47]

In addition to challenges related to psychosocial functioning, health-related behaviors may become increasingly compromised as children grow older. Treatment burden is high during this period, with preteen children spending more than an hour per day completing treatment-related tasks.[48] The time-intensive nature of disease management may increasingly interfere with school- and peer-related demands of childhood. A recent study used diary data assessment methods to document ACT adherence in school-age children and found only 51% of the recommended ACT were completed, and of those completed, 64% lasted the recommended duration.[49] In this same study, diary data showed that adherence to enzymes and nebulized medications was less than 50%.[49] Several barriers to adherence have been identified, such as lack of knowledge of CF in general and of individual treatment recommendations, disagreement with provider recommendations, complexity of treatment, psychological issues (on the part of the parent and the child), forgetting, oppositional behaviors, difficulty with time management, and child's low level of disease symptoms.[50–52]

Research targeting improved adherence to CF treatment has reported the short-term benefits of behavioral interventions for school-age children with CF. In a recent multisite randomized clinical trial comparing a behavioral versus nutrition-only intervention, children in the behavioral treatment group had nearly double the daily caloric intake than did the children in the nutrition group after the 9-week treatment. Between-group differences disappeared at the 2-year follow-up, at which point all the children maintained approximately 120% DRI. Analysis of the nutrition intervention suggests that this treatment included important behavioral components such as weekly monitoring of intake, successive approximation toward goals, and individualized goal plans, suggesting that behavioral approaches, whether implemented in strictly psychological interventions or integrated into the work of other disciplines, are successful at improving health behavior for school-age children.[53] Single-subject studies have documented the efficacy of behavioral interventions for increasing at-home exercise[54] and ACT.[55,56] A randomized clinical trial investigating a self-administered education program based on the cognitive-behavioral and social learning models was shown to be effective in improving adherence to prescribed aerosol treatment in this age group, with an improvement in ACT only on the days that the child was feeling unwell.[57]

There are few studies examining the effect of CF on the family of the school-age child. However, a recent study of a clinic sample of parents of children in this age range revealed increased rates of anxiety and depression in mothers and fathers, with rates of anxiety approaching 50%. Overall, however, parents reported a positive quality of life.[58] Correlates of better parent adjustment have been shown to include less self-blame, less avoidant coping, and more social support for parents, family cohesion, and parental hope for positive outcomes for their children.[12,59] These correlates seem to differ between mothers and fathers.[59] As might be predicted, parents are particularly concerned with and affected by their child's worsening disease status and possibility of death.[58] Systematic interventions directly targeting the mental health of CF parents are sparse, despite the relationship between child and parental distress. However, one study examined the benefit of massage therapy for school-age children with CF and their parents. Compared with a group that only read together, child and parent anxiety were improved in the massage group, as was child peak air flow.[60]

Clinical Implications

The peer- and treatment-related challenges and evolving cognitive development that the school-age years bring to the child with CF offer a tremendous opportunity for children to develop or enhance critical psychosocial skills that are important for adjustment. For example, helping children develop effective means of handling awkward social situations related to their CF can expand their social behavior repertoire, leading to greater confidence in navigating social situations. In addition, using behavioral methods to enhance adherence and track relevant outcomes can increase children's sense of involvement, control, and self-efficacy, essential components of self-management across the life span.[61] As parent perception of their child's vulnerability may affect child self-perception, it is important also to work with parents to identify if these perceptions are present. Normalizing these reactions yet also encouraging parents to have developmentally appropriate expectations for behavior and allowing children the opportunity to learn from their mistakes are important to keep child development on course. The cognitive growth during this period, in conjunction with evolving social skills, makes this an optimal time to engage children fully in collaboration with health care providers. Working with children to clarify what would be personally motivating in terms of physical or psychosocial outcomes and then realistically linking health behaviors to the child's own values likely promote goal-driven behavior as well as helping children make the connection between self-management and goal attainment in multiple arenas.

ADOLESCENCE

Adolescence is a period of rapid social, cognitive, and physiologic changes. The proportion of time spent with peers increases relative to family time, with peers also becoming more influential.[31] Adolescence is characterized by persistent movement toward increasing autonomy and separation from parents, and adolescent-parent relationships are frequently characterized by conflict.[28] Cognition becomes more abstract and self-concept continues to be refined though experiences such as trying on different roles and behaviors, which sometimes has negative health implications. Concomitant with puberty, sexual exploration adds another level of complexity to social relationships.[28] At the same time as this tremendous developmental growth, CF typically worsens during adolescence, particularly for females, and the presence of more frequent symptoms (especially cough and fatigue) and pulmonary exacerbations (intense period of disease activity) corresponds with greater illness burden.[62]

Thus, the interface between biopsychosocial development and disease progression can make this time period particularly challenging for the adolescent with CF. When they would typically be gaining more independence, immersing themselves in the company of their peers and thinking about the future, their worsening disease may cause them to be isolated from peers because of the need to be home-bound or admitted to hospital, to be more reliant on family, and to have a heightened sense of a foreshortened future.[63] This situation may be particularly salient for females, who have been shown to have a higher mortality and poorer health-related quality of life than males.[64] Declines in pulmonary function start earlier for girls, and the relative risk of survival for females compared with males is lower up to the age of 20 years. Several factors are believed to be related to this gender difference, including girls' reported tendencies to be less adherent to the high-fat diet and other aspects of treatment, to suppress coughing because of the greater public self-consciousness seen in females, to use passive coping more frequently, the normative reduction in physical activity noted for adolescent females, and higher levels of strain reported by females.[65]

Research has examined the effect of CF on some developmental processes. For instance, Meijer and colleagues[66] examined peer interactions in a chronically ill adolescent sample comprised of 98 adolescents (1 of 4 with CF). Compared with healthy norms, females with a chronic illness were significantly less socially engaged but as socially skilled. Females with CF were notable for higher levels of assertiveness. Males with a chronic illness displayed fewer problematic social behaviors, with a trend toward being less socially engaged. Duration of illness was positively associated with social skills and assertiveness, suggesting that one possible benefit of the chronic illness experience is developing a greater facility for negotiation. Perhaps the need to manage symptoms and interface with health care providers from a young age helps young people become more adept at identifying their needs and getting them met.

Other studies have looked at the supportive behaviors of peers and families in adolescents with CF and suggest that families provide more tangible support and peers provide more emotional and companionship support. However, unsupportive family behaviors seem to be particularly problematic for adolescent adjustment.[67] Peer support may serve as a buffer for negative family interactions, whereas families do not seem to protect against the effect of strained peer relationships.[68]

CF has also been examined in the area of teenage risky behaviors. For example, although chronically ill young people have been shown to have an increased rate of risky behaviors relative to healthy peers,[69] young people with CF report fewer risky behaviors related to alcohol, tobacco, and marijuana relative to healthy peers. However, 20% of young people with CF report having smoked, a concerning statistic given the effect smoking has on nutrition and pulmonary function.[70] The prevalence of eating disorders, which typically begin in adolescence, is another risky health behavior with particular relevance to CF because of the relationship between nutritional status and mortality.[71] A recent study using rigorous diagnostic methods for eating disorders did not find an increased prevalence of adolescents with CF meeting full criteria for an eating disorder relative to the general population. However, subclinical levels of eating disturbance were increased compared with the general population, with 53% of the adolescents with CF indicating disturbed eating attitudes versus 40% to 47% of adolescents in the general population. A total of 18.8% of the females and 7.1% of the males reported engaging in weight-loss behaviors despite the average BMI in the sample being just at the lower limit of the healthy weight range.[71] Although CF imposes a modest delay on puberty, sexual libido is not affected and some, but not all, research suggests that these young people have similar onset of sexual behaviors.[70,72]

The limitations of CF notwithstanding, most adolescents report a high quality of life.[6] Recent research has begun to investigate cognitive factors related to adjustment in this population, which may be particularly relevant during adolescence because of evolving cognitive development. One such variable is hopefulness. Szyndler and colleagues[6] examined several variables related to quality of life and psychopathologic distress in an adolescent CF sample and found that hopefulness was correlated with better physical, social, and emotional functioning. One newer line of research in late adolescent and emerging adulthood development is the effect of chronic illness on goal pursuit, termed health-related hindrance.[73] In a recent study of 18- to 28-year-olds with chronic illness (divided between patients with CF and cancer), the more that the illness impeded goal pursuit, the more psychological distress and the less subjective well-being the individuals experienced.[73]

Another variable that has been recently studied in adolescents with CF is the concept of acceptance. Acceptance reflects an individual's ability to acknowledge and tolerate aversive thoughts and emotions even as they work toward achieving meaningful goals related to their values, and is a key component of the acceptance and commitment model of therapy.[74] Although the full model has not been researched in CF, Casier and colleagues[75] explored the idea of acceptance in a sample of adolescents with CF and found that adolescents who believed that they had the ability to live with CF and manage the associated negative consequences scored lower on measures of anxiety, depression, and functional disability. Similarly, Abbott and colleagues[76] also found that optimistic acceptance (ie, accepting the CF diagnosis, using problem-focused coping, and staying optimistic about the future) was related to better psychosocial quality of life in a sample of young adults, whereas distraction (ie, attempting to forget about CF) was related to worse quality of life. Despite the movement toward more autonomy from family, family variables such as organization, cohesion, and emotional expressiveness have been shown to be associated with better psychological functioning in adolescents.[6]

Research on the level of psychopathology in adolescents with CF is conflicting. Whereas some studies have not shown a higher risk for psychological distress in this population,[6] others have. For instance, in a recent study using structured diagnostic interviews with children with CF ranging from 9 to 17 years of age, 57% met DSM (*Diagnostic and Statistical Manual of Mental Disorders*) criteria for at least 1 psychiatric disorder. Anxiety was the most prevalent disorder, with 30% of the young people with CF meeting criteria.[52] A very low rate of depression was noted in this study, with only 2% of the young people meeting criteria. Higher rates of depression have been noted in other studies of adolescents with CF, although anxiety consistently seems to be the more prevalent of the two disorders.[39] As seen in the child literature, cognitive-behavioral therapy (CBT) has been shown to be effective in the general population for adolescent anxiety and depression.[44,77] Interpersonal therapy (IPT) has also been successfully used with adolescent depression, and the combination of medication with CBT or IPT may be most effective for some adolescents.[44] Given the importance of weight maintenance as well as the compromised function of multiple organs secondary to CF, the side effect of psychopharmacologic mediations must be carefully monitored. Although between-group studies have not been conducted exploring the use of evidence-based psychological treatment to improve psychological functioning in the adolescent CF population, case studies suggest that CBT can be effective in improving adjustment in adolescents with CF.[78]

Just as development may affect variables related to psychosocial outcomes, developmental processes are also related to changes in health behaviors important to management of CF. Research consistently reports that CF-related adherence worsens once children become adolescents, with up to 50% doing less than their prescribed treatment and up to 30% not doing any treatment.[79] Cognitive factors are influential in this arena as well. For example, adolescents who believed that their treatments were necessary and that CF was responsive to treatment had better adherence, with indications that these beliefs mediate the relationship between age and adherence.[80] Family factors and psychological distress are also believed to influence treatment decisions and behaviors. Adherence has also been shown to be associated with self-reported family cohesion and flexibility as well as observation-based ratings of overall positive family interactions, especially for tasks that are more challenging and require more family resources.[52,81] Although some research suggests that psychopathology negatively affects adherence, a recent study revealed that anxiety may improve adherence, perhaps reflecting a greater preoccupation with the illness.[52]

The relationships between adherence and the shift to greater autonomy for CF-related tasks have been of great interest in recent years because adolescents with CF are no longer so sick as they were 30 years ago, and have the opportunity to reach older developmental milestones if they successfully manage their disease. Recent research in this area has shown that responsibility for self-management increases throughout development, with periods of regression often found during illness exacerbations.[82] A study using computerized telephone diaries showed that parents gradually decreased their time involved in their child's CF-related activities from preadolescent to later adolescent years, although their involvement in other types of activities remained the same.[83] In this study, more supervision, particularly by mothers, correlated with better adherence regardless of patient age.[83]

Adolescent-focused outpatient adherence interventions are lacking in this population, but several approaches seem to be promising. One newer approach that has been shown to be effective in other pediatric behavioral health issues is motivational interviewing (MI).[84] MI targets enhancing motivation to engage in healthy behaviors rather than developing specific adherence-related skills. This approach takes an accepting attitude to patients' ambivalence to change and collaborates through goal clarification and increasing self-efficacy for those behaviors that the patient thinks are important. This approach may be particularly appealing to adolescents, who are themselves in the process of refining self-concept and individuation. Another approach is Internet-based health interventions incorporating psychoeducation, cognitive restructuring and problem-solving which have also shown promise in enhancing the self-management of adolescents with chronic illness. This approach may be appealing for adolescents who have grown up with great facility with Web-based applications. Other innovative approaches using developmentally appropriate technology such as cell phones are in development.[85]

The transition to more autonomy in issues related to health care goes beyond adherence behaviors for adolescents with cystic fibrosis. Unlike their peers 30 years ago, many adolescents age out of the pediatric setting and are expected to move to adult providers. Research exploring transition to adult CF clinics has shown that although the median age of transfer to adult care is 19 years, transition-related discussions are not typically initiated until 17 years of age. In addition, as of 2008, only one-quarter of CF centers offered transition-focused visits.[86] As noted earlier, evidence suggests that school-age children may not be optimally involved in patient–health care team collaboration[30]; thus, young people may suddenly find themselves expected to take responsibility for their health interactions in adult CF clinics without having been adequately prepared. In addition, anticipating leaving home or going to university may raise concerns about access to health care.[63] Earlier involvement in health care collaboration, addressing individual-specific concerns for the future, showing collaboration between pediatric and adult providers, and occasional pediatric follow-up during the year of transition have been shown to be effective.

Clinical Implications

Given the precipitous decline in disease status often shown in adolescence, engaging adolescents in self-management is of primary concern. Although typical adolescent autonomy is developed in part by being allowed the chance to experiment and learn from mistakes, the mistake of not caring for one's health can be life-threatening with CF. Thus, for maximum health benefits, parents may need to stay involved in supervising their adolescent's health activities for longer than they might have expected, but will need to shift to strategies that are more collaborative. Behavioral strategies such as successive approximation (eg, having the adolescent independently manage 1 small aspect of treatment) tied to natural consequences such as more freedom may help keep the transition developmentally appropriate but still closely monitored. In addition, the notion of acceptance may be particularly relevant to the adolescent with CF, for whom escape is clearly not an option because of daily treatment burdens and symptoms. Acceptance-based skills such as learning to perform treatment recommendations even although they are aversive, or staying engaged with friends even when fatigued, may help adolescents with CF continue to achieve important developmental tasks and meaningful goals as they move into adulthood.

SPECIFIC MEDICAL MILESTONES
CF Complications

The onset of CF-related diabetes (CFRD) is a medical milestone, which typically occurs during late adolescence and affects 10% to 15% of adults with CF. CFRD is often precipitated by a worsening of CF symptoms and is associated with earlier mortality.[87] The additional treatment burden brought on by a second chronic illness complicates an already involved treatment regimen and requires learning a new set of health management skills. Some research suggests that those who manage their CF well may already have in place self-management systems conducive to effective integration of the new treatment burden into their daily life.[87] In addition, although the new CFRD diagnosis initially may be experienced as overwhelming, most people adjust to the new treatment issues. However, when the development of CFRD coincides with significant CF disease progression, this second diagnosis can provoke a sense of powerlessness and psychological distress.[87]

Another particularly distressing consequence of CF is CF-related pain. In a recent study, at least one episode of pain in the previous month was reported for 59% of children aged 1 to 18 years and 89% of adults with CF, with the duration of pain exceeding 6 months for 55% of the children and 73% of adults.[3] Multiple pain locations were common. Pain was reported to significantly affect quality of life in 50% of the children and 70% of the adults. Approximately two-thirds of children and adults indicated that their medical treatment improved their pain. Procedural pain was also highly prevalent, with approximately 80% of children and adults reporting at least one episode during the past month, with high rates found in patients with severe disease. More than one-quarter of children reported pain during ACT.[3] Pain from blood-sticks was also significant, with 90% of all patients reporting anticipatory fear. Pain medication did not sufficiently treat the pain in one-third of all individuals in this study,[3] suggesting that other pain management strategies are indicated. Chest pain seems to be particularly distressing for children, and may have negative implications for their ability and willingness to complete ACT, thus posing a health risk.[88] CF-related pain has been shown to be related to physical and emotional functioning, as well as overall quality of life.[88] Nonpharmacologic cognitive-behavioral interventions have been shown to be helpful for procedural pain[17] and chronic pain across the life span,[89] and should be readily introduced to patients with pain.

Hospitalizations

The clinical course of CF is characterized by pulmonary exacerbations that frequently necessitate hospitalization for intensive ACT and intravenous antibiotic treatment. The effect of hospitalization on overall adjustment is not known, but has been believed to negatively affect quality of life. In one study, inpatients with CF reported significantly worse quality of life than did outpatients despite having similar lung functioning, suggesting that there may be factors other than objective health status that account for CF-related admission.[62] Research has suggested that as many as two-thirds of frequently admitted chronically ill children have major psychosocial factors contributing to the admission, such as somatization of personal/family difficulties, lack of appropriate living situations, and medical or psychological issues in the parent.[90] A randomized clinical trial exploring the benefits of a brief written self-disclosure intervention for adolescents and adults with CF found that the intervention group had fewer hospitalization days than did the control group, despite there being no between-group differences in psychological or physiologic outcomes. No specific mechanism for this effect could be identified by the study design. However, the investigators postulate that the process of writing may have promoted more active engagement and coping with disease-related issues, thereby causing these young adults to rely less on health care providers for support.[91]

Despite the disruption that hospitalizations pose, they seem to offer psychosocial benefits as well. Postpulmonary exacerbation psychosocial quality of life was better for individuals with CF treated in the hospital versus those who were treated at home, suggesting that factors such as increased 24-hour support by inpatient health care providers, greater improvement in fatigue, or respite for parents may have longer-term psychosocial profit.[92] Inpatients with CF are, in effect, a captive audience for the 1- to 3-week typical admission duration, which provides an often-unexploited opportunity to enhance coping and self-management. Cognitive-behavioral interventions can be used effectively with hospitalized patients to enhance stress management, coping with pain, sleep challenges, and other health-related challenges, which patients can also apply at home.[93] In addition, CF-specific health behaviors can be enhanced by incorporating psychoeducation and evidence-based behavioral strategies into routine inpatient treatment. For example, the authors' institution recently used quality improvement strategies to promote best-practice ACT on our adolescent unit. Evidence-based best-practice protocols were developed for a variety of ACT modalities, then patients were educated on proper technique per protocol, and collaborated with their respiratory therapist to identify the ACT modality that was the best fit for them. Behavioral strategies were implemented by unit staff that focused on positive reinforcement for ACT behaviors that met best-practice criteria. This program has resulted in significant increases in the quantity and quality of the ACT in which patients participated.[94] Generalization of optimal utilization of ACT from hospital to the home setting needs to be studied. Thus, the inpatient admission may be an opportunity for more in-depth assessment and intervention for important psychosocial and health behavior issues.

End-stage Lung Disease

The current median age of death from CF is approximately 25 years and most individuals die from end-stage lung disease (ESLD).[1] Lung transplantation is the most aggressive treatment available for advanced lung disease, and is considered when predicted survival with transplant surpasses predicted survival without. Approximately 120 to 150 individuals with CF receive a transplant per year,[95] and higher quality of life after transplant has been reported.[96] Five-year survival rate is 50% to 60% for patients with CF who receive a transplant,[95] and estimates suggest that up to 25% of patients with CF die while on the waiting list.[96] Thus, even with the prospect of lung transplant, many teenagers and young adults are faced with confronting end-of-life issues.

There is little research on psychosocial aspects related to end of life in the CF population. However, there is some evidence to suggest that having survived multiple pulmonary exacerbations throughout the course of the illness, patients with CF in ESLD may perceive CF to be beatable,[97] and the possibility of lung transplantation may contribute to this perspective.[98] In addition, the chronic and progressive course of CF sometimes makes it challenging to know when it is the right time to have end-of-life discussions; they are sometimes timed with transition to adult care providers or at annual review meetings with CF providers, which is preferable than during periods of disease acuity.[97,98] There is typically a short time period between institution of a do-not-resuscitate order and time of death (eg, 5 days), suggesting that patients with CF continue with life-preserving measures within hours of death.[98] Instituting palliative care treatment plans in conjunction with lung transplantation treatment plans may afford patients with CF the maximum comfort even as they await transplantation and at time of death.[98] Honest communication maximizing provision of care options and emotional support, family involvement, attending to spiritual and psychosocial needs of patients, and comprehensive symptom management are the cornerstones of end-of life care.[99] Once a death has occurred, follow-up support to the bereaved family is also indicated, including referral for counseling for instances of complicated grief.[99]

SUMMARY

CF may complicate some of the processes inherent in psychosocial development, and there is more research to be done clarifying the interface between developmental processes, psychosocial variables, and health for the child with CF. The increasing focus on self-management and adherence from a developmental perspective can have a significant effect on meaningful health outcomes in this population. There is also exciting newer research focusing on positive correlates of psychosocial adjustment, such as hopefulness, acceptance, and the importance of achieving meaningful goals despite CF. These variables relate to the concept of positive psychology, which is the field of psychology that explores the adaptive, more affirmative experiences of the human experience.[100] Although positive psychology has been understudied in pediatric psychology, it may be particularly relevant to understanding why many children and adolescents with CF report high quality of life despite the treatment burden of their illness. In addition, understanding if young people with CF undergo posttraumatic growth (ie, experience meaningful benefits from their CF-related experiences) may point the field toward a clearer understanding of the full scope of the psychosocial experience related to this illness and may help elucidate the processes that promote living a full, meaningful, and productive life within the context of a life-limiting illness.[100]

ACKNOWLEDGMENTS

The authors would like to thank Dr John M. Ernst for helpful editorial assistance.

REFERENCES

1. Cystic Fibrosis Foundation. Patient Registry 2007 Annual Data Report. Available at: http://www.cff.org/treatments/LungTransplantation/. Accessed December 21, 2009.
2. Boucher RC. Cystic fibrosis. In: Fauci AS, Braunwald E, Kasper DL, et al, editors, Harrison's principles of internal medicine, vol. 17. New York: McGraw-Hill Medical; 2008. p. 1632–5.
3. Sermet-Gaudelus I, De Villartay P, de Dreuzy P, et al. Pain in children and adults with cystic fibrosis: a comparative study. J Pain Symptom Manage 2009;38(2): 281–90.
4. Duff A, Brownlee K. Psychosocial aspects of newborn screening programs for cystic fibrosis. Child Health Care 2008;37(1):21–37.
5. Stallings VA, Stark LJ, Robinson KA, et al. Evidence-based practice recommendations for nutrition-related management of children and adults with cystic fibrosis and pancreatic insufficiency: results of a systematic review. J Am Diet Assoc 2008;108(5):832–9.
6. Szyndler JE, Towns SJ, van Asperen PP, et al. Psychological and family functioning and quality of life in adolescents with cystic fibrosis. J Cyst Fibros 2005;4(2):135–44.
7. Gleason MM. Relationship assessment in clinical practice. Child Adolesc Psychiatr Clin N Am 2009;18(3):581–91.
8. Tluczek A, Koscik RL, Farrell PM, et al. Psychosocial risk associated with newborn screening for cystic fibrosis: parents' experience while awaiting the sweat-test appointment. Pediatrics 2005;115(6):1692–703.
9. Glasscoe C, Lancaster GA, Smyth RL, et al. Parental depression following the early diagnosis of cystic fibrosis: a matched, prospective study. J Pediatr 2007;150(2):185–91.

10. Berge J, Patterson J. Cystic fibrosis and the family: a review and critique of the literature. Fam Syst Health 2004;22:74–100.
11. Solomon C, Breton J. Early warning signals in relationships between parents and young children with cystic fibrosis. Child Health Care 1999;28(3):221–40.
12. Wong MG, Heriot SA. Parents of children with cystic fibrosis: how they hope, cope and despair. Child Care Health Dev 2008;34(3):344–54.
13. Collins V, Halliday J, Kahler S, et al. Parents' experiences with genetic counseling after the birth of a baby with a genetic disorder: an exploratory study. J Genet Couns 2001;10(1):53–72.
14. Grasso MC, Button BM, Allison DJ, et al. Benefits of music therapy as an adjunct to chest physiotherapy in infants and toddlers with cystic fibrosis. Pediatr Pulmonol 2000;29(5):371–81.
15. Myant KA, Williams JM. Children's concepts of health and illness: understanding of contagious illnesses, non-contagious illnesses and injuries. J Health Psychol 2005;10(6):805–19.
16. Harbord MG, Cross DG, Botica F, et al. Children's understanding of cystic fibrosis. Aust Paediatr J 1987;23(4):241–4.
17. Slifer KJ, Tucker CL, Dahlquist LM. Helping children and caregivers cope with repeated invasive procedures: how are we doing? J Clin Psychol Med Settings 2002;9(2):131–52.
18. Ward C, Massie J, Glazner J, et al. Problem behaviours and parenting in preschool children with cystic fibrosis. Arch Dis Child 2009;94(5):341–7.
19. Powers SW, Patton SR, Byars KC, et al. Caloric intake and eating behavior in infants and toddlers with cystic fibrosis. Pediatrics 2002;109(5):E75.
20. Stark LJ, Jelalian E, Mulvihill MM, et al. Eating in preschool children with cystic fibrosis and healthy peers: behavioral analysis. Pediatrics 1995;95(2):210–5.
21. Mitchell MJ, Powers SW, Byars KC, et al. Family functioning in young children with cystic fibrosis: observations of interactions at mealtime. J Dev Behav Pediatr 2004;25(5):335–46.
22. Spieth LE, Stark LJ, Mitchell MJ, et al. Observational assessment of family functioning at mealtime in preschool children with cystic fibrosis. J Pediatr Psychol 2001;26(4):215–24.
23. Hobbs S, Schweitzer J, Cohen L, et al. Maternal attributions related to compliance with cystic fibrosis treatment. J Clin Psychol Med Settings 2003;10(4):273–7.
24. Powers S, Jones J, Ferguson K, et al. Randomized clinical trial of behavioral and nutrition treatment to improve energy intake and growth in toddlers and preschoolers with cystic fibrosis. Pediatrics 2005;116(6):1442.
25. Quittner AL, Opipari LC, Espelage DL, et al. Role strain in couples with and without a child with a chronic illness: associations with marital satisfaction, intimacy, and daily mood. Health Psychol 1998;17(2):112–24.
26. Sharpe D, Rossiter L. Siblings of children with a chronic illness: a meta-analysis. J Pediatr Psychol 2002;27(8):699–710.
27. Quittner AL, Opipari LC. Differential treatment of siblings: interview and diary analyses comparing two family contexts. Child Dev 1994;65(3):800–14.
28. Smetana JG, Campione-Barr N, Metzger A. Adolescent development in interpersonal and societal contexts. Annu Rev Psychol 2006;57:255–84.
29. McClellan CB, Cohen LL, Moffett K. Time out based discipline strategy for children's non-compliance with cystic fibrosis treatment. Disabil Rehabil 2009;31(4):327–36.
30. Savage E, Callery P. Clinic consultations with children and parents on the dietary management of cystic fibrosis. Soc Sci Med 2007;64(2):363–74.

31. Reis HT, Collins WA, Berscheid E. The relationship context of human behavior and development. Psychol Bull 2000;126(6):844–72.
32. D'Auria J, Christian B, Richardson L. Through the looking glass: children's perceptions of growing up with cystic fibrosis. Can J Nurs Res 1997;29(4):99.
33. Berlin KS, Sass DA, Hobart Davies W, et al. Cystic fibrosis disclosure may minimize risk of negative peer evaluations. J Cyst Fibros 2005;4(3):169–74.
34. Plante WA, Lobato D, Engel R. Review of group interventions for pediatric chronic conditions. J Pediatr Psychol 2001;26(7):435–53.
35. Zuckerman JB, Seder DB. Infection control practice in cystic fibrosis centers. Clin Chest Med 2007;28(2):381–404.
36. Waine DJ, Whitehouse J, Honeybourne D. Cross-infection in cystic fibrosis: the knowledge and behaviour of adult patients. J Cyst Fibros 2007;6(4):262–6.
37. Griffiths AL, Armstrong D, Carzino R, et al. Cystic fibrosis patients and families support cross-infection measures. Eur Respir J 2004;24(3):449–52.
38. Russo K, Donnelly M, Reid AJ. Segregation–the perspectives of young patients and their parents. J Cyst Fibros 2006;5(2):93–9.
39. Cruz I, Marciel KK, Quittner AL, et al. Anxiety and depression in cystic fibrosis. Semin Respir Crit Care Med 2009;30(5):569–78.
40. Thompson RJ Jr, Gustafson KE, Gil KM, et al. Illness specific patterns of psychological adjustment and cognitive adaptational processes in children with cystic fibrosis and sickle cell disease. J Clin Psychol 1998;54(1):121–8.
41. Bennett D, Snooks Q, Llera S, et al. Monitoring and internalizing symptoms among youths with cystic fibrosis. Child Health Care 2008;37(4):278–92.
42. Carpentier M, Mullins L, Wagner J, et al. Examination of the cognitive diathesis-stress conceptualization of the hopelessness theory of depression in children with chronic illness: the moderating influence of illness uncertainty. Child Health Care 2007;36(2):181–96.
43. Mullins LL, Wolfe-Christensen C, Pai AL, et al. The relationship of parental over-protection, perceived child vulnerability, and parenting stress to uncertainty in youth with chronic illness. J Pediatr Psychol 2007;32(8):973–82.
44. Birmaher B. Practice parameter for the assessment and treatment of children and adolescents with depressive disorders. J Am Acad Child Adolesc Psychiatry 2007;46(11):1503–26.
45. Rapee RM, Schniering CA, Hudson JL. Anxiety disorders during childhood and adolescence: origins and treatment. Annu Rev Clin Psychol 2009;5:311–41.
46. Christian BJ, D'Auria JP. Building life skills for children with cystic fibrosis: effectiveness of an intervention. Nurs Res 2006;55(5):300–7.
47. Davis MA, Quittner AL, Stack CM, et al. Controlled evaluation of the STAR-BRIGHT CD-ROM program for children and adolescents with cystic fibrosis. J Pediatr Psychol 2004;29(4):259–67.
48. Ziaian T, Sawyer MG, Reynolds KE, et al. Treatment burden and health-related quality of life of children with diabetes, cystic fibrosis and asthma. J Paediatr Child Health 2006;42(10):596–600.
49. Modi AC, Lim CS, Yu N, et al. A multi-method assessment of treatment adherence for children with cystic fibrosis. J Cyst Fibros 2006;5(3):177–85.
50. Eiser C, Zoritch B, Hiller J, et al. Routine stresses in caring for a child with cystic fibrosis. J Psychosom Res 1995;39(5):641–6.
51. Modi AC, Quittner AL. Barriers to treatment adherence for children with cystic fibrosis and asthma: what gets in the way? J Pediatr Psychol 2006;31(8):846–58.
52. White T, Miller J, Smith GL, et al. Adherence and psychopathology in children and adolescents with cystic fibrosis. Eur Child Adolesc Psychiatry 2009;18(2):96–104.

53. Stark LJ, Quittner AL, Powers SW, et al. Randomized clinical trial of behavioral intervention and nutrition education to improve caloric intake and weight in children with cystic fibrosis. Arch Pediatr Adolesc Med 2009;163(10):915–21.
54. Bernard RS, Cohen LL, Moffett K. A token economy for exercise adherence in pediatric cystic fibrosis: a single-subject analysis. J Pediatr Psychol 2009; 34(4):354–65.
55. Hagopian LP, Thompson RH. Reinforcement of compliance with respiratory treatment in a child with cystic fibrosis. J Appl Behav Anal 1999;32(2):233–6.
56. Stark LJ, Miller ST, Plienes AJ, et al. Behavioral contracting to increase chest physiotherapy: a study of a young cystic fibrosis patient. Behav Modif 1987; 11(1):75–86.
57. Downs JA, Roberts CM, Blackmore AM, et al. Benefits of an education programme on the self-management of aerosol and airway clearance treatments for children with cystic fibrosis. Chron Respir Dis 2006;3(1):19–27.
58. Driscoll KA, Montag-Leifling K, Acton JD, et al. Relations between depressive and anxious symptoms and quality of life in caregivers of children with cystic fibrosis. Pediatr Pulmonol 2009;44(8):784–92.
59. Dewey D, Crawford S. Correlates of maternal and paternal adjustment to chronic childhood disease. J Clin Psychol Med Settings 2007;14(3):219–26.
60. Hernandez-Reif M, Field T, Krasnegor J, et al. Children with cystic fibrosis benefit from massage therapy. J Pediatr Psychol 1999;24(2):175–81.
61. Wahl AK, Rustoen T, Hanestad BR, et al. Self-efficacy, pulmonary function, perceived health and global quality of life of cystic fibrosis patients. Soc Indic Res 2005;72(2):239–61.
62. Hegarty M, Macdonald J, Watter P, et al. Quality of life in young people with cystic fibrosis: effects of hospitalization, age and gender, and differences in parent/child perceptions. Child Care Health Dev 2009;35(4):462–8.
63. Iles N, Lowton K. Young people with cystic fibrosis' concerns for their future: when and how should concerns be addressed, and by whom? J Interprof Care 2008;22(4):436–8.
64. Arias Llorente RP, Bousono Garcia C, Diaz Martin JJ. Treatment compliance in children and adults with cystic fibrosis. J Cyst Fibros 2008;7(5):359–67.
65. Patterson JM, Wall M, Berge J, et al. Associations of psychosocial factors with health outcomes among youth with cystic fibrosis. Pediatr Pulmonol 2009; 44(1):46–53.
66. Meijer S, Sinnema G, Bijstra J, et al. Peer interaction in adolescents with a chronic illness. Pers Individ Dif 2000;29(5):799–813.
67. Graetz BW, Shute RH, Sawyer MG. An Australian study of adolescents with cystic fibrosis: perceived supportive and nonsupportive behaviors from families and friends and psychological adjustment. J Adolesc Health 2000;26(1):64–9.
68. Herzer M, Umfress K, Aljadeff G, et al. Interactions with parents and friends among chronically ill children: examining social networks. J Dev Behav Pediatr 2009;30(6):499–508.
69. Suris JC, Michaud PA, Akre C, et al. Health risk behaviors in adolescents with chronic conditions. Pediatrics 2008;122(5):e1113–8.
70. Britto MT, Garrett JM, Dugliss MA, et al. Risky behavior in teens with cystic fibrosis or sickle cell disease: a multicenter study. Pediatrics 1998;101(2):250–6.
71. Bryon M, Shearer J, Davies H. Eating disorders and disturbance in children and adolescents with cystic fibrosis. Child Health Care 2008;37(1):67–77.
72. Roberts S, Green P. The sexual health of adolescents with cystic fibrosis. J R Soc Med 2005;98(Suppl 45):7–16.

73. Schwartz LA, Drotar D. Health-related hindrance of personal goal pursuit and well-being of young adults with cystic fibrosis, pediatric cancer survivors, and peers without a history of chronic illness. J Pediatr Psychol 2009;34(9): 954–65.

74. Hayes SC, Luoma JB, Bond FW, et al. Acceptance and commitment therapy: model, processes and outcomes. Behav Res Ther 2006;44(1):1–25.

75. Casier A, Goubert L, Huse D, et al. The role of acceptance in psychological functioning in adolescents with cystic fibrosis: a preliminary study. Psychol Health 2008;23(5):629–38.

76. Abbott J, Hart A, Morton A, et al. Health-related quality of life in adults with cystic fibrosis: the role of coping. J Psychosom Res 2008;64(2):149–57.

77. Sauter FM, Heyne D, Michiel Westenberg P. Cognitive behavior therapy for anxious adolescents: developmental influences on treatment design and delivery. Clin Child Fam Psychol Rev 2009;12(4):310–35.

78. Hains AA, Davies WH, Behrens D, et al. Cognitive behavioral interventions for adolescents with cystic fibrosis. J Pediatr Psychol 1997;22(5):669–87.

79. DiGirolamo AM, Quittner AL, Ackerman V, et al. Identification and assessment of ongoing stressors in adolescents with a chronic illness: an application of the behavior-analytic model. J Clin Child Psychol 1997;26(1):53–66.

80. Bucks RS, Hawkins K, Skinner TC, et al. Adherence to treatment in adolescents with cystic fibrosis: the role of illness perceptions and treatment beliefs. J Pediatr Psychol 2009;34(8):893–902.

81. DeLambo KE, Ievers-Landis CE, Drotar D, et al. Association of observed family relationship quality and problem-solving skills with treatment adherence in older children and adolescents with cystic fibrosis. J Pediatr Psychol 2004;29(5): 343–53.

82. Williams B, Mukhopadhyay S, Dowell J, et al. From child to adult: an exploration of shifting family roles and responsibilities in managing physiotherapy for cystic fibrosis. Soc Sci Med 2007;65(10):2135–46.

83. Modi A, Marciel K, Slater S, et al. The influence of parental supervision on medical adherence in adolescents with cystic fibrosis: developmental shifts from pre to late adolescence. Child Health Care 2008;37(1):78–92.

84. Erickson SJ, Gerstle M, Feldstein SW. Brief interventions and motivational interviewing with children, adolescents, and their parents in pediatric health care settings: a review. Arch Pediatr Adolesc Med 2005;159(12):1173–80.

85. Marciel KK, Saiman L, Quittell LM, et al. Cell phone intervention to improve adherence: cystic fibrosis care team, patient, and parent perspectives. Pediatr Pulmonol 2010;45(2):157–64.

86. McLaughlin SE, Diener-West M, Indurkhya A, et al. Improving transition from pediatric to adult cystic fibrosis care: lessons from a national survey of current practices. Pediatrics 2008;121(5):e1160–6.

87. Collins S, Reynolds F. How do adults with cystic fibrosis cope following a diagnosis of diabetes? J Adv Nurs 2008;64(5):478–87.

88. Palermo TM, Harrison D, Koh JL. Effect of disease-related pain on the health-related quality of life of children and adolescents with cystic fibrosis. Clin J Pain 2006;22(6):532–7.

89. Palermo TM, Eccleston C, Lewandowski AS, et al. Randomized controlled trials of psychological therapies for management of chronic pain in children and adolescents: an updated meta-analytic review. Pain 2010;148:387–97.

90. Kelly AF, Hewson PH. Factors associated with recurrent hospitalization in chronically ill children and adolescents. J Paediatr Child Health 2000;36(1):13–8.

91. Taylor L, Wallander J, Anderson D, et al. Improving health care utilization, improving chronic disease utilization, health status, and adjustment in adolescents and young adults with cystic fibrosis: a preliminary report. J Clin Psychol Med Settings 2003;10(1):9–16.
92. Yi MS, Tsevat J, Wilmott RW, et al. The impact of treatment of pulmonary exacerbations on the health-related quality of life of patients with cystic fibrosis: does hospitalization make a difference? J Pediatr 2004;144(6):711–8.
93. Spirito A, Russo DC, Masek BJ. Behavioral interventions and stress management training for hospitalized adolescents and young adults with cystic fibrosis. Gen Hosp Psychiatry 1984;6(3):211–8.
94. Ernst MM, Wooldridge JL, Conway E, et al. Using quality improvement science to implement a multidisciplinary behavioral intervention targeting pediatric inpatient airway clearance. J Pediatr Psychol 2010;35(1):14–24.
95. Cystic Fibrosis Foundation. Cystic fibrosis. Available at: http://www.cff.org/treatments/LungTransplantation/. Accessed December 21, 2009.
96. Hadjiliadis D. Special considerations for patients with cystic fibrosis undergoing lung transplantation. Chest 2007;131(4):1224–31.
97. Chapman E, Landy A, Lyon A, et al. End of life care for adult cystic fibrosis patients: facilitating a good enough death. J Cyst Fibros 2005;4(4):249–57.
98. Philip JA, Gold M, Sutherland S, et al. End-of-life care in adults with cystic fibrosis. J Palliat Med 2008;11(2):198–203.
99. Kang T, Hoehn KS, Licht DJ, et al. Pediatric palliative, end-of-life, and bereavement care. Pediatr Clin North Am 2005;52(4):1029–46, viii.
100. Barakat LP, Pulgaron ER, Daniel LC. Positive psychology in pediatric psychology. In: Roberts MC, Steele RG, editors. Handbook of pediatric psychology. 4th edition. New York: The Guilford Press; 2009.

Psychiatric Issues in Pediatric Organ Transplantation

Margaret L. Stuber, MD

KEYWORDS

• Child • Adolescent • Transplant • Psychiatric

The field of solid organ transplantation has grown enormously since 1983, when the widespread availability of effective immunosuppression made what had been surgically possible a viable clinical reality. In the United States, 23,846 solid organ transplants were performed between January and October 2009.[1] As of January 18, 2010, 105,239 people were listed as awaiting transplants in the United States.[1] This article addresses the types of transplants now commonly performed for children, assessment and support of children and families undergoing transplantation, the long-term impact of organ transplantation on children, and new developing areas in organ transplantation.

Pediatric solid organ transplants are still relatively rare. Fewer than 8% of the recipients of solid organ transplants in the United States annually are younger than 18 years according to the 2008 report from the OPTN/SRTR.[1] The annual number of pediatric solid organ transplants has been approximately 2000 children since 1998. Although the wait for an organ that is a match for size and blood type may be longer for young children, the 5-year survival is similar in children and young adults (**Tables 1** and **2**).[1]

Immunosuppression is the critical element in survival of most solid organ transplant recipients.[2,3] Organs vary as to their levels of immune activity, and subsequently some require more exact matching with the donor and more or different types of immunosuppression. Kidney transplants proved to be feasible in identical twins (for whom immunosuppression was not needed) as early as the 1950s.[4] In the 1960s, non-twin kidney transplants were successful using a combination of azathioprine and prednisone.[5] However, even with immunosuppression, liver transplants almost always

A version of this article was previously published in the *Child and Adolescent Psychiatric Clinics of North America, 19:2.*

This work was supported in part by a grant from the Astellas Company (PI: Margaret L. Stuber, MD), and a grant from the Maternal and Child Health Bureau (Title V, Social Security Act), Health Resources and Services Administration, Department of Health and Human Services (R40 MC00120) (PI: Margaret L. Stuber, MD).

Department of Psychiatry and Biobehavioral Sciences, Semel Institute, David Geffen School of Medicine at UCLA, 760 Westwood Plaza, Room 48-240, Los Angeles, CA 90024-1759, USA
E-mail address: mstuber@mednet.ucla.edu

Pediatr Clin N Am 58 (2011) 887–901
doi:10.1016/j.pcl.2011.06.011
0031-3955/11/$ – see front matter
© 2011 Elsevier Inc. All rights reserved.

Table 1
One-year survival rates according to age at transplantation

Organ	Age (y)			
	<1	1–5	6–10	11–17
Heart	82.8%	85.9%	86.8%	89.7%
Liver	81.1%	78.1%	84.4%	87.4%
Kidney	a	92.7%	94.7%	94.1%
Intestine	63.8%	75.6%	66.7%	80.0%
Lung	a	a	88.0%	78.0%

[a] Graft survival not computed because the number of subjects was <10. One-year survival rate is based on 2002–2004 transplants, 3-year survival rates were based on 1999–2002 transplants, 5-year survival rates were based on 1997–2000 transplants.

Data from a graph from the Organ Procurement and Transplantation Network (OPTN). All Kaplan-Meier Graft survival rates for transplants performed between 1997 and 2004. Based on OPTN data as of January 8, 2010.

resulted in rejection until the introduction of cyclosporine in 1983.[6] Since then, tacrolimus and sirolimus have added options for organ transplantation immunosuppression, and have led to decreased use of prednisone, azathioprine, and cyclosporine.[7] However, posttransplant lymphoproliferative disorder (PTLD), nephrotoxicity, and de novo autoimmune hepatitis remain possible complications of these medications, in addition to the usual risks for decreased immune function.[8] The growth problems associated with chronic steroids have led to attempts to reduce or remove it as a component in immunosuppression regimens for pediatric recipients.[9]

KIDNEY

Kidney transplants were the earliest of the solid organ transplants to be successful, and they continue to have the best long-term survival.[1] Today the 5-year survival rate for pediatric kidney transplants is more than 90%. Kidney transplantation has several advantages over other solid organ transplantations.

First, kidney transplantation has a mechanical alternative, dialysis, which can keep a person alive while awaiting a matched organ. Hemodialysis requires visits to an

Table 2
Five-year survival rates according to age at transplantation

Organ	Age (y)			
	<1	1–5	6–10	11–17
Heart	68.0%	71.1%	75.1%	67.8%
Liver	66.9%	75.31%	67.0%	64.2%
Kidney	100%	84.2%	82.2%	a
Intestine	30.8%	34.7%	69.2%	a
Lung	a	a	40.7%	34.6%

[a] Graft survival not computed because the number of subjects was <10. One-year survival rate is based on 2002–2004 transplants, 3-year survival rates were based on 1999–2002 transplants, 5-year survival rates were based on 1997–2000 transplants.

Data from a graph from the Organ Procurement and Transplantation Network (OPTN). All Kaplan-Meier Graft survival rates for transplants performed between 1997 and 2004. Based on OPTN data as of January 8, 2010.

outpatient center three times a week, for hours at a time, and peritoneal dialysis requires connection to an elaborate, sterile set of equipment in the home for 10 hours a night. Patients undergoing dialysis must still watch their salt intake, and the intermittent nature of the dialysis cannot replicate the constant detoxification of a working kidney. Therefore, although both types of dialysis have risks, and impact a patient's work and social life, dialysis is the reason that, with kidney transplantation, graft failure is not usually equivalent to recipient death.[10]

Second, kidneys are paired organs, and humans can generally function well with just one, which means that living-related kidney donation has been possible. Using relatives as donors allows better immunologic matching, and therefore decreased risk for rejection. Living-related kidney donation also means the donated organ is taken from a healthy person, and is available when the recipient needs it, not when a matched cadaver is found. Although kidney donation is a major surgical procedure, the risk to the donor is relatively small.

Additionally, because kidneys are paired organs, two recipients can receive organs from one cadaver donor, which has helped to decrease the waiting list relative to other types of solid organ transplants. Anything that decreases the wait time improves the outcome of surgery because it allows the recipient to be healthier at transplantation.[11]

Third, kidneys are less immune active than some other organs. Although matching of organs by blood type (A, B, AB, or O) and Rh factor (negative or positive) is important, the more-specific HLA typing used for liver and heart transplants seems to be less important in graft rejection for kidney transplants. The difference in 10-year deceased donor kidney survival between the best and worst HLA-matched combinations was 10%, with half-lives ranging from 11.6 to 8.6 years.[12] Some renal transplant recipients have been able to stop taking immunosuppressant medication altogether.[13]

Fourth, most pediatric kidney transplantations are performed in children older than 6 years,[1] partly because of the illnesses that lead to kidney failure in this population, and partly because of the option of dialysis. This later age at transplantation allows larger organs to be used than would be possible in younger and smaller children, expanding the number of potential donors.

A result of these differences from other organ transplantations is that kidney transplantation has been practiced since the 1950s, and is therefore well established at many centers. More programs are authorized to provide kidney transplantations because more have performed and continue to perform the required number of procedures to be considered "expert." The number of kidney transplantations in adults related to diabetic nephrology led to combined pancreas and kidney transplantations, primarily in adults. These are now successful, with a 1-year graft survival rate of 85% and 3-year patient survival rate of 90%.[14] Joint kidney and liver transplantations are also relatively common.[15]

LIVER

Liver transplantation does not have many of the advantages of kidney transplantation. No mechanical substitute is available for the liver, and the liver is not a paired organ. The liver is active immunologically and must be matched carefully to prevent rejection. Most liver transplantations in children are performed on those younger than 5 years, and most of these are for congenital illness, such as alpha 1-antitrypsin deficiency or biliary atresia.[16] Therefore, the children are small and cannot accommodate an adult liver.

However, the liver is an organ with individual lobes, and people can survive with less than a complete functional liver. Thus, for the reasons described earlier, once the surgical techniques were found to be feasible, partial livers were used for children. Removing just one lobe of the liver allowed donors to continue a healthy life, allowed better-matched relatives to be donors, produced a smaller organ to fit young children, and gave an option to children who would not survive the wait for a deceased donor.[17]

However, one problem was the coercion inherent in being a potential living-related donor. Although this had also been an issue for kidney transplantation, the availability of dialysis reduced some of the time urgency and increased the likelihood of finding another donor. For parents of very small children experiencing liver failure, very few options were available. Programs responded to this by requiring careful assessments of potential donors to see that they qualified as giving true informed consent. That is, they needed to understand the problem, the various alternative treatments (including doing nothing), and the potential consequences of each option, and had to be consenting without undue influence. In reality, parents rarely felt comfortable refusing to be a donor.

Living-related partial liver donation is now uncommon except in areas with little access to deceased donor organs.[18] Although mortality was very low for donors, it was not zero, and the morbidity could be significant, if only involving the loss of a month of employment. New techniques using one cadaver liver for multiple recipients made the use of parental donors less necessary.[19]

Although liver transplantation is performed at major centers worldwide, it is specialized enough that not all medical centers have programs. To maintain a contract with the United Network for Organ Sharing, which oversees distribution of organs, a center must perform a minimum number of transplants and meet criteria on survival, complications, and services provided. Liver transplantation is therefore usually performed at a regional center, with long-term follow-up coordinated though the regional center at the local hospital or clinics.[20]

HEART

Hearts are neither paired nor lobed, and are very immunologically active. But an unexpected aspect of heart transplantation has led to some of the most serious concerns about pediatric heart transplants. Although initial survival was excellent, and improving technique led to dramatic improvements in 1-year survival rates after cardiac transplantation, long-term graft survival has been limited by what is called *accelerated transplant coronary artery disease* or *cardiac graft vasculopathy*. This condition is an immunologically mediated chronic rejection characterized by progressive fibroproliferative disease, resulting in intimal thickening and occlusion of the grafted coronary vessels.[21] Lipid accumulation in allograft arteries is prominent, with lipoprotein entrapment in the subendothelial tissue, through interactions with proteoglycans.[22] The hope that pediatric organ transplant recipients could undergo just one transplantation and live with that heart for their normal life expectancy is lessened by evidence that significant atherosclerotic disease can be seen in as few as 5 years. This area is one of intense research.[23]

LUNG AND HEART/LUNG

Cystic fibrosis is one of the most common indications for lung transplantation worldwide, and certainly the most common indication for all pediatric lung transplantations and for bilateral lung transplantation irrespective of age.[24] Outcomes are outstanding when compared with other indications for lung transplantation, and an increasing number of centers now report mean survival of greater than 10 years posttransplant.[1]

Pediatric lung or heart/lung transplantation is also performed to treat congenital heart disease, primary pulmonary hypertension, or pulmonary fibrosis, and has not generally been performed in very young children. Bronchiolitis obliterans remains the major late complication.[25] Survival has not been as good as with liver and heart transplants, but has been improving, at least for some underlying illnesses.[26] Reduced-size transplantation has proven successful, allowing smaller children to undergo transplantation despite the scarcity of small donors.[27] Combined heart and lung transplantation has comparable success with lung transplantation.[28]

SMALL BOWEL OR MULTIVISCERAL

Transplantation of the small bowel is performed when the intestine cannot provide the body with sufficient nutrition or hydration. The most common reasons for intestinal failure in children are necrotizing enterocolitis, gastroschisis, intestinal atresia, volvulus, psycho-obstruction, and aganglionosis. Although short-gut syndrome, secondary to surgical correction of the conditions listed earlier, is the most common cause of intestinal failure, short intestinal length is neither necessary nor sufficient to require transplantation.[29]

Transplantation of the small bowel in children had a high initial rate of complications, resulting in a relatively low 5-year survival rate.[30] Although the 1-year survival rate in adults who have undergone small bowel transplantation is now comparable to that of those who have undergone liver and heart transplantations, survival in children is still much less nationally.[1] However, specific centers report 1- and 5-year survival rates of 90% and 77%, respectively.[30] Transplantation of the small bowel has been performed when parenteral nutrition failed.[29] Multivisceral grafts can include donor spleen, large intestine, and small bowel. These patients frequently require intensive care preoperatively and have unique intensive care needs postoperatively.[31] With increasing survival rates, intestinal and multivisceral transplantation have reached the mainstream of medical care. Indications now include neoplastic disease, extensive splanchnic thrombosis, and abdominal catastrophes.[32] Living-donor intestinal transplantation is also being explored as an alternative to minimize death of potential recipients while on the waitlist.[33]

TRANSPLANT EVALUATIONS

Organs for transplantation are a scarce resource, and therefore allocation is carefully monitored and regulated. Teams of physicians from various specialties assess candidates to ascertain if they are sick enough to need a transplant, well enough to survive the transplant, and able to follow the medical instructions necessary to keep the graft alive. Once patients are listed as good candidates, priority is given to the sickest person in the region on the list who matches the donor organ. The list must be regularly updated to remove anyone who is too sick, lest an organ be "wasted." For adult patients, the role of the psychiatrist is primarily to evaluate the patient for suitability to be on the list. The psychiatrist generally determines if patients demonstrates signs that they will be nonadherent. In addition to frank psychopathology, determining a history of smoking, illicit drugs, or alcohol abuse requires particular attention.[34]

For most pediatric candidates, because they are young, nonadherence assessment focuses primarily on the parents. This assessment is often performed by social workers rather than psychiatrists or psychologists. Referral for psychiatric assessment in pediatric organ transplantation primarily occurs with adolescents. A Pediatric

Transplant Rating Instrument was developed for use in these settings, which assesses the following domains[35]:

1. Knowledge and motivation regarding the transplant
2. History of adherence with medications, appointments, and risks for nonadherence
3. Patient and parental psychiatric and substance abuse history
4. Parental supervision, family conflict, and communication style
5. Financial, logistical, and psychosocial support
6. Relationship with the medical team.

Child psychiatrists or psychologists may also be asked to assess a potential candidate for solid organ transplantation in several other situations.

Suicide Attempt

The classic version of this situation would be a teenager who has taken a handful of acetaminophen and is in acute liver failure. In this case, the acute injury may resolve without need for transplantation, but the assessment must be performed while the patient is alert, before hepatic encephalopathy makes it impossible to assess the situation adequately. The primary goal of this assessment is to determine whether this suicide attempt was serious or a gesture that is unlikely to be repeated. A careful history and mental status examination, with collaboration from family members, can usually determine if the teen has a chronic psychiatric problem. In most cases involving suicide attempts, the psychiatric assessment is advisory, guiding the post-transplant care rather than advising against placing the patient on the list.

Need for a "Family Transplant"

Some unfortunate children have chaotic family situations in addition to a life-threatening illness. Examples of these cases could include young teens who have hepatitis from rape by a stepfather or older teens who has viral endocarditis from their heroin-dealing mother. Although the odds are high that these children will be nonadherent later, many teams have difficulty condemning them to death because of the sins of their parents. The immediate need is to find them a safe place and support system for the pretransplantation waiting period, but this can be difficult because these children generally require more medical care than can be provided in regular foster care settings. Even more difficult is helping these children with long-term survival; evidence suggests that problematic early childhoods are predictive of poor adherence.[36] The family is an important component of transplantation success.[37]

PRETRANSPLANT PSYCHIATRIC CONSIDERATIONS

Consultation–liaison child psychiatrists are familiar with most of the psychiatric and psychological issues in the pretransplant phase of care to because they are similar to those seen in families dealing with other life-threatening childhood illnesses.[38]

Guilt

Guilt can be a significant issue for parents of infants struggling with a genetic illness, the cause of which they were usually previously unaware. It is also an issue for people whose children have infectious diseases, particularly if the cause is associated with travel. However, the parental wish to protect their children from all that is harmful means that some feelings of guilt will almost always be present.

Anger and Blame

When people want to find a reason for something that is apparently random, they may feel guilt or blame, or a mixture of both. Anger and blame can be generalized or very specific, with parents most commonly blaming each other or one or more of the doctors they have seen.

Depression and Helplessness

Parents are typically advocates for their ill or hospitalized children. However, sometimes the parents withdraw. This behavior does not necessarily mean that they do not care about their children, although often staff will interpret it as abandonment.

The best intervention for all psychiatric and psychological issues is obviously a quick and successful transplantation. However, given the lengthy time that many children are on the list awaiting a transplant, some work is often necessary to help parents deal with their guilt, anger, and helplessness, and for the staff to manage what they may perceive as difficult parents. Particularly problematic are the parents who deal with their own emotional distress by trying to take control. These parents can range from those who will only allow certain people in the child's hospital room, to those who actually readjust settings on intravenous drips or ventilators. Setting up limits while acknowledging the parents' need for some control in an overwhelming situation requires work with the entire extended treatment team but can be very effective.[39]

For less-problematic but distressed parents, helping them find and use a social support network can be very helpful. Some transplant programs will have groups for parents. Internet-based programs can also be helpful, such as the Experience Journal (experincejournal.org).[40] This very user-friendly Web site has stories written by parents and children dealing with pediatric liver transplantation and congenital heart disease, and features interviews with doctors and other medical information.

TRANSPLANT HOSPITALIZATION

The actual transplantation is usually a surprise. After days to months of waiting, a sudden disruption of life occurs when an organ is available. It is an exciting event, but frightening. This effect is amplified if the organ is coming from a living-related donor. In these cases, two family members are at risk during the surgery, and two who need support afterward. For very young children, who do not understand the concept of short-term pain for long-term gain, the transplant hospitalization, pain, procedures, and intensive care unit, can be traumatic. Other children may not be able to appreciate that this hospitalization will be different from others.

Transplant hospitalizations can be brief, despite the major surgery and usually lengthy illness that preceded the event. However, the surgery is often associated with complications. What a surgeon considers minimal, such as a return to the operating room to deal with a small bleed, may feel overwhelming to the family or child. Although everyone is warned otherwise, they usually have some hope that the transplant will result in immediate improvement in the child's condition. Children do experience quick response, and many are out of intensive care in days after an organ transplantation. However, the initial course is often rocky, particularly if the child has been seriously ill, and parents are well advised to use their extended families and other social support networks.[41]

POSTTRANSPLANT

The first year posttransplantation is often difficult. Children and parents learn that they have traded a life-threatening illness for a chronic condition, which requires daily medications, regular doctor visits, and caution regarding exposure to infectious disease. In addition, the child will likely experience at least one episode of rejection while the medical team is adjusting their immunosuppressant regime. Not all recipients will be hospitalized during the year after transplantation, but many will. A qualitative study of pediatric heart transplant recipients found that they considered the limitations on their activities with friends and family and at school major obstacles to quality of life.[42]

Family must also make adjustments. Children who have been seen as fragile must gradually be allowed to encounter normal developmental challenges. Parents (and school personnel) may be reluctant to allow children to return to school, engage in physical activities, and play with friends. Parents have the challenge of finding a new equilibrium in being safe but not overprotective as the child reenters the growth curve.[43] Parents often underestimate the impact of the transplant on the child, focusing on how much healthier the child is and not noticing how depressed the child may have become.[44]

One question for families is who will oversee the medication. With very young children, obviously parents must assume responsibility for ordering, obtaining, and administering the medication. For a parent to say that a 2 year old "doesn't want to take the medication" is understandable, but is not an acceptable reason for the child to not receive the necessary immunosuppressant medications. However, as children get older they should assume more responsibility for their lives, including self-care. Surveys have shown that at approximately 9 years of age, children begin assuming some ownership of their medication regimens.[45] That is, at this age children start taking the medication on their own, rather than taking it when given by parents. Parents are still responsible for monitoring when more medications are needed, calling in prescriptions, and picking up the medications. They may also check with the child to ensure the medication has been taken. As children get older, they can and should assume more of the tasks associated with medication self-care, with parental monitoring.

This transition can be daunting to parents and children. However, the alternatives are problematic. Children who assume no responsibility until adolescence are likely to see the medications as something outwardly imposed by adults, and are more likely to resist them. But even when teens are passively compliant, this does not prepare them well for the eventual transition to care by an internist rather than a pediatrician. Pediatricians and their offices are more likely to follow-up on patients who do not schedule, cancel, or do not show up for appointments than are doctors and offices that care for adult patients. Studies have shown that this transition can be difficult for children and adolescents who have chronic conditions.[46] One approach to this has been to have pediatric practices continue to follow up with teens until their mid-20s, when most are functioning independently.[47] Other programs have created transition clinics for teens and young adults, which specifically focus on helping young people take control of their own health care.[48]

ADHERENCE

One of the most complicated problems in all types of pediatric transplants is that of nonadherence to medical instruction. Although some types of transplant, such as heart, have specific expectations regarding diet and exercise, consistent use of immunosuppression is the primary behavioral challenge to survival after organ transplantation.

Nonadherence with medications is very common, with studies repeatedly showing that only approximately half of the people prescribed medication take at least 80% of the medications as prescribed.[49] The complexity of the regimen is associated with the likelihood of adherence; that is, medications that must be taken several times a day, or in specific relationship to food or milk, are less likely to be taken regularly.[34] Medications that have adverse effects are less likely to be taken, but so are medications that are largely preventative and have no immediate adverse impact when not taken. An example is antihypertensive medications, which can cause sexual side effects and often create no immediate perceivable adverse effects when stopped.

Physicians are often surprised that transplant recipients would ever stop immunosuppressant medications; after all, the transplant saved them from death, why would they do anything to put themselves at risk. The reasons are multiple.

Complex regimens are the most likely to lead to poor adherence, and immunosuppressant regimens almost always involve more than one medication, taken more than once a day. Medications that can be paired with a morning or evening regimen are simpler than those that need to be taken at school. Students are almost never allowed to carry medication with them at school and must go to the nurse's office to get it, increasing the probability that they will forget or try to avoid the embarrassment of a trip to the nurse's office.

> Medication that causes adverse effects is less likely to be taken. The weight gain and impact on the face and abdomen associated with steroids makes them aversive to children and adolescents. Cyclosporine can lead to increased gum growth, and darker, thicker arm hair, which are cosmetic concerns. Recipients learn that these effects diminish if they reduce or stop their medication.
>
> Recipients who decrease or stop their medications also note the absence of immediate adverse consequences. In fact, some recipients can successfully stop immunosuppressive medications and not experience rejection of the grafted organ. Unfortunately, who those fortunate individuals are, or exactly why it occurs, is not yet known and so this cannot be predicted. Other recipients will experience a relatively quick response of acute rejection, which can be recognized, but may still result in loss of the graft. However, most recipients will simply intermittently take the immunosuppression medication, resulting in a smoldering chronic rejection, which can also ultimately result in graft failure.
>
> Adolescents are particularly prone to nonadherence with medical advice. This phenomenon is partly because of their developmentally appropriate questioning of authority and desire to make their own decisions. It is also caused by what is now known to be immaturity of the prefrontal cortex, resulting in poor judgment in emotionally charged situations. The issues of transitions of care contribute to adolescent nonadherence.

Usual interventions, such as education about the consequences of nonadherence, are ineffective at changing behavior in some adolescents. More intensive interventions, such as reminder cell phone calls or texts might be successful, but would be unnecessary and expensive to do with all recipients. However, targeting those who might require interventions has been difficult. Several studies have shown that clinicians are not effective in predicting or identifying pediatric recipients who are or will be nonadherent.

Studies using self-report, pilling-counting, and computerized pill bottle tops have not been able to predict who will experience biopsy-proven rejection.[50] However, studies of tacrolimus levels in pediatric liver transplant recipients have identified one promising possibility. Three programs have found that the standard deviation between at least three routine blood levels can be used to differentiate between those who will experience biopsy-proven rejection and those who will not.[51] These results have been replicated, showing that intermittent use of immunosuppression is seen in these widely varying levels.[52] Interventions to help decrease nonadherence have been piloted, including one using text messaging to remind teens to take their medication[53] and targeted interventions with those who have high fluctuations in tacrolimus levels[54] or symptoms of posttraumatic stress.[55]

POSTTRAUMATIC STRESS

Life-threatening illness and the painful and invasive interventions that are often required have recently been shown to be traumatic, causing symptoms of posttraumatic stress disorder (PTSD) in adults,[56] children,[57] and parents.[58,59] A study of the primary caregivers of 170 pediatric liver, heart, and kidney transplant recipients found that anxiety and clinical norms for depression did not differ significantly from those of a healthy comparison group. However, 27.1% of the parents met criteria for a diagnosis of PTSD 1 to 3 years after successful transplantation.[58] Another study of 52 parents of pediatric heart transplant recipients showed somewhat similar results, with 10 of the 52 reporting symptoms consistent with a diagnosis of PTSD.[59] In a study of 104 adolescent recipients of liver, heart, or kidney transplants, 16% met all symptoms criteria for PTSD at least 1 year posttransplant.[57]

LONG-TERM QUALITY OF LIFE

Quality of life is difficult to assess in young children, and measures used for children differ significantly from those used for adolescents. However, long-term quality of life in adults who underwent solid organ transplantation as children or adolescents is generally favorable. Most data are from kidney, liver, and heart transplantation. Children have been able to resume growing and return to school, and report that they are relatively physically, socially, and psychologically healthy.[60] Individuals who underwent pediatric organ transplantation report a better quality of life than those who have chronic illness, including patients on dialysis for renal failure, but not as good a quality of life as healthy controls. However, long-term effects of immunosuppressive medication are a significant problem and the major predictor of perceived quality of life. These concerns range from minor issues, such as vaccinations[61]; to moderate issues, such as infections[62,63]; to life-threatening issues, such as renal failure[64] or cancer.[65]

Neuropsychological studies of pediatric organ transplant recipients suggest that not all of the neuropsychological sequelae of renal, cardiac, or liver failure are reversible. A recent review reported normal intelligence but significantly impaired gross and fine motor skills in school-aged kidney transplant recipients, and that 27% of liver transplant recipients who had chronic liver disease in early infancy had intelligence scores more than 2 standard deviations below test norms.[66] In one study, pediatric heart transplant recipients had a mean overall IQ of 86.7, 46% had low scores on expressive language, 63% had visual-motor deficits, and 48% had fine motor deficits.[67] These deficits can obviously present problems in school, both before and after transplantation.[68]

LATER COMPLICATIONS OF TRANSPLANTATION

Malignancy, sepsis, and PTLD account for more than 65% of deaths occurring more than 1 year after pediatric liver transplantation.[69] Kidney transplant recipients have been found to have more than three times the risk of most types of cancer as the general population. Most of these cancers were of known or suspected viral origin.[70] PTLD occurs in 1% to 20% of organ recipients after solid organ transplantation.[71] It can manifest as anything from a benign infectious mononucleosis-like illness to non-Hodgkin's lymphomas with nodal and extranodal site involvement, with a death rate as high as 33%.[72] PTLD risk factors include recipient pretransplant Epstein-Barr virus

(EBV)–negative serostatus, type of transplant, intensity of immunosuppression, and age.[73] Minimizing immunosuppression burden and using antiviral agents active against EBV are useful strategies to prevent PTLD. PTLD treatment may require reduction of immunosuppression, radiation, surgical excision, monoclonal antibodies, interferon-alfa, and chemotherapy.[74]

PREGNANCY POSTTRANSPLANT

The first person to become pregnant after a solid organ transplant was a 21-year-old woman in 1956 who had received a kidney from her identical twin sister.[4] Most pregnancies followed in individuals posttransplant have been in those who underwent kidney transplantation, but data are now available on pregnancies after liver transplantation.[75] Carrying a pregnancy does not seem to be associated with significant structural problems, despite the presence of an abdominal kidney (the original kidneys are usually not removed during a kidney transplant, and the allograft is placed in the abdomen rather than the pelvis). Although some immunosuppression is a normal part of pregnancy, transplant recipients must continue to take immunosuppressive medications during pregnancy. Long-term follow-up suggests that the rate of learning disabilities, attention deficit disorder, and malformations is no higher in children born to mothers treated with cyclosporine, azathioprine, or prednisone than in the general population.[4] Currently fairly limited long-term information is available on pregnancy outcomes of recipients taking tacrolimus or sirolimus.[75]

FUTURE DIRECTIONS

As immunosuppression improves, increasingly complex transplants are being attempted. Successful transplantation of the face[76] and hand have now been reported.[77] Although the surgical techniques are already well developed, very few programs are attempting theses procedures in the United States, and either of these are unlikely to be attempted soon for children or adolescents. The immunosuppressant regimen is still not well established, which is critical because, unlike most solid organ transplants, face and hand transplants are not performed to treat a life-threatening condition. Therefore ethically justifying exposure of the recipient to potentially toxic drugs and the risks associated with being immunocompromised is more difficult.[78]

From a psychiatric standpoint, a disfigured face or missing hand presents major problems in terms of identity, self-image, and quality of life. However, these visible types of transplantation also present challenges. In addition, these complex transplants require a great deal of rehabilitation for the patient to use the new part successfully. Although the recipient of a new hand will not be as ill as someone receiving a new liver, the level of adherence and commitment to frequent and intense rehabilitation regimens is much greater for the hand, at least initially.[78] The loss of the graft is also not equivalent to the loss of life. These types of issues will be confronting child psychiatrists in the not so distant future.

SUMMARY

Solid organ transplantation has become highly successful for children who have kidney, liver, or heart failure, and is becoming increasingly successful for end-stage pulmonary and intestinal diseases. Psychiatric challenges include consultation to transplant teams regarding candidate selection, support for families during the wait for transplant, enhancing adherence to medication posttransplant, and addressing long-term problems such as posttraumatic stress responses. New ethical challenges are on the horizon, as transplantation moves to organs critical for psychological well-being but not for survival, such as faces and hands. A clear understanding of the developmental and family aspects of transplantation are necessary as child and adolescent psychiatrists attempt to keep up with the growing number of immunosuppressive drugs and approaches to the pediatric transplant recipient.

REFERENCES

1. Available at: http://www.unos.org/Data/. Accessed January 18, 2010.
2. Woodroffe R, Yao GL, Meads C, et al. Clinical and cost-effectiveness of newer immunosuppressive regimens in renal transplantation: a systematic review and modelling study. Health Technol Assess 2005;9(21):1–179, iii–iv.
3. Sarwal M, Pascual J. Immunosuppression minimization in pediatric transplantation. Am J Transplant 2007;7(10):2227–35.
4. Armenti VT, Constantinescu S, Moritz MJ, et al. Pregnancy after transplantation. Transplant Rev (Orlando) 2008;22(4):223–40.
5. Asberg A, Midtvedt K, Line PD, et al. Calcineurin inhibitor avoidance with daclizumab, mycophenolate mofetil, and prednisolone in DR-matched de novo kidney transplant recipients. Transplantation 2006;82(1):62–8.
6. Dell-Olio D, Kelly DA. Calcineurin inhibitor minimization in pediatric liver allograft recipients. Pediatr Transplant 2009;13(6):670–81.
7. Flechner SM, Kobashigawa J, Klintmalm G. Calcineurin inhibitor-sparing regimens in solid organ transplantation: focus on improving renal function and nephrotoxicity. Clin Transplant 2008;22(1):1–15.
8. Gibelli NE, Tannuri U, Pinho-Apezzato ML, et al. Sirolimus in pediatric liver transplantation: a single-center experience. Transplant Proc 2009;41(3):901–3.
9. Sarwal MM. Out with the old, in with the new: immunosuppression minimization in children. Curr Opin Organ Transplant 2008;13(5):513–21.
10. Cecka JM. The OPTN/UNOS renal transplant registry. Clin Transpl 2005;1:1–16.
11. Cecka JM. Kidney transplantation in the United States. Clin Transpl 2008;1:1–18.
12. Knoll G. Trends in kidney transplantation over the past decade. Drugs 2008;68(Suppl 1):3–10.
13. Traum AZ, Ko DS, Kawai T. The potential for tolerance in pediatric renal transplantation. Curr Opin Organ Transplant 2008;13(5):489–94.
14. Gruessner AC, Sutherland DE, Gruessner RW. Pancreas transplantation in the United States: a review. Curr Opin Organ Transplant 2010;15(1):93–101.
15. Sutherland SM, Alexander SR, Sarwal MM, et al. Combined liver-kidney transplantation in children: indications and outcome. Pediatr Transplant 2008;12(8):835–46.
16. Bucuvalas JC, Alonso E. Long-term outcomes after liver transplantation in children. Curr Opin Organ Transplant 2008;13(3):247–51.
17. Spada M, Riva S, Maggiore G, et al. Pediatric liver transplantation. World J Gastroenterol 2009;15(6):648–74.
18. Chan KL, Fan ST, Lo CM, et al. Pediatric liver transplantation in Hong Kong-a domain with scarce deceased donors. J Pediatr Surg 2009;44(12):2316–21.
19. Hong JC, Yersiz H, Farmer DG, et al. Longterm outcomes for whole and segmental liver grafts in adult and pediatric liver transplant recipients: a 10-year comparative analysis of 2,988 cases. J Am Coll Surg 2009;208(5):682–9 [discussion: 689–91].
20. Brown RS, Belton AM, Martin JM, et al. Evolution of quality at the Organ Center of the Organ Procurement and Transplantation Network/United Network for Organ Sharing. Prog Transplant 2009;19(3):221–6.

21. Hornick P, Rose M. Chronic rejection in the heart. Methods Mol Biol 2006;333: 131–44.
22. Rahmani M, Cruz RP, Granville DJ, et al. Allograft vasculopathy versus atherosclerosis. Circ Res 2006;99(8):801–15.
23. Raichlin E, Bae JH, Kushwaha SS, et al. Inflammatory burden of cardiac allograft coronary atherosclerotic plaque is associated with early recurrent cellular rejection and predicts a higher risk of vasculopathy progression. J Am Coll Cardiol 2009;53(15):1279–86.
24. Morton J, Glanville AR. Lung transplantation in patients with cystic fibrosis. Semin Respir Crit Care Med 2009;30(5):559–68.
25. Sweet SC. Pediatric lung transplantation. Proc Am Thorac Soc 2009;6(1):122–7.
26. Grady RM, Gandhi S, Sweet SC, et al. Dismal lung transplant outcomes in children with tetralogy of Fallot with pulmonary atresia compared to Eisenmenger syndrome or pulmonary vein stenosis. J Heart Lung Transplant 2009;28(11):1221–5.
27. Kirk R, Edwards LB, Aurora P, et al. Registry of the international society for heart and lung transplantation: twelfth official pediatric heart transplantation report-2009. J Heart Lung Transplant 2009;28(10):993–1006.
28. Aurora P, Edwards LB, Christie JD, et al. Registry of the international society for heart and lung transplantation: twelfth official pediatric lung and heart/lung transplantation report-2009. J Heart Lung Transplant 2009;28(10):1023–30.
29. Vianna RM, Mangus RS. Present prospects and future perspectives of intestinal and multivisceral transplantation. Curr Opin Clin Nutr Metab Care 2009;12(3):281–6.
30. Mazariegos GV, Squires RH, Sindhi RK. Current perspectives on pediatric intestinal transplantation. Curr Gastroenterol Rep 2009;11(3):226–33.
31. Mazariegos GV. Intestinal transplantation: current outcomes and opportunities. Curr Opin Organ Transplant 2009;14(5):515–21.
32. Hauser GJ, Kaufman SS, Matsumoto CS, et al. Pediatric intestinal and multivisceral transplantation: a new challenge for the pediatric intensivist. Intensive Care Med 2008;34(9):1570–9.
33. Vianna RM, Mangus RS, Tector AJ. Current status of small bowel and multivisceral transplantation. Adv Surg 2008;42:129–50.
34. Telles-Correia D, Barbosa A, Mega I, et al. Adherence correlates in liver transplant candidates. Transplant Proc 2009;41(5):1731–4.
35. Fung E, Shaw RJ. Pediatric transplant rating instrument—a scale for the pretransplant psychiatric evaluation of pediatric organ transplant recipients. Pediatr Transplant 2008;12(1):57–66.
36. Shemesh E, Annunziato RA, Yehuda R, et al. Childhood abuse, nonadherence, and medical outcome in pediatric liver transplant recipients. J Am Acad Child Adolesc Psychiatry 2007;46(10):1280–9.
37. DeMaso DR, Douglas Kelley S, Bastardi H, et al. The longitudinal impact of psychological functioning, medical severity, and family functioning in pediatric heart transplantation. J Heart Lung Transplant 2004;23(4):473–80.
38. Melnyk BM, Alpert-Gillis L, Feinstein NF, et al. Creating opportunities for parent empowerment: program effects on the mental health/coping outcomes of critically ill young children and their mothers. Pediatrics 2004;113(6):e597–607.
39. Green A, Meaux J, Huett A, et al. Constantly responsible, constantly worried, constantly blessed: parenting after pediatric heart transplant. Prog Transplant 2009;19(2):122–7.
40. DeMaso DR, Gonzalez-Heydrich J, Erickson JD, et al. The experience journal: a computer-based intervention for families facing congenital heart disease. J Am Acad Child Adolesc Psychiatry 2000;39(6):727–34.

41. Burra P, De Bona M. Quality of life following organ transplantation. Transpl Int 2007;20(5):397–409.

42. Green A, McSweeney J, Ainley K, et al. In my shoes: children's quality of life after heart transplantation. Prog Transplant 2007;17(3):199–207.

43. Shemesh E, Annunziato RA, Shneider BL, et al. Parents and clinicians underestimate distress and depression in children who had a transplant. Pediatr Transplant 2005;9(5):673–9.

44. Shemesh E. Assessment and management of psychosocial challenges in pediatric liver transplantation. Liver Transpl 2008;14(9):1229–36.

45. Annunziato RA, Emre S, Shneider B, et al. Adherence and medical outcomes in pediatric liver transplant recipients who transition to adult services. Pediatr Transplant 2007;11(6):608–14.

46. Annunziato RA, Parkar S, Dugan CA, et al. Brief report: deficits in health care management skills among adolescent and young adult liver transplant recipients transitioning to adult care settings. J Pediatr Psychol 2009. [Epub ahead of print].

47. McDonagh JE. Growing up and moving on: transition from pediatric to adult care. Pediatr Transplant 2005;9(3):364–72.

48. Annunziato RA, Emre S, Shneider BL, et al. Transitioning health care responsibility from caregivers to patient: a pilot study aiming to facilitate medication adherence during this process. Pediatr Transplant 2008;12(3):309–15.

49. Dew MA, Dabbs AD, Myaskovsky L, et al. Meta-analysis of medical regimen adherence outcomes in pediatric solid organ transplantation. Transplantation 2009;88(5):736–46.

50. Shemesh E, Shneider BL, Savitzky JK, et al. Medication adherence in pediatric and adolescent liver transplant recipients. Pediatrics 2004;113(4):825–32.

51. Stuber ML, Shemesh E, Seacord D, et al. Evaluating non-adherence to immunosuppressant medications in pediatric liver transplant recipients. Pediatr Transplant 2008;12(3):284–8.

52. Dobbels F, Van Damme-Lombaert R, Vanhaecke J, et al. Growing pains: nonadherence with the immunosuppressive regimen in adolescent transplant recipients. Pediatr Transplant 2005;9(3):381–90.

53. Miloh T, Annunziato R, Arnon R, et al. Improved adherence and outcomes for pediatric liver transplant recipients by using text messaging. Pediatrics 2009; 124(5):e844–50.

54. Shemesh E, Annunziato RA, Shneider BL, et al. Improving adherence to medications in pediatric liver transplant recipients. Pediatr Transplant 2008;12(3):316–23.

55. Shemesh E, Lurie S, Stuber ML, et al. A pilot study of posttraumatic stress and nonadherence in pediatric liver transplant recipients. Pediatrics 2000;105(2):E29.

56. Shemesh E, Yehuda R, Milo O, et al. Posttraumatic stress, nonadherence, and adverse outcome in survivors of a myocardial infarction. Psychosom Med 2004; 66(4):521–6.

57. Mintzer LL, Stuber ML, Seacord D, et al. Traumatic stress symptoms in adolescent organ transplant recipients. Pediatrics 2005;115(6):1640–4.

58. Young GS, Mintzer LL, Seacord D, et al. Symptoms of posttraumatic stress disorder in parents of transplant recipients: incidence, severity, and related factors. Pediatrics 2003;111(6 Pt 1):e725–31.

59. Farley LM, DeMaso DR, D'Angelo E, et al. Parenting stress and parental posttraumatic stress disorder in families after pediatric heart transplantation. J Heart Lung Transplant 2007;26(2):120–6.

60. Kaller T, Boeck A, Sander K, et al. Cognitive abilities, behaviour and quality of life in children after liver transplantation. Pediatr Transplant 2010. [Epub ahead of print].

61. Prelog M, Zimmerhackl LB. Varicella vaccination in pediatric kidney and liver transplantation. Pediatr Transplant 2010;14(1):41–7.
62. Fonseca-Aten M, Michaels MG. Infections in pediatric solid organ transplant recipients. Semin Pediatr Surg 2006;15(3):153–61.
63. Kotton CN. Update on infectious diseases in pediatric solid organ transplantation. Curr Opin Organ Transplant 2008;13(5):500–5.
64. Mueller-Ehmsen J, Schmid C, Vogeser M, et al. Mycophenolate and sirolimus as calcineurin inhibitor-free immunosuppression improves renal function better than calcineurin inhibitor-reduction in late cardiac transplant recipients with chronic renal failure. Transplantation 2009;87(5):726–33.
65. Groetzner J, Kaczmarek I, Schulz U, et al. Cancer incidence and risk factors after solid organ transplantation. Int J Cancer 2009;125(8):1747–54.
66. Alonso EM, Sorensen LG. Cognitive development following pediatric solid organ transplantation. Curr Opin Organ Transplant 2009;14(5):522–5.
67. Uzark K, Spicer R, Beebe DW. Neurodevelopmental outcomes in pediatric heart transplant recipients. J Heart Lung Transplant 2009;28(12):1306–11.
68. Weil CM, Rodgers S, Rubovits S. School re-entry of the pediatric heart transplant recipient. Pediatr Transplant 2006;10(8):928–33.
69. Bucuvalas J. Long-term outcomes in pediatric liver transplantation. Liver Transpl 2009;15(Suppl 2):S6–11.
70. Vajdic CM, McDonald SP, McCredie MR, et al. Cancer incidence before and after kidney transplantation. JAMA 2006;296(23):2823–31.
71. Ohta H, Fukushima N, Ozono K. Pediatric post-transplant lymphoproliferative disorder after cardiac transplantation. Int J Hematol 2009;90(2):127–36.
72. Uribe M, Hunter B, Alba A, et al. Posttransplant lymphoproliferative disorder in pediatric liver transplantation. Transplant Proc 2009;41(6):2679–81.
73. Lim WH, Russ GR, Coates PT. Review of Epstein-Barr virus and post-transplant lymphoproliferative disorder post-solid organ transplantation. Nephrology (Carlton) 2006;11(4):355–66.
74. Schubert S, Renner C, Hammer M, et al. Relationship of immunosuppression to Epstein-Barr viral load and lymphoproliferative disease in pediatric heart transplant patients. Heart Lung Transplant 2008;27(1):100–5.
75. Coffin CS, Shaheen AA, Burak KW, et al. Pregnancy outcomes among liver transplant recipients in the United States: a nationwide case-control analysis. Liver Transpl 2010;16(1):56–63.
76. Siemionow M, Papay F, Alam D, et al. Near-total human face transplantation for a severely disfigured patient in the USA. Lancet 2009;374(9685):203–9.
77. Ravindra KV, Buell JF, Kaufman CL, et al. Hand transplantation in the United States: experience with 3 patients. Surgery 2008;144(4):638–43.
78. Gordon CR, Siemionow M. Requirements for the development of a hand transplantation program. Ann Plast Surg 2009;63(3):262–73.

Inflammatory Bowel Disease

Eva Szigethy, MD, PhD[a,b,*], Laura McLafferty, BS[a], Alka Goyal, MD[b]

KEYWORDS

- Inflammatory bowel disease • Chronic physical illness
- Depression • Anxiety • Psychotherapy
- Health-related quality of life

Crohn disease (CD) and ulcerative colitis (UC) are the two types of inflammatory bowel disease (IBD). Although UC and CD share some clinical features, they are considered separate entities. About 25% of cases are diagnosed in childhood and adolescence.[1] Affected children face a lifelong battle with troublesome symptoms such as abdominal pain, bloody diarrhea, and fatigue. Other frequently associated problems include delayed puberty, short stature, undesirable medication side effects, and isolation from peers. To date, there is no cure for IBD. Patients control symptoms of the disease with medications and surgical intervention for severe disease and complications.

Many patients have a genetic predisposition to IBD that can manifest as an overactive immune response to bacteria located in the gastrointestinal tract.[2–4] Current opinion regarding the etiology of IBD states that in a genetically susceptible host, an environmental trigger (eg, infection, medication, smoking) may be the inciting event. This trigger enables the luminal gut bacteria to cross the epithelial barrier leading to uncontrolled downstream signaling among the gut immune cells, resulting in recruitment and differentiation of T-cell lymphocytes.[5] Different T-cell subtypes are thought to be involved in the exaggerated immune response to resident gut bacteria in CD and UC.[3,6]

A growing number of different genes have been implicated in the etiopathogenesis of both CD and UC. In CD, many of the implicated genes are involved in innate immunity which, when defective, plays a key role in IBD-related inflammation. In addition to a compromised innate immunity, these patients also display heightened adaptive

A version of this article was previously published in the *Child and Adolescent Psychiatric Clinics of North America, 19:2.*

Funding support: Dr Szigethy's research is funded by an NIH Director's Innovator Award, 1DP2OD001210, and NIMH-funded R01, MH077770.

[a] Department of Psychiatry, University of Pittsburgh School of Medicine, 3811 O'Hara Street, Pittsburgh, PA 15213, USA

[b] Division of Pediatric Gastroenterology, Children's Hospital of Pittsburgh, 4401 Penn Avenue, Pittsburgh, PA 15224, USA

* Corresponding author. Division of Pediatric Gastroenterology, Children's Hospital of Pittsburgh, 4401 Penn Avenue, Pittsburgh, PA 15224.

E-mail address: szigethye@upmc.edu

doi:10.1016/j.pcl.2011.06.007
pediatric.theclinics.com
0031-3955/11/$ – see front matter © 2011 Elsevier Inc. All rights reserved.

immunity, which keeps the inflammatory process in an active state. Innate immunity refers to various specific defense mechanisms that come into play immediately or within hours of an antigen's appearance in the body. Adaptive immunity involves a more complex antigen-specific immune response mediated by various cytokines.

Cytokines consist of a complex family of inflammatory proteins released during IBD-related immune system activation. The mechanisms of cytokine-mediated inflammation in IBD are complex and beyond the scope of this review.[3,4,7] It seems that CD and UC have very different types of cytokines involved in the inflammation; however, new evidence is emerging that there is some overlap.[8,9] For example, it is hypothesized that the T-helper (Th1) cellular immune system is the major player in mediating inflammation in CD, whereas the predominant means of inflammation in UC is via the Th2 humoral immune system. More recent data have shown that a newly discovered subset of T cells, Th17 cells, plays a critical role in inflammation in both forms of IBD, independent of either Th1 or Th2 pathways.

Three specific examples of gene mutations associated with susceptibility to IBD and their role in disease pathogenesis are described in more detail later.[2–4] The Nucleotide Oligomerization Domain (NOD)-2 gene mutations affect the recognition and handling of bacteria that are vital to the innate immune system and linked to increased risk of CD. Three mutations (leu1007insC, Gly908Arg, and Arg702Trp) in the NOD2 gene were identified in 2001 and shown to increase the risk of developing CD but not UC. Patients carrying 1 NOD2 mutation have a two- to four-fold increased risk whereas the likelihood increases to 20 to 40 times in patients carrying 2 mutations. Furthermore, patients with NOD2 risk alleles develop CD at a younger age and have fibrostenosing disease involving the terminal ileum.

As described above, NOD receptors recognize bacterial peptidoglycans, components of the bacterial cell wall that lead to the production of various cytokines and antimicrobial peptides. Chronic stimulation of these receptors in healthy hosts is critical for the process of tolerance to the gut bacterial flora. It is speculated that in patients carrying gene mutations of NOD2 receptors, the process of tolerance is defective and bacterial exposure to the intestinal epithelium could lead to nuclear factor (NF)-κB mediated excessive interleukin (IL)-12 production, which favors Th1 polarization of naïve T cells, leading to CD. In addition, decreased production of antimicrobial peptides may weaken the defensive barrier of the intestinal epithelium.

Several autophagy genes have also been associated with CD, specifically ATG16L1 and immunity-related GTPase M protein (IRGM). Autophagy is an important player in the gut innate immune system. Autophagy is a process through which the intestinal cells can degrade and clear various intracellular components including microbes, organelles, and apoptotic bodies. Some of the degraded products can also attach to HLA class II molecules for antigen presentation. The autophagy pathway also contributes to T-cell tolerance. Recently, mutations in IL-23 receptor were found to be associated with risk of developing both CD and UC. Carriers of Arg381Gln mutation are 2 to 3 times less likely to develop IBD. IL-23 affects the IL-17 pathway, which is a mediator in the Th17 lineage of T cells involved in pathogenesis of IBD. In summary, these advances in the understanding of both the genetics and pathophysiology of the illness have aided in the development of treatment targets for IBD.

CLINICAL MANIFESTATIONS

CD and UC have overlapping clinical features including abdominal pain, diarrhea, weight loss, hematochezia, malnutrition, anemia, fatigue, fevers, mouth ulcers, joint pain or swelling, and characteristic skin lesions such as erythema nodosum or pyoderma gangrenosum. Other extra intestinal manifestations seen in both UC and CD include uveitis, sclerosing cholangitis, gallstones, and renal stones. Although CD and UC share many symptoms and characteristics, there are numerous genetic, anatomic, and histologic features that differentiate the 2 illnesses.

Crohn Disease

CD usually has a more insidious onset (possibly due to delayed diagnosis) and can affect any part of the gut from the mouth to the anus. On histopathological examination, the inflammation is usually transmural and can be characterized by "skip" lesions. The hallmark finding of granulomas is, however, present in only a few patients. The most common region of involvement is ileocolonic, followed by colonic, small bowel, or gastroduodenal disease. The most common presenting symptoms are abdominal pain (86%), diarrhea (78%), or hematochezia (49%). In the pediatric population, the patient may be diagnosed with CD while being evaluated for malnutrition, short stature, delayed puberty, fatigue, or sometimes fistulizing disease. Fistulas are connections formed in gastrointestinal regions affected by ulceration to other parts of the organ or the surface of a nearby skin, seen in CD but not UC. Patients with CD have been misdiagnosed as having anorexia nervosa, or even sexual abuse. Other clinical manifestations include drainage, abscess (intra-abdominal or perianal), pain, or malnutrition. Patients with CD are at risk for having a stricture or obstruction in the small bowel or colon. As a result, they may present with bowel obstruction or even perforation leading to peritonitis.[1,10,11]

Ulcerative Colitis

Symptoms of UC can include diarrhea, abdominal cramping, and hematochezia. Due to the presence of bloody stools, medical attention is sought much earlier than in CD. In contrast to CD, patients with UC have primarily colonic involvement confined to the mucosal layer without skip lesions, although patients can have gastritis or distal colitis. Children present with pancolitis more frequently than adults. Other extraintestinal manifestations such as weight loss, malnutrition, and delayed puberty are less commonly observed. Anemia and hypoalbuminemia are common in both types of IBD, but other inflammatory markers such as sedimentation rate and C-reactive protein may be relatively normal in UC whereas they may be elevated in CD.[1,11,12]

EPIDEMIOLOGY

The prevalence of CD in North America ranges from 26.0 to 198.5 per 100,000 persons and that of UC varies from 37.5 to 229 cases per 100,000. Incidence rates of CD are 3.1 to 14.6 per 100,000 patient-years and for UC are 2.2 to 14.3 cases per 100,000 person-years.[13] About 1.4 million Americans suffer from inflammatory bowel disease.[6] Approximately 25% of new cases of IBD are diagnosed during childhood and adolescence, and peak incidence of diagnosis occurs in the second and third decades. The incidence of CD in children appears to be increasing while that of UC has remained relatively stable.[14] UC at any age and CD in older populations are evenly distributed between the two sexes. However, in children younger than 15 to 17 years, males with CD outnumber females by a ratio of 1.2:1 to 1.5:1. Pediatric IBD is also unique compared with adult onset in being more extensive at the time of presentation and undergoing continued progression within the first 5 to 7 years after diagnosis. CD tends to have a predominantly colonic involvement in children younger than 8 years. Family history is positive in 30% of patients diagnosed with CD before 20 years of age, compared with 18% at 20 to 29 years and 13% after 40 years.[11,15,16]

TREATMENT

The treatment paradigm in IBD has shifted from symptom control to mucosal healing, which is likely to result in prevention of disease progression, fewer complications, and reduction in the need for surgery. Other considerations in the treatment of children with IBD are optimization of nutrition, achievement of normal pubertal development and growth spurt, facilitation of emotional and social development, and prevention of long-term complications and disability while minimizing unwanted side effects.

Crohn Disease

The treatment of CD depends on the location, type of disease (inflammatory, stricturing, or perforating), and presence of fistulas or abscesses. Mesalamines are often used because they are safe; however, they are unlikely to induce disease remission on their own. At present, steroids are used as first-line therapy for induction of CD remission. If disease is confined to the terminal ileum and cecum, oral budesonide can be used instead of systemic steroids because it has the advantage of being released directly into these gastrointestinal regions. Budesonide also has the added advantage of extensive first-pass metabolism in the liver, making systemic side effects unlikely. For maintenance of remission immunomodulators, including mercaptopurine and methotrexate, can be used in those who cannot be weaned from steroids or who experience relapse of their CD after steroid withdrawal. Both agents have a similar mode of action but are used judiciously due to side effects, including an increased risk of lymphoma. Infliximab has been found to be helpful in both the induction and maintenance of disease remission. Other biologic agents approved for CD include adalimumab, certolizumab, and natalizumab. The latter agent works by preventing migration of plasma leukocytes and extracellular matrix proteins to the site of inflammation in the gut. There is a high risk of infection, as natalizumab is not specific for the gut.

In children, nutritional therapy is also a desirable first-line treatment because it is only slightly inferior to steroids in efficacy, and it has added advantages of promoting mucosal healing and optimizing growth.[17–19] The more palatable newer formulas can be taken orally, but some patients may require placement of nasogastric or a gastrostomy tube. Nutritional therapy has no side effects, but adherence to a strict diet for 8 weeks on polymeric formula alone is often prohibitive, particularly during adolescence when peer imitation is an important driver of identify formation. Although the exact mechanism of action is not well understood, various possibilities include enhancement of the innate immune system as a result of better nutritional status, reduced antigenic load in the distal intestine, and altered gut flora. Surgery in patients with CD is used mainly for complications such as stricture, abscess, perforation, or fistulizing disease. Surgery is not curative for CD because of a high risk of postoperative disease recurrence.[20,21]

Ulcerative Colitis

For mild to moderate disease severity, oral and rectal mesalamines are the mainstay of therapy. Most preparations are formulated to be released in both the terminal ileum and colon, or just the colon. These agents are now also available in once-daily dosing options to improve adherence. Mesalamines work by inhibition of NF-κB and leukotriene synthesis, modification of neutrophil-mediated tissue damage, and scavenging of reactive oxygen species. Patients who fail to respond to mesalamines or who have severe disease can be treated with oral or intravenous steroids. Steroids have a general anti-inflammatory effect and also inhibit cell-mediated immunity, but prolonged use can lead to unacceptable side effects including short stature, weight gain, moon facies, and skin striae. If a patient is unresponsive or becomes steroid dependent, then immunomodulators such as mercaptopurine may be used, and biologic agents such as infliximab, a cytokine antagonist targeting tumor necrosis factor α (TNF-α), have been effective in avoiding or at least delaying the need for surgery. TNF-α is a key cytokine involved in the pathogenesis of IBD. As a last resort, surgery can be curative in UC as the disease is confined to the colon, although it requires the surgical placement of an ostomy, either temporarily or permanently.[20–22]

INCIDENCE OF PSYCHOLOGICAL/BEHAVIORAL DISORDERS IN CHILDREN WITH IBD
Adjustment Disorder/Depression and Anxiety

The diagnosis of a chronic illness such as IBD during childhood can involve a grieving process that begins with shock and disbelief and proceeds through feelings of anguish (sadness) and protest (anger) toward the gradual assimilation of illness information and adjustment to the implications of the disease. In both children and adolescents, the diagnosis of IBD can involve a sense of loss in any one of the following areas: independence, sense of control, privacy, body image, healthy self, peer relationships, roles inside and outside the family, self-confidence, productivity, future plans, familiar daily routines, ways of expressing sexuality, and pain-free existence. The child's reaction to IBD, including the degree of perceived loss, is moderated by developmental factors, disease severity, and environmental/social factors (eg, family reaction). For example, adolescents with severe physical illness may have fragile self-esteem due to delays in physical growth or pubertal maturation, shame associated with fecal incontinence, or steroid-induced weight gain, and thus have a more challenging adjustment to the disease.[23] There are, however, conflicting reports as to what extent self-esteem is affected by IBD. Some studies suggest that self-esteem in adolescents with IBD is comparable with that of healthy controls,[24] contradicting others that found self-esteem worse in those affected with IBD.[25–27] One factor that seems to negatively affect self-esteem is more severe disease activity and having separated parents.[24]

Children with IBD may experience overwhelming psychological distress including guilt for being a burden to caretakers, threats to narcissistic integrity and self-esteem, regressive fear of strangers on whom the patient must rely, separation anxiety, fear of loss of love and approval, fear of loss of control of bodily functions, and fear of pain and humiliation. Invasive medical procedures can result in traumatization and reactions ranging from dissociation, emotional blunting, anxiety, and anger (Szigethy and Siegle, unpublished observations, 2009). Although initially most children deny that IBD interferes with their lives, with persistent questioning many admit frustration and anger about their IBD symptoms and treatment.[28] Children with IBD also exhibit concern about fatigue, body image, and lack of control over activities (eg, school, sports, and work).[25,29–31]

Several studies have found that adolescents with IBD are more depressed than adolescents with other diseases,[26,32–34] with rates of depression as high as 25%.[35] In a study by Mackner and colleagues,[25] children with IBD and depression were at an increased risk of anxiety.[36] Anxiety disorders have also been described in adolescents with IBD.[37] Externalizing disorders (eg, disruptive behavioral disorders, conduct disorder) and attention deficit hyperactivity disorder (ADHD) have been less well studied in these children. Disordered eating (eg, severe restriction often secondary to abdominal pain) is commonly seen in clinic but the rate of eating disorders has not been studied. The temporal relationship between mood and anxiety disorders and IBD has also not been systematically examined. Children diagnosed at a younger age appear to adjust better than older teenagers. Whether this is due to a more flexible sense of self-identity, cognitive maturation, or differences in the grieving process or processing of illness experience has not been studied.

Influence of Physiologic Changes of IBD on Psychological Functioning

Physiologic changes associated with the disease process itself (eg, cytokine-induced inflammation, steroid treatment) may affect the brain, thereby resulting in emotional and behavioral changes that further compromise the child's adjustment.[38] Szigethy and colleagues[35] found in a study of 102 youths with IBD that those who had moderate to severe IBD-related symptoms had significantly greater depressive severity than youths with inactive disease. Furthermore, depressive severity has been strongly associated with the degree of pain and diarrhea, as well low plasma albumin levels.[39] Hypoalbuminemia may be a marker for both chronic inflammation and malnutrition. In another study, pediatric patients with inactive IBD or with mild disease for at least 1 year reported normal emotional/behavioral functioning, similar to that of healthy children.[40] In children with IBD, exogenous steroids used to treat IBD have been associated with impairment in mood, executive function, and short-term memory.[35,41]

In adults with IBD, there was a significant inverse correlation between sleep quality and IBD severity,[42] and abnormal sleep patterns were reported even in patients with inactive IBD compared with normal controls. Because they often need more sleep, sleep disturbances could have an even greater impact on adolescents and adversely affect their quality of life (QOL), psychological functioning, and coping ability. Given that sleep is critical for disease healing, studies are needed to determine how IBD affects sleep architecture, duration, and quality, so that better treatments for insomnia and fatigue can be developed.

Functional Abdominal Pain

Even in remission, IBD patients may still experience severe gastrointestinal symptoms similar to those present in irritable bowel syndrome (IBS), including abdominal pain, bloating, abdominal distention, diarrhea, urgency, loose stools, constipation, hard stools, and incomplete bowel movements. In adults, approximately one-third of patients with UC and two-thirds of patients with CD report these symptoms, possibly from the visceral hypersensitivity or autonomic dysfunction induced by chronic inflammation.[43] In adult patients with UC in remission, the prevalence of IBS-like symptoms is about 3 times higher than in healthy controls, and these patients had impaired health-related quality of life (HRQOL) similar to that of patients whose UC was in the active phase.[44] In children with quiescent CD, rectal sensory threshold for pain (RSTP) was significantly decreased in comparison with that of healthy controls, and was similar to the RSTP of children with functional gastrointestinal disorders.[45]

IMPACT
Medication Adherence

Because medications are critical to the management of IBD, medical adherence is particularly important for children with IBD. Although having to take daily medication can adversely affect QOL, the consequences of nonadherence can lead to more severe disease and QOL outcomes, including an increase risk for surgery.[46] Adherence can be especially problematic during adolescence. One study found that medication adherence rates in pediatric IBD were 38% according to parents and 48% according to the children studied.[47] Family dysfunction and poor child coping strategies were associated with worse adherence. In a sample of 44 patients 10 to 21 years old who had IBD, there was a significant relationship between age and dietary adherence, with younger children more likely to report better dietary adherence.[48] In another study, medication adherence was assessed in 36 adolescents with IBD via interviews, pill counts, and biologic assays. Nonadherence to 6-mercaptopurine/azathioprine (6-MP/AZA) was related to poorer self-reported physical health QOL. In contrast, greater adherence to 5-aminosalicylate (5-ASA) was related to poorer psychological health QOL, especially social functioning, on the Pediatric Quality of Life Inventory.[49] These results may be related to the child's perceptions that taking multiple pills is related to poorer QOL, particularly in social realms. The interaction between social functioning and treatment adherence was also illustrated in a recent study showing that positive social relationships buffered the negative effects of peer victimization on treatment adherence in youth with IBD.[50]

Disease Outcomes

In adults with IBD, depression and life stressors have been associated with a more refractory course of IBD; however, this has not been studied in children. Camara and colleagues[51] found that 13 of 18 prospective studies conducted since 1980 reported a statistically significant association between stress and worsened IBD outcomes in adults. In another review, Singh and colleagues[52] found strong evidence for an association between perceived stress levels and IBD flares. There is evidence that the course of IBD is worse in depressed patients,[53] and in an animal model of colitis, induction of a depressive episode in mice reactivated the colitic inflammation.[54]

Illness Perception

Several studies have probed illness perception in children and adolescents. In response to questions that explored the impact of IBD on their daily lives, children with IBD aged 7 to 19 years, themes of discomfort from symptoms and treatment, vulnerability, diminished control over their lives and future, and seeing themselves as different from healthy peers were commonly discussed.[55] Additional difficulties noted were lack of energy, food restriction, medication side effects, diminished self-perception, and less social interaction.

In a study consisting of 50 depressed adolescents, qualitative illness narrative analysis of perception of IBD experience was conducted using responses to 10 questions in a structured interview to probe themes of pessimism, contingency (ie, a sense the child could control their disease), and coping with IBD. This study found that IBD severity was inversely correlated with positive contingency as well as positive feelings about IBD medications. In addition, depressive severity was associated with negative self-competence and sense of damaged self (McLafferty and Szigethy, unpublished observations, 2010). These correlations were not affected by age or gender. In another study examining how 17 adolescents (age 11–17 years) with IBD responded to their parents' concern for them, ambivalence was the most prevalent theme described. There was an oscillation between seeking close contact with one's parents and pushing them away. The other theme categories that emerged were ability/inability, compliance/resistance, and trust/distrust, suggesting that it is important to have an awareness of the simultaneous existence of conflicting attitudes, reactions, and emotions.[56]

There are several reports of shame and embarrassment in the literature concerning adolescents with IBD. Nicholas and colleagues[57] interviewed 80 children and adolescents (7–19 years old) with IBD, concerning the impact of IBD on their lives. The interviewees revealed negative body-image perceptions from the disease process (short stature, weight loss, physical weakness) and side effects from treatment (weight gain, acne, visible nasogastric tube). There is also embarrassment related to using public bathrooms.[55] In another study of 20 adolescents with ostomies or J-pouches, embarrassment and shame were recurring themes that led to hesitance about revealing their ostomy,[57] and fear that it would be discovered. Adolescents were able to develop acceptance of their ostomies over variable amounts of time, particularly with more education and independence in the care of the ostomy.

Psychosocial Functioning/Quality of Life

HRQOL is a concept that consists of the physical, emotional, and social aspects of health perception and health functioning. Several instruments are now available to measure IBD-related HRQOL, including generic and disease-specific types. Generic assessments are multidimensional problem lists designed to be applied to any population, and they are able to compare QOL in populations with different diseases. Generic measures have been used in HRQOL studies in both adults[58,59] and children with IBD.[35,60]

Disease-specific instruments focus on concerns relevant to a particular illness. Unlike generic measures, they can measure changes in HRQOL over time or with treatment.[58,61] One disease-specific measure developed and validated for children is the IMPACT questionnaire, designed for use in youths 10 years or older. Its most recent form, IMPACT-III, consists of 35 questions encompassing 6 domains: IBD symptoms, body image, functional/social impairment, emotional impairment, treatment/interventions, and systemic impairment. The patient's current health status is believed to have the greatest influence on responses to the IMPACT questionnaire.[62,63] This pediatric IBD-specific measure accomplishes 3 tasks: (1) documenting the effects of health care interventions on patient outcomes; (2) providing a more complete picture of the patient than that available from pediatric IBD disease indices alone; and (3) helping to identify the needs of the child with IBD and success of medical management.[64]

In pediatric IBD, adolescents with IBD symptom exacerbation are more likely to express greater psychosocial difficulty,[65–67] but steroid exposure, hospitalizations, and time from IBD diagnosis did not significantly impact HRQOL in children with IBD.[67] In young adult patients who were diagnosed with IBD as children or adolescents, HRQOL was significantly decreased when compared with healthy age-matched controls.[68] Indeed, compared with healthy controls, children with IBD have decreased psychosocial health, social functioning, and school functioning.[25,69]

Family Functioning/Interactions

Interviews with adolescents with CD stress the importance of achieving a balance between adequate social support and time for self-reflection.[70] One area of the physically ill adolescent's life in which this balance can be difficult to achieve is family functioning. Children with IBD who have good mental health reported a good family climate and open social network,[27] and positive affect in mothers of adolescents with IBD is inversely correlated with the adolescents' depression.[71] Family conflict and low QOL have been positively correlated with pain, fatigue, depression, and lower QOL in children with IBD. Collectively, studies suggest that family functioning is an important component of how children cope with chronic illness. In addition, parents of children with IBD reported significantly less social support and mothers reported greater distress compared with parents of healthy children.[72] The lack of social support, but not parental distress, was correlated with increased behavioral problems in children with IBD. If it is possible that a family's dynamic is influencing the adolescent's health status, therapy should be implemented to examine and potentially improve family functioning and parental affect.

Transition to Adulthood

Even without the presence of a chronic physical illness, adolescence is a challenging life phase with significant changes in both physiologic (eg, emotional regulation, cognitive processing, maturation of self-image) and physical (eg, pubertal changes, growth) realms. The transition from adolescence to adulthood may be particularly challenging for youth with a chronic disease such as IBD. In individual interviews 6 patients 19 to 24 years old with UC and a temporary ostomy identified several themes present in their experiences living with UC and an ostomy: embarrassment, feeling different, and unpredictability/sense of loss of control.[73] In a study of 22 patients 15 to 21 years old who have a chronic illness (23% had IBD), most adolescents anticipating their transfer to adult care identified only negatives about the transition and felt unprepared at the time of their interview with Tuchman and colleagues.[74] College students with active IBD have significantly poorer adjustment to college and students with IBD had lower physical QOL compared with healthy controls,[75] suggesting that this transition is important to monitor. The goals of successful transition to adulthood include the acquisition of skills to manage their illness, including further education/knowledge about their illness as well as relaxation techniques to manage stress,[76] to continue striving for autonomy and self-regulation and for identity formation by learning from trial and error.

COMMON TREATMENT MODALITIES
Medication

Psychotropic medications are often used to treat patients with IBD, although they should only be considered after a thorough psychological assessment has been completed and behavioral therapy has been deemed inadequate or unavailable. In a survey of 18 gastroenterologists, Mikocka-Walus and colleagues[77] found that 78% had prescribed antidepressants for their IBD patients for the purpose of treating pain, depression, anxiety, and insomnia. In a review by Mikocka-Walus and colleagues,[78] 10 of 12 nonrandomized studies involving adults with IBD suggested that paroxetine, bupropion, and phenelzine were effective in the treatment of psychological and somatic symptoms in these patients. Amitriptyline was found to be ineffective for treating somatic symptoms of IBD, and mirtazapine was not recommended for use in IBD patients. Desipramine attenuated the susceptibility of a murine model of depression to colitis,[79] and in adults with IBD, bupropion improved depression and IBD severity, and was particularly effective for fatigue and concentration difficulties.[80] Whether the newer proinflammatory cytokine antagonists being used to treat IBD will prevent depression remains to be determined. Of note, most psychotropic medications have the potential for serious side effects (eg, increased suicidal ideation), may have drug-drug interactions with IBD-related medications, and require careful monitoring. Thus, the first-line approach to psychological problems is psychosocial intervention, discussed next in this article.[81] Factors used to determine which medication in this class to initiate include symptom complex, family history of medication response, and gastrointestinal tolerability.

Educational Resources

In a study by Casellas and colleagues,[82] IBD patients were surveyed about the health care they receive, and virtually all patients in that survey considered having adequate information about their disease process as very important. Of note, only half of those patients thought they had sufficient information. Having inadequate information was found to result in poorer reported QOL.[83] In one study, 69 adults with IBD were randomly assigned to either an educational intervention focused on IBD or treatment as usual.[84] The educational group had greater knowledge about IBD, increased satisfaction, and improved medication adherence, but there was no significant difference in HRQOL between the 2 groups. In another study, 49 adult patients with IBD who received 8 sessions of educational intervention did not exhibit any significant change in anxiety at 6-month follow-up visit, or any significant changes over time in bowel symptoms, systemic symptoms, emotional or social functioning portions of the Inflammatory Bowel Disease Questionnaire (IBDQ), or in generic HRQOL (as measured by SF-36).[85] Educational interventions employed include written information, interactive computer learning models, social skills, and disease management training.

Self-management training was shown to improve HRQOL.[86,87] In one study of 700 adults with IBD, patients randomized to a self-management approach to illness (by being provided with information designed to promote patient choice and decreased health care visits) reported better QOL and increased confidence in being able to cope with their IBD compared with those in the usual treatment group.[86] A brief psychosocial group intervention consisting of education and group therapy versus usual medical treatment in 44 adults with inactive IBD resulted in no significant improvement in HRQOL or coping ability over a 12-month period.[88]

The social, educational, and long-term vocational goals of adolescence, as well as the goals of achieving autonomy, self-regulation, and identity formation, can be enhanced by the acquisition of skills to manage the illness. Grootenhuis and colleagues[89] studied 22 adolescents with IBD who received psychoeducational intervention that included training in information-seeking skills, relaxation, social competence, and positive thinking, and found that the intervention had a positive effect on coping, feelings of competence, and HRQOL.

Cognitive Behavioral Therapy

In adolescents, results from psychotherapy studies are positive. Depressed youth with IBD who received cognitive behavioral therapy (CBT) with focus on illness perception had significant improvements in depression and perceived control over IBD compared with those receiving their usual medical treatment. Such was the case even after controlling for change in IBD severity and steroid burden that may have precipitated some depressive features.[90,91] In addition, the benefits of CBT on depressive symptoms and global functioning persisted 1 year after treatment.[34] The model of CBT used was focused on helping adolescents determine the appropriate locus of control and adjusting their behaviors and thoughts accordingly.[92] Adolescents with IBD have also been found to benefit from cognitive reappraisal and developing interest in activities that can exist within the limitations of their disease process (eg, crafts).[55] The more positive effects of psychotherapy in adolescents may be due to their more flexible behavioral repertoires and less-engrained maladaptive coping strategies.

Narrative Therapy

Narrative therapy emphasizes the patient's personal story or narrative of their illness, and has been shown to be strongly associated with psychological adaptation. The therapist encourages the patient to relate his or her illness narrative, which in children typically centers on 5 pervasive themes: (1) identity (the symptoms the child sees as part of their illness); (2) cause (the child's personal ideas about the etiology of their illness); (3) time-line (how long the child feels that the illness will last); (4) consequences (the child's anticipated effects of the illness); (5) cure and control (how the child expects to recover from or control the illness).[93] Although the sharing of illness narratives on appropriate Web sites (eg, http://www.experiencejournal.com) has not been tested for efficacy, children with chronic physical illness have found online communities that promote real-time sharing of narratives to be both safe and enjoyable.[94]

It is feasible to implement narrative strategies using a family systems perspective. The illness narrative becomes the family's story of their child's illness and its impact on the family system. De Maso and colleagues[95] found that computer-based narrative sharing was helpful for families of depressed children in increasing familial understanding of the child's illness, increasing hope, and augmenting positive reactions in the children's caretakers.

Hypnosis

Relaxation and hypnosis have been used to target symptoms of anxiety and abdominal pain, and to improve immune functioning. Hypnotherapy was shown to have promising effects on IBD course and QOL in 15 adults with severe IBD refractory to corticosteroid treatment,[96] and Keefer and Keshavarzian[97] found that after hypnotherapy, 8 female patients with IBD reported a significant improvement in QOL. Yet in another study, 2 female patients with CD, 1 with CD in active phase and the other in remission, reported improved coping and psychological state but no change in IBD symptoms or QOL after receiving hypnotherapy.[98] In patients with UC, hypnotherapy was shown to significantly improve IBD-related inflammation.[99] Shaoul and colleagues[100] found that hypnotherapy improved clinical symptoms of IBD and decreased inflammatory markers in 6 children with IBD. Hypnotherapy was also shown to decrease abdominal pain in pediatric IBS.[101] Given the higher susceptibility to hypnosis of children compared with adults, the therapeutic use of hypnosis holds promise for treatment of abdominal pain and emotional symptoms in pediatric IBD.

Social Support/Support Groups

In adult IBD patients, social support has been shown to have a positive impact on QOL.[102] Support from family members and friends has been shown to have a positive effect on coping in children with IBD.[55] Social support from other adolescents with IBD can also be valuable. Adolescents who attended a summer IBD camp experienced improved social functioning, improved total QOL, and better acceptance of IBD symptoms[103]; this may act to normalize the illness experience. Female adolescents with IBD and their mothers who participated in monthly support groups for 1 year consisting of education and social interaction reported that the sessions were helpful, and the adolescents showed significant improvement in the emotional and social functioning subscales of IMPACT-III from baseline to post-treatment.[104] There are several Web-based interactive Internet sites available for children and adolescents with IBD that also provide educational materials and opportunities for social interaction and sharing IBD experiences. These sources include http://www.ccfa.org; http://www.myibdu.org; http://www.experiencejournal.com/ib/index.shtml; http://www.ibdsf.com; http://www.starlight.org; and http://www.ucandcrohns.org. Future studies are needed to assess these promising interventions for efficacy using randomized controlled trials.

School Planning

It is critical that all children and adolescents with IBD have an educational plan in place in case they need to miss school due to IBD flare-ups or treatment (eg, hospitalization). A 504 Plan is a federally mandated document that public schools are required to follow. This plan indicates that any child with a chronic illness or disability who misses school due to their condition or its treatment needs to be provided with an individualized educational plan to catch up without penalty.[105] Although such plans are individualized based on the specific needs of each student, common requests include discrete bathroom access, tutoring for missed classes, and extra time to catch up on examinations and assignments without penalty. Even though private schools are not mandated to follow such plans, often they cooperate with a letter from a physician requesting such services. The 504 Plan can also be used to educate school officials and teachers about IBD so they can better adjust the educational plan.

SUMMARY

Pediatric-onset IBD is a lifelong chronic illness with high medical morbidity and associated psychological and psychosocial challenges. Depression and anxiety are particularly prevalent and have a multifaceted etiology, including IBD-related factors and psychosocial stress. Youth with active IBD or receiving treatment with steroids, social isolation, family conflict, or showing impaired social or academic functioning would particularly benefit from screening for psychiatric comorbidities, especially anxiety and depression. Furthermore, exploring a child's illness perceptions and experiences can also inform providers of targets for psychosocial interventions. Fortunately, there are a growing number of empirically supported treatments, such as CBT, to help with coping with IBD as well as the related psychological and psychosocial difficulties. While there is convincing evidence that such interventions can help improve anxiety, depression, and HRQOL, their effects on IBD severity and course await further study. Further studies are also needed to assess developmental and cultural factors in treatments aimed at improving QOL and decreasing suffering in this chronic illness population until a cure can be found.

ACKNOWLEDGMENTS

The authors would like to thank Maggie Kirshner for her administrative assistance with the manuscript and David Benhayon, MD, PhD, Christine Karwowski, MD, Melissa Newara, MS, Patricia Delaney, LCSW, and Amy Levine, MSW, PhD for their editorial comments.

REFERENCES

1. Griffiths AM. Specificities of inflammatory bowel disease in childhood. Best Pract Res Clin Gastroenterol 2004;18:509–23.
2. Achkar JP, Duerr R. The expanding universe of inflammatory bowel disease genetics. Curr Opin Gastroenterol 2008;24:429–34.
3. Shih DQ, Targan SR, McGovern D. Recent advances in IBD pathogenesis: genetics and immunobiology. Curr Gastroenterol Rep 2008;10:568–75.
4. Silverberg MS, Cho JH, Rioux JD, et al. Ulcerative colitis-risk loci on chromosomes 1p36 and 12q15 found by genome association-wide study. Nat Genet 2009;41:216–20.
5. Kugathasan S, Amre D. Inflammatory bowel disease-environmental modification and genetic determinants. Pediatr Clin North Am 2006;53:727–49.
6. Abraham C, Cho JH. Inflammatory bowel disease. N Engl J Med 2009;361: 2066–78.
7. Kanai T, Nemoto Y, Kamada N, et al. Homeostatic (IL-7) and effector (IL-17) cytokines as distinct but complementary target for an optimal therapeutic strategy in inflammatory bowel disease. Curr Opin Gastroenterol 2009;25:306–13.

8. Xavier RJ, Podolsky DK. Unravelling the pathogenesis of inflammatory bowel disease. Nature 2007;448:427–34.
9. Abraham C, Cho J. Interleukin-23/Th17 pathways and inflammatory bowel disease. Inflamm Bowel Dis 2009;15:1090–100.
10. Sawczenko A, Sandhu B. Presenting features of inflammatory bowel diseases in children. Arch Dis Child 2003;88:995–1000.
11. Vernier–Massouille G, Balde M, Salleron J. Natural history of pediatric Crohn's disease. A population-based cohort study. Gastroenterology 2008;135:1106–13.
12. Hyams JS, Davis P, Grancher K. Clinical outcome of ulcerative colitis in children. J Pediatr 1996;129:81–8.
13. Loftus EV, Sandborn WJ. Epidemiology of inflammatory bowel disease. Gastroenterol Clin North Am 2002;31:1–20.
14. Turunen P, Kolho KL, Auvinen A, et al. Incidence of inflammatory bowel disease in Finnish children, 1987–2003. Inflamm Bowel Dis 2006;12:677.
15. Van Limbergen J, Russell RK, Drummond HE, et al. Definition of phenotypic characteristics of childhood-onset inflammatory bowel disease. Gastroenterology 2008;135:1114–22.
16. Sauer CG, Kugathasa Subra. Pediatric inflammatory bowel disease: highlighting pediatric differences in IBD. Gastroenterol Clin North Am 2009;38:611–28.
17. Smith PA. Nutritional therapy for active Crohn's disease. World J Gastroenterol 2008;14:4420–3.
18. Borrelli O, Cordischi L, Cirulli M, et al. Polymeric diet alone versus corticosteroids in the treatment of active pediatric Crohn's disease: a randomized controlled open-label trial. Clin Gastroenterol Hepatol 2006;4:744–53.
19. Zachos M, Tondeur M, Griffiths AM. Enteral nutritional therapy for induction of remission in Crohn's disease. Cochrane Database Syst Rev 2007;(1):CD000542.
20. Schwartz M, Cohen R. Optimizing conventional therapy for inflammatory bowel disease. Curr Gastroenterol Rep 2008;10:585–90.
21. Rutgeerts P, Vermeire S, Van Assche G. Biological therapies for inflammatory bowel diseases. Gastroenterology 2009;136:1182–97.
22. Devlin SM, Panaccione R. Evolving inflammatory bowel disease treatment paradigms: top-down versus step-up. Gastroenterol Clin North Am 2009;38:577–94.
23. Mamula P, Markowitz JE, Baldassano RN. Inflammatory bowel disease in early childhood and adolescence: special considerations. Gastroenterol Clin North Am 2003;32:967–95.
24. Lindfred H, Saalman R, Nilsson S, et al. IBD and self-esteem in adolescence. Acta Paediatr 2008;97:201–5.
25. Mackner LM, Crandall W, Szigethy EM. Psychosocial functioning in pediatric inflammatory bowel disease. Inflamm Bowel Dis 2006;12:239–44.
26. Engstrom I. Mental health and psychological functioning in children and adolescents with inflammatory bowel disease: a comparison with children having other chronic illnesses and with healthy children. J Child Psychol Psychiatry 1992;33:563–82.
27. Engstrom I. Inflammatory bowel disease and social interaction in families with children with inflammatory bowel disease. J Pediatr Gastroenterol Nutr 1999;28:S28–33.
28. Akobeng AK, Suresh-Babu MV, Firth D, et al. Quality of life in children with Crohn's disease: A Pilot Study. J Pediatr Gastroenterol Nutr 1999;29:S37–9.

29. Griffiths AM, Nicholas D, Smith C, et al. Development of a quality-of-life index for pediatric inflammatory bowel disease: dealing with differences related to age and IBD type. J Pediatr Gastroenterol Nutr 1999;28:S46–52.

30. Rabbett H, Elbadri A, Thwaites R, et al. Quality of life in children with Crohn's disease. J Pediatr Gastroenterol Nutr 1996;23:528–33.

31. Lavigne JV, Faier-Routman J. Psychological adjustment to pediatric physical disorders: a meta-analytic review. J Pediatr Psychol 1992;17:133–57.

32. Burke P, Meyer V, Kocoshis S, et al. Depression and anxiety in pediatric inflammatory bowel disease and cystic fibrosis. J Am Acad Child Adolesc Psychiatry 1989;28:948–51.

33. Burke P, Kocoshis SA, Chandra R, et al. Determinants of depression in recent onset pediatric inflammatory bowel disease. J Am Acad Child Adolesc Psychiatry 1990;29:608–10.

34. Raymer D, Weininger O, Hamilton JR. Psychological problems in children with abdominal pain. Lancet 1984;1:439–40.

35. Szigethy E, Levy-Warren A, Whitton S, et al. Depressive symptoms and inflammatory bowel disease in children and adolescents: a cross-sectional study. J Pediatr Gastroenterol Nutr 2004;39:395–403.

36. Mackner LM, Crandall W. Psychological factors affecting pediatric inflammatory bowel disease. Curr Opin Pediatr 2007;19:548–52.

37. Szigethy E, Carpenter J, Baum E, et al. Case study: longitudinal treatment of adolescents with depression and inflammatory bowel disease. J Am Acad Child Adolesc Psychiatry 2006;45:396–400.

38. Szigethy E, Low C. Cytokines and depression. In: Ingram RE, editor. International encyclopedia of depression. New York: Springer Publishing Co; 2009. p. 200–4.

39. Karwowski C, Richardson A, Kirshner MA, et al. Characterizing depression in children with inflammatory bowel disease. J Pediatr Gastroenterol Nutr 2009; 49(Suppl 1):E60.

40. Mackner LM, Crandall WV. Long-term psychosocial outcomes reported by children and adolescents with inflammatory bowel disease. Am J Gastroenterol 2005;100:1386–92.

41. Mrakotsky C, Bousvaros A, Chriki L, et al. Impact of acute steroid treatment on memory, executive function, and mood in pediatric inflammatory bowel disease. J Pediatr Gastroenterol Nutr 2005;41:540–1.

42. Ranjbaran Z, Keefer L, Farhadi A, et al. Impact of sleep disturbances in inflammatory bowel disease. J Gastroenterol Hepatol 2007;22:1748–53.

43. Ananthakrishnan AN, Issa M, Barboi A, et al. Impact of autonomic dysfunction on inflammatory bowel disease. J Clin Gastroenterol 2009, Sept 1 [online].

44. Ansari R, Attari F, Razjouyan H, et al. Ulcerative colitis and irritable bowel syndrome: relationships with quality of life. Eur J Gastroenterol Hepatol 2008;20:46–50.

45. Faure C, Giguère L. Functional gastrointestinal disorders and visceral hypersensitivity in children and adolescents suffering from Crohn's disease. Inflamm Bowel Dis 2008;14:1569–74.

46. Kane SV. Systematic review: adherence issues in the treatment of ulcerative colitis. Aliment Pharmacol Ther 2006;23:577–85.

47. Mackner L, Crandall W. Oral medication adherence in pediatric inflammatory bowel disease. Inflamm Bowel Dis 2005;11:1006–12.

48. Vlahou CH, Cohen LL, Woods AM, et al. Age and body satisfaction predict diet adherence in adolescents with inflammatory bowel disease. J Clin Psychol Med Settings 2008;15:278–86.

49. Hommel K, Davis C, Baldassano R. Medication adherence and quality of life in pediatric inflammatory bowel disease. J Pediatr Psychol 2008;33:867–74.
50. Janicke DM, Gray WN, Kahhan NA, et al. Brief report: the association between peer victimization, prosocial support, and treatment adherence in children and adolescents with inflammatory bowel disease. J Pediatr Psychol 2009;34: 769–73.
51. Camara RJ, Ziegler R, Begré S, et al. The role of psychological stress in inflammatory bowel disease: quality assessment of methods 18 prospective studies and suggestions for future research. Digestion 2009;80:129–39.
52. Singh S, Graff LA, Bernstein CN. Do NSAIDs, antibiotics, infections, or stress trigger flares in IBD? Am J Gastroenterol 2009;104:1298–313.
53. Graff LA, Walker JR, Bernstein CN. Depression and anxiety in inflammatory bowel disease: a review of comorbidity and management. Inflamm Bowel Dis 2009;15:1105–18.
54. Ghia JE, Blennerhassett P, Deng Y, et al. Reactivation of inflammatory bowel disease in a mouse model of depression. Gastroenterology 2009;136: 2280–8.
55. Nicholas DB, Otley A, Smith C, et al. Challenges and strategies of children and adolescents with inflammatory bowel disease: a qualitative examination. Health Qual Life Outcomes 2007;5:28.
56. Reichenberg K, Lindfred H, Saalman R. Adolescents with inflammatory bowel disease feel ambivalent towards their parents' concern for them. Scand J Caring Sci 2007;21:476–81.
57. Nicholas DB, Swan SR, Gerstle TJ, et al. Struggles, strengths, and strategies: an ethnographic study exploring the adolescents living with an ostomy. Health Qual Life Outcomes 2008;6:114.
58. Irvine EJ. Quality of life issues in patients with inflammatory bowel disease. Am J Gastroenterol 1997;92(Suppl 12):18S–24S.
59. Boye B, Jahnsen J, Mokleby K, et al. The INSPIRE study: are different personality traits related to disease-specific quality of life (IBDQ) in distressed patients with ulcerative colitis and Crohn's disease? Inflamm Bowel Dis 2008;14:680–6.
60. Maunder R, Esplen MJ. Facilitating adjustment to inflammatory bowel disease: a model of psychosocial intervention in non-psychiatric patients. Psychother Psychosom 1999;68:230–40.
61. Guyatt G, Mitchell A, Irvine EJ, et al. A new measure of health status for clinical trials in inflammatory bowel disease. Gastroenterology 1989;96:804–10.
62. Griffiths AM, Otley AR, Hyams J, et al. A review of activity indices and end points for clinical trials in children with Crohn's disease. Inflamm Bowel Dis 2005;11:185–96.
63. Perrin JM, Kuhlthau K, Chughtai A, et al. Measuring quality of life in pediatric patients with inflammatory bowel disease: psychometric and clinical characteristics. J Pediatr Gastroenterol Nutr 2008;46:164–71.
64. Blank C, Switzer G. The use of questionnaires in pediatric inflammatory bowel disease. Curr Gastroenterol Rep 2006;8:242–5.
65. Taft T, Keefer L, Leonhard C, et al. Impact of perceived stigma on inflammatory bowel disease patient outcomes. Inflamm Bowel Dis 2009;15:1224–32.
66. Drossman DA, Patrick DL, Mitchell CM, et al. Health-related quality of life in inflammatory bowel disease. Functional status and patient worries and concerns. Dig Dis Sci 1989;34:1379–86.
67. Otley AR, Griffiths AM, Hale S, et al. Healthy-related quality of life in the first year after diagnosis of pediatric inflammatory bowel disease. Inflamm Bowel Dis 2006;12:684–91.

68. Turunen P, Ashorn M, Auvinen A, et al. Long-term health outcomes in pediatric inflammatory bowel disease: a population-based study. Inflamm Bowel Dis 2009;15:56–62.

69. Upton P, Eiser C, Cheung I, et al. Measurement properties of the UK-English version of the Pediatric Quality of Life Inventory 4.0 (PedsQL) generic core scales. Health Qual Life Outcomes 2005;3:22.

70. Lynch T, Spence D. A qualitative study of youth living with Crohn's disease. Gastroenterol Nurs 2008;31:224–30.

71. Tojek TM, Lumley MA, Corlis M, et al. Maternal correlates of health status in adolescents with inflammatory bowel disease. J Psychosom Res 2002;52: 173–9.

72. Engstrom I. Parental distress and social interaction in families with children with inflammatory bowel disease. J Am Acad Child Adolesc Psychiatry 1991;30: 904–12.

73. Savard J, Woodgate R. Young peoples' experience of living with ulcerative colitis and an ostomy. Gastroenterol Nurs 2009;32:33–41.

74. Tuchman LK, Slap GB, Britto MT. Transition to adult care: experiences and expectations of adolescents with a chronic illness. Child Care Health Dev 2008;34:557–63.

75. Adler J, Raju S, Beveridge AS, et al. College adjustment in University of Michigan students with Crohn's and colitis. Inflamm Bowel Dis 2008;14:1281–6.

76. Fletcher P, Schneider M, Van Ravenswaay V, et al. I am doing the best that I can!: living with inflammatory bowel disease and/or irritable bowel syndrome (part II). Clin Nurse Spec 2008;22:278–85.

77. Mikocka-Walus AA, Turnbull DA, Moulding NT, et al. "It doesn't do any harm, but patients feel better": a qualitative exploratory study on gastroenterologists' perspective on the role of antidepressants in inflammatory bowel disease. BMC Gastroenterol 2007;7:38.

78. Mikocka-Walus AA, Turnbull DA, Moulding NT, et al. Antidepressants and inflammatory bowel disease: a systematic review. Clin Pract Epidemol Ment Health 2006;2:24.

79. Varghese AK, Verdù EF, Berick P, et al. Antidepressants attenuate increased susceptibility to colitis in a murine model of depression. Gastroenterology 2006;130:1743–53.

80. Kane S, Altschuler EL, Kast RE. Crohn's disease remission on bupropion. Gastroenterology 2003;125:1290.

81. Karwowski CA, Keljo D, Szigethy EM. Strategies to improve quality of life in adolescents with inflammatory bowel disease. Inflamm Bowel Dis 2009;15: 1755–64.

82. Casellas F, Fontanet G, Borruel N, et al. The opinion of patients with inflammatory bowel disease on healthcare received. Rev Esp Enferm Dig 2004;96: 174–84.

83. Moser G, Tillinger W, Sachs G, et al. Disease-related worries and concerns: a study on out-patients with inflammatory bowel disease. Eur J Gastroenterol Hepatol 1995;7:853–8.

84. Waters BM, Jensen L, Fedorak RN. Effects of formal education for patients with inflammatory bowel disease: a randomized controlled trial. Can J Gastroenterol 2005;19:235–44.

85. Larsson K, Sundberg HM, Karlborn U, et al. A group-based patient education programme for high-anxiety patients with Crohn disease or ulcerative colitis. Scand J Gastroenterol 2003;38:763–9.

86. Kennedy AP, Nelson E, Reeves D, et al. A randomised controlled trial to assess the effectiveness and cost of a patient orientated self management approach to chronic inflammatory bowel disease. Gut 2004;53:1639–45.

87. Garcia-Vega E, Fernandez-Rodriguez C. A stress management program for Crohn's disease. Behav Res Ther 2004;42:367–83.

88. Oxelmark L, Magnusson A, Löfberg R, et al. Group-based intervention program in inflammatory bowel disease patients: effects on quality of life. Inflamm Bowel Dis 2007;13:182–90.

89. Grootenhuis MA, Maurice-Stam H, Derkx BH, et al. Evaluation of a psychoeducational intervention for adolescents with inflammatory bowel disease. Eur J Gastroenterol Hepatol 2009;21:430–5.

90. Szigethy E, Kenney E, Carpenter J, et al. Cognitive behavioral therapy for adolescents with inflammatory bowel disease and subsyndromal depression. J Am Acad Child Adolesc Psychiatry 2007;46:1290–8.

91. Szigethy E, Craig AE, Iobst EA, et al. Profile of depression in adolescents with inflammatory bowel disease: implications for treatment. Inflamm Bowel Dis 2009;15:69–74.

92. Weisz JR, McCabe MA, Dennig MD. Primary and secondary control among children undergoing medical procedures: adjustment as a function of coping style. J Consult Clin Psychol 1994;62:324–32.

93. Weinman J, Petrie KJ, Moss-Morris R, et al. The illness perception questionnaire: a new method for assessing the cognitive representation of illness. Psychol Health 1996;11:431–40.

94. Bers MU, Gonzalez-Heydrich J, Demaso DR. Use of a computer-based application in a pediatric hemodialysis unit: a pilot study. J Am Acad Child Adolesc Psychiatry 2003;42:493–6.

95. De Maso DR, Marcus NE, Kinnamon C, et al. Depression experience journal: a computer-based intervention for families facing childhood depression. J Am Acad Child Adolesc Psychiatry 2006;45:158–65.

96. Miller V, Whorwell PJ. Treatment of inflammatory bowel disease: a role for hypnotherapy? Int J Clin Exp Hypn 2008;56:306–17.

97. Keefer L, Keshavarzian A. Feasibility and acceptability of gut-directed hypnosis on inflammatory bowel disease: a brief communication. Int J Clin Exp Hypn 2007;55:457–66.

98. Emami MH, Gholamrezaei A, Daneshgar H. Hypnotherapy as an adjuvant for the management of inflammatory bowel disease: a case report. Am J Clin Hypn 2009;51:255–62.

99. Mawdsley E, Jenkins DG, Macey MG, et al. The effect of hypnosis on systemic and rectal mucosal measures of inflammation in ulcerative colitis. Am J Gastroenterol 2008;103:1460–9.

100. Shaoul R, Sukhotnik I, Mogilner J. Hypnosis as an adjuvant treatment for children with inflammatory bowel disease. J Dev Behav Pediatr 2009;30:268.

101. Vlieger AM, Menko-Frankenhuis C, Wolfkamp SC, et al. Hypnotherapy for children with functional abdominal pain or irritable bowel syndrome: a randomized controlled trial. Gastroenterology 2007;133:1430–6.

102. Oliveira S, Zaltman C, Elia C, et al. Quality-of-life measurement in patients with inflammatory bowel disease receiving social support. Inflamm Bowel Dis 2007;13:470–4.

103. Shepanski MA, Hurd LB, Culton K, et al. Health-related quality of life improves in children and adolescents with inflammatory bowel disease after a camp sponsored by the Crohn's and Colitis Foundation of America. Inflamm Bowel Dis 2005;11:164–70.

104. Szigethy E, Hardy D, Craig AE, et al. Girls connect: effects of a support group for teenage girls with inflammatory bowel disease and their mothers. Inflamm Bowel Dis 2009;15:1127–8.

105. Jaff JC, Arnold J, Bousvaros A. Effective advocacy for patients with inflammatory bowel disease: communication with insurance companies, school administrators, employers, and other health care overseers. Inflamm Bowel Dis 2006;12: 814–23.

Psychological Considerations of the Child with Asthma

Todd E. Peters, MD[a],*, Gregory K. Fritz, MD[a,b,c]

KEYWORDS

• Children • Asthma • Anxiety • Depression • Review

Asthma is a chronic lung disease defined by paroxysmal cough, wheezing, and dyspnea. Physiologically, asthma is defined as reversible obstruction of airflow caused by inflammation and hyperresponsiveness of the airways.[1] This obstruction is shown by the presence of inflammatory cells, such as neutrophils, mast cells, and eosinophils, targeting the alveolar tissue of the lungs. These cells excrete multiple cytokines and other mediators of inflammation that can be detected by lavage of alveolar secretions.[2] In addition, airways of asthmatic patients are more prone to constrict in response to stimuli such as cold air, histamine, or environmental allergens. These changes lead to decreased expiratory airflow, as shown by lower forced expiratory volume after 1 second (FEV_1). Obstruction in asthma is defined as an FEV_1 less than 80% of predicted for a child's age and size along with an FEV_1 to forced vital capacity (FVC) ratio of less than 0.8. Asthma can be misdiagnosed because of a similar triad of symptoms seen in other disease processes, such as congestive heart failure, pneumonia, foreign-body aspiration, pertussis, or cystic fibrosis.[3,4] In addition, mental health professionals need to be aware of vocal cord dysfunction (VCD), a syndrome that presents as intractable asthma symptoms but does not involve the lungs. Accurate diagnosis is critical because VCD responds to speech therapy, relaxation training, and supportive psychotherapy, and not to asthma medications.[5]

Asthma is the most common chronic illness diagnosed in children and adolescents in the United States and Europe,[1] with variance in the prevalence seen worldwide.[6] In reviewing data from 2001 to 2003, the United States Centers for Disease Control and Prevention (CDC) reported an annual rate of 6.2 million children with asthma in the United States, with a higher prevalence in children than in adults (8.5% vs 6.5%).

A version of this article was previously published in the *Child and Adolescent Psychiatric Clinics of North America, 19:2.*

[a] Division of Child and Adolescent Psychiatry, Alpert Medical School of Brown University, Providence, RI, USA

[b] E.P. Bradley Hospital, 1011 Veteran's Memorial Highway, East Providence, RI 02915, USA

[c] Rhode Island Hospital/Hasbro Children's Hospital, Providence, RI, USA

* Corresponding author. Department of Child and Adolescent Psychiatry, Brown University, E.P. Bradley Hospital, 1011 Veteran's Memorial Highway, East Providence, RI 02915.

E-mail address: Todd_Peters@brown.edu

Pediatr Clin N Am 58 (2011) 921–935

doi:10.1016/j.pcl.2011.06.006

pediatric.theclinics.com

0031-3955/11/$ – see front matter © 2011 Elsevier Inc. All rights reserved.

The CDC's 2006 National Health Interview Study shows a lifetime prevalence of asthma in children of 13.5%.[7] Studies have documented a progressive increase in asthma prevalence from 1980 to 1996 along with an increased rate of asthma-related deaths during this time.[8] However, asthma prevalence rates have not changed to a discernable degree during the last 10 years, with the rate of deaths decreasing each year since 2000.[1] In addition, there are prominent disparities in the prevalence of childhood asthma in racial and socioeconomic subgroups. In the United States, there is a higher average annual prevalence of asthma in black (12.5%) and Puerto Rican (18.7%) children compared with white children (7.7%).[1,9] Based on recent data, these disparities remain throughout life.[7]

Because of high prevalence rates and prolonged natural course, asthma has a size-able economic and societal effect. A recent systematic review of the economic burden of asthma[10] detailed the effect of asthma on populations throughout the world. Asthma-related costs are direct and indirect. Direct costs, such as hospitalizations and medications, are strongly related to asthma severity. Most children have significant disability, leading to increased indirect costs as described by an overall decrease in productivity. This decreased productivity is a result of many missed school days by children and associated parental absenteeism from work. This gross financial effect is often in excess of $1000 per year for children, a rate that increases substantially with age and asthma severity.[10] In addition, a correlation was found between comorbid conditions and higher costs and resource use. Therefore, it is vital for treatment professionals to discuss asthma severity with those affected along with potential comorbid illnesses, such as stress and psychiatric illness.

HISTORICAL PERSPECTIVE OF ASTHMA AND PSYCHIATRIC ILLNESS

Before the advent of modern immunology and the development of the concept of atopy, asthma was considered primarily a nervous disease. In some early medical textbooks, this disease process was called asthma nervosa. In the 1940s to 1950s, psychoanalytic theorists (most notably Franz Alexander) described asthma as 1 of the 7 classic psychosomatic diseases caused by specific emotional conflicts. The conflict of asthma was between strong dependency wishes and a concomitant fear of separation; the wheeze was seen as a "suppressed cry for the mother."[11] Although this concept was intriguing, particularly from the perspective of an analyst envisioning a long-term treatment course, empiric investigations over the years failed to support this etiologic theory.

Over the past several decades, transformations in the field have emphasized a complex bidirectional integration of biologic and psychological factors, which are related to the course and functional outcomes of asthma. The onset and severity of asthma is currently believed to be predicted by a combination of genetics, environmental variables including exposure to infections, allergens, or irritants, and psychosocial influences such as maternal distress, psychological illness, and stress.[2,12,13] Recent evidence shows that maternal anxiety during pregnancy has been linked to significantly increased rates of asthma at approximately 7 years of age (odds ratio 1.64).[14] Maternal depression has also been consistently linked to asthma in childhood, resulting in higher morbidity as shown by more severe asthma symptoms,[15] higher number of unscheduled visits to physicians, and more frequent emergency room visits,[16] all resulting in a higher number of inpatient medical hospitalizations.[17–19] Furthermore, parental/caregiver stress has been linked to higher likelihood of wheezing[20] and associated respiratory infections[21] in early childhood; caregiver stress often results in family relationship issues and parenting difficulties, which can lead to more prevalent asthma symptoms and diagnosis in early childhood.[19,22]

In children suffering from asthma, it is apparent that dyspnea, paroxysmal cough, and wheezing induce prominent distress in those affected and can lead to emergency room visits and subsequent hospitalizations. Conversely, dyspnea and shortness of breath are central symptoms of panic attacks, which can lead to hyperventilation and ultimately worsen bronchoconstriction. However, there has been considerable debate as to whether or not children with asthma have more behavioral problems or psychiatric disturbance than healthy peers, with results of individual studies supporting both positions.

ASTHMA AS A PREDISPOSING FACTOR TO PSYCHIATRIC ILLNESS IN YOUNG PEOPLE

Recent studies have demonstrated an increased diagnosis of psychiatric illness in children with asthma compared with healthy controls. A rigorous meta-analysis of all such studies concluded that children with asthma have a small but consistent increased risk for behavioral difficulties relative to healthy children.[23] This study found a direct link between asthma severity and worse behavioral issues and reported a prevalence of internalizing symptoms (anxiety and depression) compared with externalizing symptoms (hyperactivity or oppositionality). These findings are consistent with a previous study by Wamboldt and colleagues,[24] which found that parental ratings of internalizing symptoms were correlated with asthma severity. In addition, Kashani and colleagues[25] in 1988 performed a small study (n = 112) of asthmatic young people and found a statistically significant increase of anxiety symptoms reported by parents of children with asthma compared with normal controls.

Asthma and its Association with Anxiety Disorders

Despite the increase in symptoms, it remained to be determined whether there was an association between asthma and increased diagnosis of internalizing disorders in children. Most research in this field has explored a link between asthma and anxiety disorders, which also demonstrated a higher level of anxiety disorders in the asthmatic population in children, as reviewed recently by Katon and colleagues[26] One of the first studies examining the prevalence of anxiety disorders in the pediatric population with asthma was reported by Bussing and colleagues[27] in 1996. This study demonstrated an increased prevalence of anxiety disorders in children with asthma (43.2%) compared with healthy controls (19.4%) in a study of 62 children. Two subsequent studies by Vila and colleagues[28,29] compared children with asthma with a similar number of children with insulin-dependent diabetes and healthy controls. These studies found that 32% to 35% of children with asthma met criteria for an anxiety disorder, with clinically increased mean scores on the State-Trait Anxiety Inventory for Children and Child Behavior Checklist in the asthmatic group compared with the diabetic group. The latter study[29] found a high prevalence of generalized anxiety disorder of 24% in the studied asthmatic population. These findings were followed by a large (n >1000) longitudinal study of children from age 3 to 21 years that determined that a diagnosis of asthma before age 18 years resulted in an increased risk for agoraphobia or panic disorder in early adulthood.[30] This research paved the way for research on a large community sample of 1285 young people called the Methods of the Epidemiology of Child and Adolescent Mental Disorders Survey. Through analysis of this population, Ortega and colleagues[31] determined a prevalence of anxiety disorders in 49.2% of those suffering from asthma compared with 37.7% of healthy controls along with clinically increased diagnosis of simple phobia, separation anxiety disorder, and overanxious disorder. Goodwin and colleagues[32] also performed a secondary analysis of this population, finding a statistically significant risk of panic attacks in the asthmatic population (odds ratio = 1.5). Similar correlations were shown in studies of a community sample of Puerto Rican children, which determined a greater risk of internalizing disorders in children affected by asthma compared with nonasthmatic Puerto Rican young people at baseline and 1-year follow-up while controlling for socioeconomic factors.[33,34] In a recent study of 200 adolescents, those who suffered life-threatening asthma symptoms had higher levels of posttraumatic stress symptoms and associated diagnosis of posttraumatic stress disorder (PTSD). In addition, a diagnosis of PTSD was found to be directly linked to asthma morbidity.[35] Within the last 5 years, 2 studies have attempted to investigate the link between social anxiety and history of asthma symptoms. These studies by Ortega and colleagues[36] and Bruzzese and colleagues[37] found no significant correlation between a lifetime diagnosis of asthma and social phobia; however, the latter study[37] demonstrated a significant link between active asthma symptoms with higher levels of social anxiety, as seen on the Social Anxiety Scale of Adolescents.

Following these initial studies, Katon and colleagues[38] conducted the largest study to date (n = 1379) of psychiatric illness in young people with asthma. This study was completed after interviewing children (aged 11–17 years) with the telephone version of the National Institute of Mental Health Diagnostic Interview Schedule for Children (NIMH DISC-4.0) and subsequent parent interview, reviewing sociodemographic factors and completing the Child Behavior Checklist (CBCL) for all participants. This study demonstrated an almost twofold increased prevalence of at least 1 anxiety or depressive disorder diagnosis in asthmatic children (16.3%) when compared with normal controls (8.6%). It was also found that several independent factors significantly increased the risk of meeting criteria for 1 or more internalizing disorders, including female gender, living with a single parent, increased report of externalizing behaviors by parents, a more recent diagnosis of asthma, and more impairment from asthma symptoms.

Asthma and its Link to Depression and Increased Risk Behaviors

Other studies have reported an increased link between negative affect, depression, and other psychiatric disorders in asthmatic children and adolescents. Blackman and Gurka[39] reviewed data taken from the National Survey of Children's Health 2003, which was designed to investigate the health of the general child population in a random selection of 102,353 children aged 0 to 17 years, including the national prevalence of emotional and behavioral issues.[40] This research found clinically increased rates of depression, attention-deficit/hyperactivity disorder (ADHD), behavioral disorders, and learning disabilities in asthmatic young people. Furthermore, a diagnosis of asthma was associated with an increased likelihood of being bullied, along with higher rates of missed school. The severity of asthma symptoms was also found to be directly linked to the likelihood of depression, learning disabilities, ADHD, and other behavioral disorders.[39] Asthma is also correlated with increased risk-taking behaviors in children, including increased substance abuse, driving without a seat belt, and dangerous sexual practices.[39,41] In 2007, Bender reviewed data on depression and substance use in asthmatic young people who participated in the CDC's 2005 Youth Risk Behavior Survey,[42] which monitors 13,917 high-school students for high-risk behaviors that can result in unintentional injuries and violence. In the 720 young people surveyed who were diagnosed with asthma (5.2% of total population), depression and rates of cigarette and cocaine use were more common than in those without asthma.[43] These findings are augmented by a recent research study on asthmatic young people that found an increased risk of cigarette use in those affected by comorbid anxiety and depressive disorders.[44]

PSYCHIATRIC ILLNESS AND ITS CORRELATION WITH ASTHMA SEVERITY IN YOUNG PEOPLE

Conversely, sadness and the diagnosis of depression and anxiety may be associated with more severe asthma symptoms. Waxmonsky and colleagues[45] monitored a group of asthmatic, inner-city children (n = 129) and found clinically increased depressive symptoms in 26% of subjects. In this depressed subgroup, children's self-reported neurovegetative symptoms strongly correlated with asthma activity, more so than either parental depression or parent/clinician ratings of the child's depression. Anxiety and depression are strongly correlated with asthma symptom burden in children and adolescents. Asthmatic children with 1 or more internalizing disorders have a higher number of days with asthma symptoms compared with asthmatic young people without an internalizing disorder.[46] Recent research demonstrates that higher negative affect scores predict increased asthma symptom severity as rated by children and their parents.[47]

Stress and emotional responses are also related to inflammation and airway resistance. Some of the early conceptualizations of asthma as psychosomatic may derive from case reports of emotions as a trigger for asthma exacerbations. Although asthma is not seen as largely caused by emotions, research does demonstrate that emotions can trigger asthma symptoms in 15% to 30% of people with asthma.[48,49] In a laboratory setting in which children with asthma were monitored while watching affectively evocative film scenes, marked emotional and autonomic responses were observed. These responses were associated with increased airway reactivity and decreased pulmonary function.[50] Experimental studies in which pulmonary function is measured before and after a patient is exposed to a stressful experience, such as performing mental arithmetic, watching emotionally charged films, or public speaking, consistently show significant bronchoconstriction in about 22% of studied asthmatic patients.[51] In addition, evidence suggests that stressful, negative life events significantly increase the risk of a new asthma attack within 2 days of the event, along with a higher potential for a delayed attack 5 to 7 weeks later.[52]

The mechanism that links emotional processes to asthma exacerbations is unclear, but autonomic mediation is likely. In addition to the direct effects of the autonomic system on bronchial smooth muscle, there are bidirectional relationships between the neuroendocrine system (including the hypothalamic-pituitary-adrenal axis) and the immune system that influence lung inflammation.[49,53–55] On a molecular level, T-cell lymphocytes have 2 different responses to microbial or allergen exposures: Th1 or proallergenic Th2 responses. In asthma and atopy, the Th1/Th2 dynamic equilibrium has been shown to be unbalanced, demonstrating increased Th2 activity and associated cytokine response, such as interleukin (IL)-4, IL-5, and IL-13.[56–62] Emotional stress produced in the laboratory setting has been associated with a greater increase in the ratio of Th2 cytokines versus Th1 in asthmatic children compared with controls, which reflects proinflammatory activity.[63] On a biochemical level, evidence suggests that the biologic link intertwining anxiety symptoms and asthma may be the brainstem respiratory sensor system as it responds to real or perceived increases in $Paco_2$ to stave off impending asphyxiation.

MANAGEMENT OF ASTHMA
Classification and Assessment of Asthma Severity

It is essential that mental health professionals working with asthmatic children be familiar with the medical management of the illness. Asthma is classified into 2 major classes based on symptom prevalence: intermittent versus persistent. Intermittent symptoms occur 2 or less days per week, cause no significant interference with normal activity, and do not cause nighttime awakenings. Persistent symptoms are classified into mild, moderate, and severe subcategories, based on lung function, the prevalence of symptoms during the daytime, nighttime awakenings, frequency of rescue-inhaler use, and frequency of severe exacerbations requiring oral glucocorticoids, as detailed in the National Asthma Education Prevention Program (NAEPP) Expert Panel Report for 2007.[64] The goals of treatment are to reduce impairment through adherence to an individualized asthma treatment plan. This plan entails providing patient/family education, monitoring lung function, controlling environmental factors and triggers, treating comorbid conditions that can exacerbate asthma, and providing proper pharmacologic therapy with quick relief and long-term, controller medications.[65]

Monitoring of asthma and pulmonary function is generally performed at home and in the medical office. Pulmonary function is most commonly assessed at home by measurement of peak expiratory flow rate (PEFR), which is decreased with obstruction seen during asthma exacerbations. A normal PEFR range is individualized for each patient and is defined as 80% to 100% of the child's best PEFR reading or 80% to 100% of an expected PEFR for a child of that age and size. PEFR can be checked as often as tolerated on inexpensive, widely available, peak flow meters and can be vital in asthma monitoring and control. However, the PEFR index is highly effort dependent and peak flow meters have their limitations. Spirometry is preferred by the NAEPP in children aged 5 years and older for studying PEFR, FEV_1, and FVC in the medical office setting; home spirometry is expensive but increasingly available. In an effort to control asthma, individual asthma triggers should be identified. Screening should focus on seasonal components versus year-round symptoms, exposure to smoke (tobacco and workplace), indoor and outdoor pollutants, and sulfites in the diet. Illnesses that may exacerbate asthma, such as upper respiratory infections, influenza, gastroesophageal reflux disease, and rhinitis, should be assessed and treated. Medications, such as β-blockers and antiinflammatory agents (such as aspirin or nonsteroidal antiinflammatory drugs), can also cause or worsen asthma symptoms.

Pharmacologic Interventions for Asthma

Pharmacologic treatment focuses on a stepwise approach based on asthma severity.[64,65] For quick relief in all classes of severity, inhaled, short-acting β2-agonists (SABA), such as albuterol, levalbuterol, or pirbuterol, should be used as needed. Intermittent asthma, by definition, should be adequately managed by use of these agents alone (step 1). Inadequate control is usually shown by use of short-acting agents more than 2 times per week, which often necessitates a step-up in treatment. Persistent asthma requires daily medication use, starting first with low-dose inhaled corticosteroid (ICS) use (step 2), using agents such as budesonide, fluticasone, beclomethasone, triamcinolone, or mometasone. Other agents, such as cromolyn, leukotriene-receptor agonists, nedocromil, or theophylline, can be used instead of inhaled steroids if there are adverse effects or sensitivities. If insufficient, subsequent titration of the ICS or addition of long-acting β2-agonist bronchodilators (LABA), such as formoterol or salmeterol, is recommended (step 3). If these changes are inadequate, the dosing of each agent is titrated (steps 4 and 5) until the addition of oral corticosteroids is warranted (step 6). If asthma is well controlled for more than 3 months on a certain step, a step-down is considered if clinically possible.

Treatment of asthma is often complicated, laden with potential risks, side effects, and adverse effects. One of the biggest complicating factors with treatment is poor patient adherence. Research has demonstrated limited adherence to controller medications in children with asthma, with a likely adherence rate across studies of approximately 50% to 60%.[66–70] Adolescents with asthma have increased knowledge about the disease process and treatment and usually have assumed greater responsibility for treatment; however, they also seem to have lower treatment compliance than younger children.[70] Although strategies of prevention of exacerbations focus on psychoeducation,[64–71] prior research has found little association between knowledge and reasoning about asthma with adherence.[70]

MANAGEMENT OF PSYCHOLOGICAL COMPONENTS OF ASTHMA
Assessment of Complicating Factors

As discussed earlier, asthma symptoms include anxiety-inducing dyspnea, which often necessitates medical interventions and hospitalizations, which in turn further provoke anxiety in a child. If repeated over time, these experiences may contribute to the development of an anxiety disorder. Conversely, dyspnea and shortness of breath are central symptoms of panic attacks, which can lead to hyperventilation. This hyperventilation, with its associated colder air moved more deeply into the lungs, has the potential to precipitate or aggravate asthmatic bronchoconstriction. In addition, evidence shows comorbid behavior problems and psychiatric disorders have been associated with limited asthma control, marked by poor adherence to the treatment regimen.[43] Psychiatric disorders in asthmatic patients are underdiagnosed, which results in increased treatment costs. The rate of recognition of anxiety and depression for children diagnosed with asthma is low; approximately 35% of depressive disorders are diagnosed, with a slightly higher recognition (43%) of major depressive disorders.[72] These low recognition rates are complicated by low agreement rates between children and parents regarding diagnosis of an internalizing disorder.[73] In addition, few children in the asthmatic population receive optimal mental health treatment.[72] An increased health care cost of approximately 50% was found in asthmatic young people with a depressive disorder with or without an associated anxiety disorder, which was also correlated with higher health care use than asthmatic young people without an internalizing disorder.[74] Furthermore, internalizing disorders seen in asthmatic patients may be exacerbated by side effects from conventional asthma treatments. Certain asthma medications, such at β_2-agonists, can increase autonomic arousal, thereby worsening anxiety symptoms. When anxiety disorders and asthma coexist, the risk of overuse of bronchodilators is considerable. Behavioral disturbances and worsening anxiety can also occur with inhaled steroids, whereas oral steroid use can be linked to worsening anxiety and depression, with the potential to lead to mania or psychosis.

Improving Symptom Perception

The corollary to these findings is that identification and effective treatment of psychiatric disorders frequently leads to better asthma management and decreased morbidity. One of the ways to improve asthma management is to focus on symptom perception in asthmatic young people.[75] An emerging literature links psychological characteristics with the ability to perceive varying degrees of respiratory compromise accurately. Recognition of early clinical symptoms prompts the early initiation of timely and appropriate self-management strategies, which in turn minimizes asthma morbidity. In the psychiatric literature on somatization, a range of characteristic individual patterns of responding to physical symptoms has been described, from extreme stoicism and denial (eg, the football player who plays an entire game with a broken hand) to those who amplify their symptoms. Those who amplify symptoms are often seen as somatizers or hypochondriacs. Prior research on limited sensitivity to resistive respiratory loads was found to increase the likelihood of near-fatal asthma attacks when compared with other people with asthma and control subjects.[76,77] Therefore, the literature on perception of asthma symptoms is relevant to our understanding of the psychiatric phenomenon of somatization, and vice versa.

Researchers have several methods to quantify perceptual accuracy of asthma in children and adults. These approaches involve individuals rating their subjective degree of compromise before objective pulmonary function testing, either in a laboratory with a methacholine challenge test or naturalistically, using a portable spirometric device that stores corresponding subjective and objective data points.[78] The accuracy of perception can be summarized by the level of correlation between the subjective judgment and the objective reality. In general, most individuals perceive pulmonary function compromise with reasonable accuracy; however, some perceptual patterns may be problematic for disease management. In several studies involving different populations of children, greater perceptual accuracy has predicted less morbidity, at baseline and at 1-year follow-up.[79] However, some children are dangerously inaccurate, ignoring or underestimating significant impairment, whereas others tend to overestimate their compromise.[80]

These patterns are illustrated by comparing 2 children of similar age and asthma severity seen in the authors' clinic. One 11-year-old boy had subjectively predicted peak flow values that were consistently lower than his actual peak flow values. His pattern was to magnify his degree of compromise, and his clinical history over the preceding year was one of high use of health care. Despite having readily controlled moderate persistent asthma, this patient had 2 inpatient hospitalizations, 10 emergency room visits, and 12 unscheduled visits to his pediatrician. His high level of sensitivity and concern led to excessive use of asthma-related medication and health care, placing him at substantial risk for side effects from overmedication and other iatrogenic problems. In contrast, a 14-year-old boy had similar symptoms and a diagnosis of moderate persistent asthma, but was accurate at perceiving his pulmonary function at any given time. This child had no history of hospitalizations, emergency department visits, or unscheduled pediatric visits in the preceding year. Although several factors, such as disease severity, family context, and health care access, are also relevant with this comparison, these cases illustrate the importance of individual variability in detecting and assessing severity of asthma symptoms.

Relaxation and Biofeedback

Psychological treatments have also proven helpful in treating physical symptoms of asthma, especially for children with asthma symptoms that are triggered emotionally, as previously reviewed by McQuaid and Nassau.[81] Early studies by Alexander[82,83] reported positive outcomes from progressive muscle relaxation, noting modest improvements in PEFR that were later replicated by Miklich.[84] The likely benefit from this intervention is related to the potential emotional triggering of asthma exacerbations. Later research by Vasquez and Buceta[85–87] showed limited benefit from relaxation alone in providing pulmonary function test improvements; however, for those children with emotionally triggered asthma symptoms, relaxation and self-management could limit the duration of asthma exacerbations. Even although they demonstrate clinically significant pulmonary function changes in the treatment groups, these studies were hampered by a small degree of improvement (<10% change) from baseline and limited long-term follow-up of results.[81,88]

In comparison, electromyogram (EMG) biofeedback has a strong, well-supported evidence base demonstrating its benefit in children with emotionally triggered asthma. The strength of biofeedback in this population centers around the core principle that a physical symptom can be influenced by continuous reporting on the physiology of that symptom. Early research in the field used biofeedback to augment relaxation training.[89,90] However, researchers began to speculate that EMG biofeedback of stress in the frontalis muscle may be related to airflow resistance via a reflexive mechanism with the trigeminal and vagus nerve systems.[81,91,92] Studies on reducing stress reflected in the frontalis muscle by EMG biofeedback reported clinical benefit in improving PEFR, exceeding benefits seen in comparative brachioradialis biofeedback.[93,94] These results led to further investigation into the short-term and long-term effects of EMG frontalis feedback. Children who were instructed to reduce frontalis muscle tension via biofeedback and continue these strategies in the home setting showed improvement in pulmonary function testing compared with children who were instructed to maintain frontalis tension.[91] These benefits of biofeedback may also translate into decreased respiratory resistance; however, evidence for this mechanism is limited to several adult studies and 1 early study in children.[95] In this study of 4 children, Feldman examined tonal feedback from forced oscillation, which is a technique used to determine airway resistance in obstructive airway diseases. This technique is performed by measurement of the velocity of returned air produced in a pulsed fashion from a sine-wave pump placed at the patient's mouth; with increased resistance, there is an associated increase in the frequency of resonated air. In this study, this higher resonated frequency correlated to a higher tonal pitch; patients were instructed to decrease the tonal pitch, thereby decreasing airway resistance. All participants demonstrated improvement in airway resistance. These intriguing findings in children have never been replicated, but would seem to merit further controlled research in a larger population.

School-based Interventions

Interventions treating the psychological aspects of asthma are not limited to laboratory testing, however. As described earlier, indirect costs of asthma are exorbitant; children with asthma miss approximately 10 million days of school each year.[64] In an effort to address this societal cost, many educational programs have been developed for parents and children with asthma. These programs were created to occur either during the day or as part of after-school education. In a recent review of these educational programs, Guevara and colleagues[96] found improvements in lung function, school absenteeism, nighttime symptoms, and visits to emergency departments. However, these programs were limited by parental availability and difficulty in accessing children's classes.[97]

In 2000, an after-school program for asthma education was developed in Providence, Rhode Island in effort to address limitations from prior studies. This program, called the Providence School Asthma Partnership, used a school-based model in an after-school setting to provide psychoeducation for inner-city families.[97] During the 3-year study period, 972 families participated in this 1-time, 2.5-hour after-school program, which focused on asthma knowledge, management of asthma triggers, and use of appropriate treatment strategies. All parents were given the opportunity to repeat this workshop as necessary along with attending a bimonthly support group, established by the program. In this study, all measured outcomes significantly improved during the 1-year treatment period. Frequency of asthma symptoms was reduced from several times per week to less than once per week. In addition, the prevalence of those children hospitalized in a given year decreased from 11% to

2% along with the frequency of emergency room visits (35% to 4%). Those children who missed school because of asthma symptoms decreased from 48% to 20%. Most importantly, this program has been sustained by private and government insurance reimbursement, providing a model that can likely be reproduced throughout the country.

SUMMARY

Asthma is a very prevalent and costly illness, affecting society in high direct and indirect costs. The triad of asthma symptoms (dyspnea, intermittent cough, and wheezing) can cause marked and potentially life-threatening distress in children suffering from asthma. As detailed in this review, the effect of asthma is not confined to respiratory distress and airway inflammation. Asthma is associated with a higher prevalence of internalizing psychiatric disorders, which in turn can further exacerbate asthma symptoms and perceived distress. The severity of self-reported neurovegetative and anxiety symptoms is directly associated with functional status, psychologically and physiologically, and can lead to worsened morbidity.[98] These findings emphasize the need for increased awareness of the association between asthma and psychiatric illness along with improved treatment strategies for asthma-related symptoms. Treatment providers should consider screening all children with asthma for depression, anxiety, and high-risk behaviors. This screening may take the form of a clinical interview in a primary care physician's office to a full psychiatric/diagnostic interview for those at highest risk.[43,99,100] In addition, mental health professionals should consider discussion of asthma control with asthmatic patients and their families seen in psychiatric clinics and hospital settings. This intervention may serve as a conduit into further psychological management and other treatment strategies. Improving asthma education and enhancing asthma control will lead to diminished psychiatric symptoms, which will ultimately decrease morbidity of this prevalent chronic disease of childhood.

REFERENCES

1. Moorman J, Rudd RA, Johnson CA, et al. National surveillance for asthma – United States, 1980–2004. MMWR Surveill Summ 2007;56(SS08):1–14, 18–54.
2. Busse WW, Lemanske RF. Asthma. N Engl J Med 2001;344(5):350–62.
3. Weinberger M, Abu-Hasan M. Pseudo-asthma: when cough, wheezing, and dyspnea are not asthma. Pediatrics 2007;120(4):855–64.
4. Weinberger M, Abu-Hasan M. Perceptions and pathophysiology of dyspnea and exercise tolerance. Pediatr Clin North Am 2009;56(1):33–48.
5. McQuaid EL, Spieth LE, Spirito A. The pediatric psychologist's role in differential diagnosis: vocal-cord dysfunction presenting as asthma. J Pediatr Psychol 1997;22(5):739–48.
6. Lai CK, Beasley R, Crane J, et al. Global variation in the prevalence and severity of asthma symptoms: phase three of the International Study of Asthma and Allergies in Childhood (ISAAC). Thorax 2009;64(6):476–83.
7. National Health Interview Survey, National Center for Health Statistics, CDC. Centers for Disease Control and Prevention website. Table 1-1 and 2-1. 2008. Available at: http://www.cdc.gov/asthma/nhis/06/data.htm. Accessed December 1, 2009.
8. Akinbami LJ, Schoendorf KC. Trends in childhood asthma: prevalence, health care utilization, and mortality. Pediatrics 2002;110(2):315–22.

9. Canino G, Koinis-Mitchell D, Ortega AN, et al. Asthma disparities in the prevalence, morbidity, and treatment of Latino children. Soc Sci Med 2006;63(11): 2926–37.

10. Bahadori K, Doyle-Waters MM, Marra C, et al. Economic burden of asthma: a systematic review. BMC Pulm Med 2009;19:9–24.

11. Alexander F. Psychosomatic medicine: its principles and application. New York: W.W. Norton & Co; 1950.

12. Kozyrskyj AL, Mustard CA, Simons FER. Socioeconomic status, drug insurance benefits, and new prescriptions for inhaled corticosteroids in schoolchildren with asthma. Arch Pediatr Adolesc Med 2001;155(11):1219–24.

13. Kozyrskyj AL, Mai X, McGrath P, et al. Continued exposure to maternal distress in early life is associated with an increased risk of childhood asthma. Am J Respir Crit Care Med 2008;177(2):142–7.

14. Cookson H, Granell R, Joinson C, et al. Mothers' anxiety during pregnancy is associated with asthma in their children. J Allergy Clin Immunol 2009;123(4): 847–53.

15. Shalowitz MU, Berry CA, Quinn KA, et al. The relationship of life stressors and maternal depression to pediatric asthma morbidity in a subspecialty practice. Ambul Pediatr 2001;1(4):185–93.

16. Bartlett SJ, Kolodner K, Butz AM, et al. Maternal depressive symptoms and emergency department use among inner-city children with asthma. Arch Pediatr Adolesc Med 2001;155:347–53.

17. Weil CM, Wade SL, Bauman LJ, et al. The relationship between psychosocial factors and asthma morbidity in inner-city children with asthma. Pediatrics 1999;104(6):1274–80.

18. Brown ES, Gan V, Jeffress J, et al. Psychiatric symptomatology and disorders in caregivers of children with asthma. Pediatrics 2006;118(6):e1715–20.

19. Chen E, Schreier HMC. Does the social environment contribute to asthma? Immunol Allergy Clin North Am 2008;28:649–64.

20. Wright RJ, Cohen S, Carey V, et al. Parental stress as a predictor of wheezing in infancy: a prospective birth-cohort study. Am J Respir Crit Care Med 2002; 165(3):358–65.

21. Klinnert MD, Nelson HS, Price MR, et al. Onset and persistence of childhood asthma: predictors from infancy. Pediatrics 2001;108(4):e69.

22. Klinnert MD, Mrazek PJ, Mrazek DA. Early asthma onset: the interaction between family stressors and adaptive parenting. Psychiatry 1994;57(1):51–61.

23. McQuaid EL, Kopel SJ, Nassau JH. Behavioral adjustment in children with asthma: a meta-analysis. J Dev Behav Pediatr 2001;22(6):430–9.

24. Wamboldt MZ, Fritz G, Mansell A, et al. Relationship of asthma severity and psychological problems in children. J Am Acad Child Adolesc Psychiatry 1998;37(9):943–50.

25. Kashani JH, König P, Shepperd JA, et al. Psychopathology and self-concept in asthmatic children. J Pediatr Psychol 1998;13(4):509–20.

26. Katon WJ, Richardson L, Lozano P, et al. The relationship of asthma and anxiety disorders. Psychosom Med 2004;66(3):349–55.

27. Bussing R, Burket RC, Kelleher ET. Prevalence of anxiety disorders in a clinic-based sample of pediatric asthma patients. Psychosomatics 1996;37(2): 108–15.

28. Vila G, Nollet-Clemençon C, Vera M, et al. Prevalence of DSM-IV disorders in children and adolescents with asthma versus diabetes. Can J Psychiatry 1999;44(6):562–9.

29. Vila G, Nollet-Clemençon C, de Blic J, et al. Prevalence of DSM IV anxiety and affective disorders in a pediatric population of asthmatic children and adolescents. J Affect Disord 2000;58(3):223–31.

30. Craske MG, Poulton R, Tsao JCI, et al. Paths to panic disorder/agoraphobia: an exploratory analysis from age 3 to 21 in an unselected birth cohort. J Am Acad Child Adolesc Psychiatry 2001;40(5):556–63.

31. Ortega AN, Huertas SE, Canino G, et al. Childhood asthma, chronic illness, and psychiatric disorders. J Nerv Ment Dis 2002;190(5):275–81.

32. Goodwin RD, Pine DS, Hoven CW. Asthma and panic attacks among youth in the community. J Asthma 2003;40(2):139–45.

33. Ortega AN, McQuaid EL, Canino G, et al. Association of psychiatric disorders and different indicators of asthma in island Puerto Rican children. Soc Psychiatry Psychiatr Epidemiol 2003;38(4):220–6.

34. Feldman JM, Ortega AN, McQuaid EL, et al. Comorbidity between asthma attacks and internalizing disorders among Puerto Rican children at one-year follow-up. Psychosomatics 2006;47(4):333–9.

35. Kean EM, Kelsay K, Wamboldt F, et al. Posttraumatic stress in adolescents with asthma and their parents. J Am Acad Child Adolesc Psychiatry 2006;45(1):78–86.

36. Ortega AN, McQuaid EL, Canino G, et al. Comorbidity of asthma and anxiety and depression in Puerto Rican children. Psychosomatics 2004;45(2):93–9.

37. Bruzzese J, Fisher PH, Lemp N, et al. Asthma and social anxiety in adolescents. J Pediatr 2009;155(3):398–403.

38. Katon W, Lozano P, Russo J, et al. The prevalence of DSM-IV anxiety and depressive disorders in youth with asthma compared to controls. J Adolesc Health 2007;41(5):455–63.

39. Blackman JA, Gurka MJ. Developmental and behavioral comorbidities of asthma in children. J Dev Behav Pediatr 2007;28(2):92–9.

40. van Dyck P, Kogan MD, Heppel D, et al. The National Survey of Children's Health: a new data resource. Matern Child Health J 2004;8(3):183–8.

41. Bender B. Risk taking, depression, adherence, and symptom control in adolescents and young adults with asthma. Am J Respir Crit Care Med 2006;173(9): 953–7.

42. Eaton DK, Kann L, Kinchen S. Youth risk behavior surveillance – United States, 2005. MMWR Surveill Summ 2006;55(5):1–108.

43. Bender BG. Depression symptoms and substance abuse in adolescents with asthma. Ann Allergy Asthma Immunol 2007;99(4):319–24.

44. Bush T, Richardson L, Katon W, et al. Anxiety and depressive disorders are associated with smoking in adolescents with asthma. J Adolesc Health 2007; 40(5):425–32.

45. Waxmonsky J, Wood BL, Stern T, et al. Association of depressive symptoms and disease activity in children with asthma: methodological and clinical implications. J Am Acad Child Adolesc Psychiatry 2006;45(8):945–54.

46. Richardson LP, Lozano P, Russo J, et al. Asthma symptom burden: relationship to asthma severity and anxiety and depression symptoms. Pediatrics 2006; 118(3):1042–51.

47. Bender B, Zhang L. Negative affect, medication adherence, and asthma control in children. J Allergy Clin Immunol 2008;122(3):490–5.

48. Isenberg SA, Lehrer PM, Hochron S. The effects of suggestion and emotional arousal on pulmonary function in asthma: a review and hypothesis regarding vagal mediation. Psychosom Med 1992;54(2):192–216.

49. Wright RJ, Rodriguez M, Cohen S. Review of psychosocial stress and asthma: an integrated biopsychosocial approach. Thorax 1998;53(12):1066–74.
50. Miller BD, Wood BL. Influence of specific emotional states on autonomic reactivity and pulmonary function in asthmatic children. J Am Acad Child Adolesc Psychiatry 1997;36(5):669–77.
51. McQuaid EL, Fritz GK, Nassau JH, et al. Stress and airway resistance in children with asthma. J Psychosom Res 2000;49(4):239–45.
52. Sandberg S, Järvenpää S, Penttinen A, et al. Asthma exacerbations in children immediately following stressful life events: a Cox's hierarchical regression. Thorax 2004;59(12):1046–51.
53. Wright RJ. Stress and atopic disorders. J Allergy Clin Immunol 2005;116(6): 1301–6.
54. Wright RJ, Cohen CT, Cohen S. The impact of stress on the development and expression of atopy. Curr Opin Allergy Clin Immunol 2005;5(1):23–9.
55. Chen E, Miller GE. Stress and inflammation in exacerbations of asthma. Brain Behav Immun 2007;21(8):993–9.
56. Robinson D, Hamid Q, Bentley A, et al. Activation of CD4+ T cells, increased TH2-type cytokine mRNA expression, and eosinophil recruitment in bronchoalveolar lavage after allergen inhalation challenge in patients with atopic asthma. J Allergy Clin Immunol 1993;92(2):313–24.
57. Boniface S, Koscher V, Mamessier E, et al. Assessment of T lymphocyte cytokine production in induced sputum from asthmatics: a flow cytometry study. Clin Exp Allergy 2003;33(9):1238–43.
58. Macaubas C, de Klerk NH, Holt BJ, et al. Association between antenatal cytokine production in the development of atopy and asthma at age 6 years. Lancet 2003;362(9391):1192–7.
59. Neaville WA, Tisler BS, Bhattacharya A, et al. Developmental cytokine response profiles and the clinical and immunologic expression of atopy during the first year of life. J Allergy Clin Immunol 2003;112(4):740–6.
60. Prescott SL, King B, Strong TL, et al. The value of perinatal immune responses in predicting allergic disease at 6 years of age. Allergy 2003;58(11):1187–94.
61. Cho S, Stanciu LA, Holgate ST, et al. Increased interleukin-4, interleukin-5, and interferon-gamma in airway CD4+ and CD8+ T cells in atopic asthma. Am J Respir Crit Care Med 2005;171(3):224–30.
62. Ngoc PL, Gold DR, Tzianabos AO, et al. Cytokines, allergy, and asthma. Curr Opin Allergy Clin Immunol 2005;5(2):161–6.
63. Nassau JH, Tien K, Fritz GK. Review of the literature: integrating psychoneuroimmunology into pediatric chronic illness interventions. J Pediatr Psychol 2008;33(2):195–207.
64. National Asthma Education and Prevention Program Expert Panel Report 3. Summary Report 2007–guidelines for the diagnosis and management of asthma. NIH Publication Number 08–5846. Available at: http://www.nhlbi.nih. gov/guidelines/asthma/asthsumm.pdf. Accessed December 1, 2009.
65. Fanta CH. Asthma. N Engl J Med 2009;360(10):1002–14.
66. Milgrom H, Bender B, Ackerson L, et al. Clinical aspects of allergic disease. J Allergy Clin Immunol 1996;98(6 Pt 1):1051–7.
67. Bender B, Milgrom H, Rand C, et al. Psychological factors associated with medication nonadherence in asthmatic children. J Asthma 1998;35(4):347–53.
68. Celano M, Geller RJ, Phillips KM, et al. Treatment adherence among low-income children with asthma. J Pediatr Psychol 1998;23(6):345–9.

69. Bender B, Wamboldt FS, O'Connor SL, et al. Measurement of children's asthma medication adherence by self report, mother report, canister weight, and Doser CT. Ann Allergy Asthma Immunol 2000;85(5):416–21.

70. McQuaid EL, Kopel SJ, Klein RB, et al. Medication adherence in pediatric asthma: reasoning, responsibility, and behavior. J Pediatr Psychol 2003;28(5): 323–33.

71. McQuaid EL, Howard K, Kopel SJ, et al. Developmental concepts of asthma: reasoning about illness and strategies for prevention. J Appl Dev Psychol 2002;23(2):179–94.

72. Katon WJ, Richardson L, Russo J, et al. Quality of mental health care for youth with asthma and comorbid anxiety and depression. Med Care 2006;44(12): 1064–72.

73. Rockhill CM, Russo JE, McCauley E, et al. Agreement between parents and children regarding anxiety and depression diagnoses in children with asthma. J Nerv Ment Dis 2007;195(11):897–904.

74. Richardson LP, Russo JE, Lozano P, et al. The effect of comorbid anxiety and depressive disorders on health care utilization and costs among adolescents with asthma. Gen Hosp Psychiatry 2008;30(5):398–406.

75. Fritz GK, McQuaid EL, Spirito A, et al. Symptom perception in pediatric asthma: relationship to functional morbidity and psychological factors. J Am Acad Child Adolesc Psychiatry 1996;35(8):1033–41.

76. Kikuchi Y, Okabe S, Tamura G. Chemosensitivity and perception of dyspnea in patients with a history of near-fatal asthma. N Engl J Med 1994;330(19): 1329–34.

77. Kifle Y, Seng V, Davenport PW. Magnitude estimation of inspiratory resistive loads in children with life-threatening asthma. Am J Respir Crit Care Med 1997;156(5):1530–5.

78. Fritz GK, Adams SK, McQuaid EL, et al. Symptom perception in pediatric asthma. Chest 2007;132(3):884–9.

79. Feldman JM, McQuaid EL, Klein RB, et al. Symptom perception and functional morbidity across a 1-year follow-up in pediatric asthma. Pediatr Pulmonol 2007; 42:339–47.

80. Koinis-Mitchell D, McQuaid EL, Seifer R, et al. Symptom perception in children with asthma: cognitive and psychological factors. Health Psychol 2009;28(2): 226–37.

81. McQuaid EL, Nassau JH. Empirically supported treatments of disease-related symptoms in pediatric psychology: asthma, diabetes, and cancer. J Pediatr Psychol 1999;24(4):305–28.

82. Alexander AB. Systematic relaxation and flow rates in asthmatic children: relationship to emotional precipitants and anxiety. J Psychosom Res 1972;16(6): 405–10.

83. Alexander AB, Miklich DR, Hershkoff H. The immediate effects of systematic relaxation training on peak expiratory flow rates in asthmatic children. Psychosom Med 1972;34(5):388–94.

84. Miklich DR, Renne CM, Creer TL, et al. The clinical utility of behavior therapy as an adjunctive treatment for asthma. J Allergy Clin Immunol 1977;60(5):285–94.

85. Vazquez MI, Buceta JM. Effectiveness of self-management programmes and relaxation training in the treatment of bronchial asthma: relationships with trait anxiety and emotional attack triggers. J Psychosom Res 1993;37(1):71–81.

86. Vazquez MI, Buceta JM. Psychological treatment of asthma: effectiveness of a self-management program with and without relaxation training. J Asthma 1993;30(3):171–83.

87. Vázquez I, Buceta J. Relaxation therapy in the treatment of bronchial asthma: effects on basal spirometric values. Psychother Psychosom 1993;60(2):106–12.

88. King NJ. The behavioral management of asthma and asthma-related problems in children: a critical review of the literature. J Behav Med 1980;3(2):169–89.

89. Davis MH, Saunders DR, Creer TL, et al. Relaxation training facilitated by biofeedback apparatus as a supplemental treatment in bronchial asthma. J Psychosom Res 1973;17(2):121–8.

90. Scherr MS, Crawford PL, Sergent CB, et al. Effect of bio-feedback techniques on chronic asthma in a summer camp environment. Ann Allergy 1975;35(5):289–95.

91. Kotses H, Harver A, Segreto J, et al. Long-term effects of biofeedback-induced facial relaxation on measures of asthma severity in children. Biofeedback Self Regul 1991;16(1):1–21.

92. Glaus KD, Kotses H. Facial muscle tension influences lung airway resistance; limb muscle tension does not. Biol Psychol 1983;17(2–3):105–20.

93. Kotses H, Glaus KD, Bricel SK, et al. Operant muscular relaxation and peak expiratory flow rate in asthmatic children. J Psychosom Res 1978;22(1):17–23.

94. Kotses H, Glaus KD, Crawford PL, et al. Operant reduction of frontalis EMB activity in the treatment of asthma in children. J Psychosom Res 1976;20(5):453–9.

95. Feldman GM. The effect of biofeedback training on respiratory resistance of asthmatic children. Psychosom Med 1976;38(1):27–34.

96. Guevara JP, Wolf FM, Grum CM, et al. Effects of educational interventions for self management of asthma in children and adolescents: systematic review and meta-analysis. BMJ 2003;326(7402):1308–9.

97. DePue JD, McQuaid EL, Koinis-Mitchell D, et al. Providence School Asthma Partnership: school-based asthma program for inner-city families. J Asthma 2007;44(6):449–53.

98. McCauley E, Katon W, Russo J, et al. Impact of anxiety and depression on functional impairment in adolescents with asthma. Gen Hosp Psychiatry 2007;29(3):214–22.

99. Vila G, Nollet-Clémençon C, de Blic J, et al. Assessment of anxiety disorders in asthmatic children. Psychosomatics 1999;40(5):404–13.

100. Gupta S, Crawford SG, Mitchell I. Screening children with asthma for psychosocial adjustment problems: a tool for health care professionals. J Asthma 2006;43(7):543–8.

The Interface of Child Mental Health and Juvenile Diabetes Mellitus

Sandra L. Fritsch, MD[a,b,]*, Mark W. Overton, MD[b],
Douglas R. Robbins, MD[a,c,d]

KEYWORDS

- Diabetes mellitus • Children • Adolescents
- Psychosocial functioning • Cognitive functioning
- Mental health

Diabetes mellitus (type 1) has long been identified as one of the most common chronic, lifelong illnesses developing in childhood. In the United States, type 2 diabetes and meta-bolic syndrome are increasing in children and adolescents at an alarming rate.[1,2] Type 1 diabetes mellitus (T1DM) has also been called insulin-dependent diabetes mellitus (IDDM) and juvenile onset diabetes mellitus. The hallmark feature of T1DM is the under production or lack of production of insulin by the beta cells of the pancreas. This lack of insulin is felt to be due to the destruction of the beta cells. The hallmark feature of type 2 diabetes is "insulin resistance." In type 2 diabetes, the pancreatic beta cells still make insulin, but cells become "resistant" to insulin and are unable to take up circulating glucose. Thus, high levels of circulating insulin and glucose are found in type 2 diabetes.[3] Risk factors for type 2 diabetes include being overweight (**Table 1**). The incidence of overweight children and adolescents (above the 95th percentile for weight) has been increasing during the last few decades, with 17.1% of all children and adolescents being defined as overweight in 2003 and 2004.[4,5] Risk factors for children and adolescents

A version of this article was previously published in the *Child and Adolescent Psychiatric Clinics of North America, 19:2.*
[a] Child and Adolescent Psychiatry, Maine Medical Center, University of Vermont College of Medicine, Tufts University School of Medicine, 22 Bramhall Street, Portland, ME 04102, USA
[b] Department of Psychiatry, Child & Adolescent Psychiatry Fellowship, Maine Medical Center, 22 Bramhall Street, Portland, ME 04102, USA
[c] Department of Psychiatry, The Glickman Family Center for Child & Adolescent Psychiatry, Maine Medical Center, 22 Bramhall Street, Portland, ME 04102, USA
[d] Department of Psychiatry, Child & Adolescent Psychiatry, Maine Medical Center, 22 Bramhall Street, Portland, ME 04102, USA
* Corresponding author. Department of Psychiatry, Child & Adolescent Psychiatry Fellowship, Maine Medical Center, 22 Bramhall Street, Portland, ME 04102.
E-mail address: fritss@mmc.org

Pediatr Clin N Am 58 (2011) 937–954
doi:10.1016/j.pcl.2011.06.008
0031-3955/11/$ – see front matter © 2011 Elsevier Inc. All rights reserved.

Table 1
Differences among T1DM, type 2 diabetes mellitus, and metabolic syndrome

Type 1 Diabetes Mellitus	Type 2 Diabetes Mellitus	Metabolic Syndrome
Onset: abrupt; often in childhood	Onset: gradual; originally adult disease, now increasing in childhood	Constellation of symptoms including:
Insulin dependent		■ Abdominal adiposity
Defect: insulin producing cells of the pancreas	Insulin resistant: hallmark feature	■ Elevated triglycerides
		■ Low HDL
	Associated with obesity, use of atypical antipsychotic medications	■ Hypertension
		■ Type 2 diabetes may be associated
	May be controlled with diet and exercise	Risk for cardiovascular disease
		May be associated with use of atypical antipsychotic medications

becoming overweight and who are at risk for metabolic syndrome or type 2 diabetes have included the increased use of atypical antipsychotics, most notably olanzapine and clozapine.[6–9]

The incidence of T1DM varies with geography, age, gender, family history, and race. Risk for developing T1DM in childhood seems to increase with distance from the equator.[10] In the United States, the highest incidence of T1DM is found in non-Hispanic white children, 23.6 per 100,000 annually.[11] Childhood-onset T1DM has a bimodal presentation for age of onset, with the first peak between ages 4 and 6 years and the second peak in early adolescence.[12]

Development of childhood-onset IDDM occurs with the destruction of the beta cells in the pancreas. The destruction is most often felt to be mediated by an autoimmune response but can also be seen in association with cystic fibrosis. In addition, there is noted genetic susceptibility as the risk for T1DM increases for first-degree relatives.[13] Thus, for genetically susceptible individuals, it is postulated that environmental exposures (proposed agents including: viral infections, immunizations, diet, vitamin D deficiency and perinatal factors) trigger an immune response, leading to the destruction of the beta cells of the pancreas. There is also an associated increased risk for celiac disease for children with T1DM. Some children and families struggle with the dietary restrictions of T1DM and the gluten-free dietary requirements for celiac disease.

The treatment regimen for T1DM includes close monitoring of blood glucose level by "finger sticks," monitoring of urine for glycosuria, diet modifications, and multiple injections of insulin per day. Some treatment centers advocate "tight" control, with blood glucose levels monitored as frequently as every 4 hours and decisions on insulin dose made as predicated by the blood glucose level. Other programs may have as "loose" a program as twice a day injections and twice a day monitoring of blood and urine glucose levels. But in the developing child with variable times of exercise, school lunches, birthday parties ensuring healthy blood glucose levels can be a challenge to the child, the family, and the care providers. Often in later adolescence, the individual with T1DM may opt (or be recommended by the treatment provider) to receive treatment from an insulin pump (subcutaneous continuous infusion of insulin). The insulin pump delivers continuous basal insulin with boluses associated with meals. Use of the insulin pump may reduce rates of hypoglycemic events, but controlled trials of pump therapy comparing injection therapy in the pediatric population are currently limited.[14,15]

There are both long-term complications of chronically high blood glucose levels on the vascular system and serious short-term problems with acute hypoglycemic events (**Box 1**). The preschool-age child may be more vulnerable to severe hypoglycemic events, and prepubertal children may be more protected from microvascular complications of T1DM. For the person with frequent "sugars running high," measurement of the glycated hemoglobin levels (A_{1c}) will be elevated. The recognized risk of hypoglycemia in younger children has led to the setting of higher HbA_{1c} target levels compared with the expectation of "stricter" metabolic control for older children and adolescents.

Shorter-term complications of diabetes include difficulties associated with hypoglycemia, ranging from tremor, confusion, and lethargy to stupor and seizures. Acute hyperglycemia can lead to polyuria, nocturnal enuresis, weight loss, and risk for diabetic ketoacidosis, which can potentially cause coma and death. Thus, diabetes can cause acute life-threatening events in addition to chronic complications. For the developing child and adolescent, effects of hypoglycemic events and hyperglycemia may cause cognition and neurodevelopmental challenges (see next section).

Longer-term complications of diabetes affect all organ systems, with the causal agent being microvascular damage. Most notable potential complications include retinopathy, nephropathy, neuropathy, cardiovascular disease, and impotence. Additional complications can include gastroparesis, menstrual difficulties, necrobiosis lipoidica, and bone changes.

EFFECT ON COGNITION AND NEUROPSYCHOLOGICAL DIFFICULTIES IN CHILDREN AND ADOLESCENTS

Children and adolescent brains continue to develop through pruning, myelinization, and other maturational processes. Childhood cognitive development is well recognized to undergo remarkable changes from barely recognizing letters to abstract thinking. The effect of hypoglycemia and hyperglycemia in the developing child on cognitive functioning and subtle neuropsychological deficits has been the subject of ongoing studies. In 2004, Desrocher and Rovet[16] provided a comprehensive review of the literature, some of the controversies, and a discussion of some of the limitations of past research. Further research since 2004 is described in the next section and in **Table 2**.

Box 1
Complications of T1DM

Short-term	Long-term
Hypoglycemia	Retinopathy
Confusion	Microvascular disease
Seizures	Nephropathy
Hyperglycemia	Neuropathy
Externalizing behaviors	Pregnancy complications
Diabetic ketoacidosis	Impotence
Coma	

Table 2
Long-term and immediate neurocognitive effects of hypoglycemia and hyperglycemia

	Hypoglycemia	Hyperglycemia
Long-term	■ Worse cognitive outcome ■ Decreased spatial intelligence ■ Delayed recall ■ Lower gray volume in left superior temporal region	■ Decreased verbal intelligence ■ Decreased gray volume in right cuneus and precuneus, smaller white volume in right posterior parietal region, increased gray matter in prefrontal region
Immediate	■ Problems with "selective attention" ■ Neuronal integrity in anterior brain seems susceptible to acute hypoglycemia	■ Increased externalizing behaviors ■ Susceptibility to cerebral edema in the frontal region associated with increased taurine

Hypoglycemia

Earlier age of onset (<5 years) has often been associated with more frequent or more severe bouts of hypoglycemia. This is thought to be secondary to individual lack of hypoglycemia awareness (or lack of verbal skills to express the acute event) and sensitivity to nocturnal hypoglycemic spells. Repeated severe bouts of hypoglycemia (more than 3 episodes) have been associated with deficits in spatial memory,[17] worse cognitive outcome and delayed recall,[18] and smaller gray matter volume in the left superior temporal region.[19] Greater exposure to severe hypoglycemia in childhood has also been associated with greater hippocampal volume,[20] and researchers postulated that this enlargement may reflect a pathologic reaction, leading to gliosis, reactive neurogenesis, or impairment of normal pruning.

A recent small study[21] tried to examine the immediate neuropsychological and neurometabolic effects of a severe hypoglycemic event (with associated seizure) in 3 prepubertal children. Immediate difficulties were noted with selective attention that improved during the subsequent 6 months, and the neuronal integrity in the anterior brain appeared particularly susceptible to acute hypoglycemia.

Hyperglycemia

Longer-term effects of chronic hyperglycemia have been noted to affect overall verbal intelligence,[18] overall brain changes including decreased gray matter volume in the right cuneus and precuneus regions, smaller white volume in the right posterior parietal region, and increased gray matter in the prefrontal region.[19]

Parents and children alike have anecdotally reported knowing when the child is running "high" glucoses by reporting changes in behavior. McDonnell and colleagues[22] studied prepubertal children with T1DM to test the potential association between glucose levels and behaviors. They, indeed, found an association between intercurrent high glycemic levels and increased externalizing behaviors, such as agitation and aggression. A recent study[23] conducted imaging studies during hyperglycemia in children with or without associated diabetic ketoacidosis, and the frontal region was notably affected with elevations of taurine associated with increased risk for cerebral edema.

Summary of Neurocognitive Effects of T1DM

T1DM has significant acute and chronic implications for the developing child and adolescent brain. Severe hypoglycemic episodes for children less than 5 years of age may later predispose the child to significant learning issues. On the other hand, chronically elevated glucose levels may predispose the child to lower verbal intelligence scores. Immediate effects of hypoglycemia may lead to problems with selective attention, whereas the child with "high sugars" may exhibit problematic externalizing behaviors. The child or adolescent and her/his family face the challenge of finding a correct balance.

PSYCHIATRIC COMORBIDITY ASSOCIATED WITH IDDM

Evidence suggests that maladjustment in children negatively affects glycemic control and subsequent metabolic functioning. Recent studies indicate elevated rates of psychiatric disorder between 33% and 42% in adolescents and young adults with diabetes,[24–26] which are 2 to 3 times higher than those found in the general population.[27–31] Diagnoses include internalizing and externalizing disorders. A recent study examined the effect of internalizing and externalizing disorders on the risk for readmission to the hospital for diabetes care, demonstrating an increased risk for readmission for adolescents (but not children) with internalizing behaviors and possibly an increased risk among those with externalizing behaviors.[32] Many studies suggest that individuals with comorbid psychiatric disorders are less likely to adhere to treatment regimens, resulting in poorer control of the illness.[30] Thus, disturbed adolescents with diabetes may be at "double jeopardy" for adverse physical and mental health outcomes.[30] An association between mood disorders in the child or adolescent with T1DM and family conflict and very "tight" metabolic control has also been reported,[33–35] raising the possibility that psychiatric symptoms may either contribute to or result from obsessive preoccupation with the demands of the diabetes treatment regimen.[30] Depression and anxiety are most commonly seen in children and adolescents with diabetes, and early adjustment disorders are more predictive of these diagnoses. Eating disorders are also common, particularly among women, and are discussed in the later section.

Adjustment Disorders

From the time of diagnosis, there is an expected pattern of adjustment because both children and families are introduced to a new world filled with challenges, constraints, and uncertainties associated with a lifelong illness. Initial adjustment to the diagnosis of diabetes is characterized by sadness, anxiety, withdrawal, and dependency,[36–39] and approximately 30% of children develop a clinical adjustment disorder in the 3 months subsequent to diagnosis.[36,40] Such difficulties often resolve within the first year, but poor adaptation in this initial phase places children at risk of later psychological difficulties.[26,30,36,38,41,42]

Depression

Studies have associated a diagnosis of depression with substantially worse glycemic control and more serious retinopathy in patients without psychiatric disorders.[43–45] Because of the overlap of symptoms such as fatigue, weight loss, and impaired memory common to both mood disorder and poor metabolic control, depression may be under diagnosed in children with diabetes.[36,43] Therefore, it is useful to reevaluate patients with symptoms of depression after glycemic control has been established. If symptoms persist, a diagnosis of depression may be indicated. Massengale[46] provides a recent review on the salient features of depression in the adolescent with T1DM. A 2003 study[47] reported that there is a 10-fold increase in the incidence of suicide and suicidal ideation in the adolescent with diabetes. In addition to other means, insulin is a potential means for self-injury.[48,49]

With nearly one-third of diabetic adolescents experiencing comorbid depression and similar numbers reported in the adult population, researchers are looking for links of brain pathology/changes caused by the illness leading to increased risk for depression. McEwen and colleagues[50] propose that the progressive atrophy of the hippocampus is seen in animals with diabetes, which is similar to changes seen in depression.

Psychotherapeutic and psychopharmacologic interventions have been found to be helpful in treating depression. Psychopharmacologic treatment should be accompanied by psychotherapy addressing the pessimistic attitudes that typically accompany depression in adolescents and that can limit the patient's willingness or ability to do what is necessary to treat the diabetes.[43]

Psychopharmacologic treatment use in conjunction with IDDM may present with unique challenges. Although the initiation of treatment with antidepressants does not usually cause serious problems, patients and parents should be alerted to the possibility of changes in blood glucose control.[43] Tricyclic antidepressants frequently stimulate appetite that can lead to hyperglycemia. Selective serotonin reuptake inhibitors can have appetite-suppressing effects and may also enhance the action of insulin, thereby inducing hypoglycemic episodes.[43,51] Because lithium carbonate seems to have effects that mimic those of insulin as well as stimulate the secretion of glucagon, either hyper- or hypoglycemia may result from its use.[43] Successful treatment of depression may also bring about changes in eating habits, exercise patterns, and the regularity of insulin injections, thereby causing unforeseen changes in blood glucose control.[43]

Anxiety Disorders

Symptoms of anxiety may also be more common in diabetic children and adolescents. As with other diagnoses, anxiety symptoms may occur in the context of poor glycemic control and must be differentiated from hypo- or hyperglycemic conditions. Self-monitoring of blood glucose concentrations can help the patients and parents discriminate between hypoglycemia and anxiety.[43,52] It is often useful to help the child discriminate internalizing symptoms of worry or persistent fears associated with anxiety from physical symptoms of palpitations or diaphoresis associated with a hypoglycemic state. Treatment with antianxiety medications may lead to improved glucose control and even to hypoglycemia.[43,52] Caution is advised when using β-blockers to treat anxiety symptoms, because they can block adrenergic symptoms that are useful in identifying the hypoglycemic state.

Eating Disorders

The coexistence of eating disorders, such as anorexia nervosa and bulimia nervosa, and diabetes has long been recognized in the clinical setting, particularly among female patients. The cause of eating disorders is multifactorial, involving psychological, biologic, genetic, family, social, and environmental factors.[53] Overall, eating disorders that meet DSM-IV diagnostic requirements are more prevalent among adolescents with T1DM than the general population. Subthreshold eating disorder, eating-related disturbances, and misuse of insulin to influence body weight, which pose an increased risk for related medical complications and eating disorders, are common in the female adolescent diabetic population.

Considering the frequency of eating disorders based on DSM-IV criteria, some studies indicate that subjects with diabetes mellitus were 2.4 times more likely to have an eating disorder than controls and 1.9 times more likely to have a subthreshold eating disorder.[54] Smith and colleagues[55] compared adolescent women with diagnoses of scoliosis and IDDM with a normal control group for an increased risk of eating disorders. Of the adolescents with T1DM, 27.5% were found to have either bulimia or binge-eating disorder based on DSM-IV criteria. Although many patients may not meet strict DSM-IV criteria for anorexia nervosa or bulimia, as indicated by refusal to maintain body weight at or above minimally normal weight for age and height and recurrent inappropriate compensatory behavior to prevent weight gain, respectively, deliberate insulin omission was cited as the most common weight loss behavior after dieting. Data suggest that between 15% and 39% of young women with diabetes manipulate their insulin to control their weight, with clinically relevant changes in eating attitudes in boys and girls occurring after their first year of treatment for diabetes.[56] Although some diabetic patients tend to be slightly more overweight than controls, it is the rapid weight gain of rehydration and the anabolic effect of insulin that may be responsible for the rapid weight gain, particularly after diagnosis. Although these changes in eating attitudes were associated with significant changes in body weight, girls were more likely to experience changes in body dissatisfaction, preoccupation with food, body image, and body shape. In relation to bulimia, rather than purging, many diabetic women reduce their dose of insulin to achieve a similar calorie-voiding effect.[57] The availability of this method of weight control, together with dietary restrictions imposed by the diabetes regimen, may explain why many diabetic patients may report less dieting to lose weight, even though they report more binge eating.[54]

Such eating disorders or disturbances in adolescents with T1DM pose a particular health risk in that they are associated with impaired metabolic control and about a 3-fold increase in the risk of diabetic retinopathy.[54] For the clinician, these findings emphasize the importance of considering an eating disorder, or at least disturbed eating, as a cause of poor control of hemoglobin HbA_{1c} control in young women with diabetes.[58]

FAMILY AND DEVELOPMENTAL FACTORS

Consideration of family functioning in families with children with IDDM has a long history. Minuchin and colleagues[59,60] in the 1970s described "psychosomatic" families. These families were described as possibly manifesting 1 of 4 maladaptive transactional patterns: enmeshment, overprotectiveness, rigidity, and lack of conflict resolution. Although the finding has not been clearly replicated, it was found that acutely stressful family interactions could lead to elevated blood glucose levels.

Since Minuchin's original work, there have been many investigations exploring the relationships of family factors mediating treatment adherence, effects of parental mental health issues on disease course, marital difficulties and its effect on the child with diabetes, and developmental aspects of the family and the child with a chronic illness. More recent work is looking at treatment approaches to the family, including multisystemic therapy (MST),[61,62] office-based parent support,[63] and the effect of psychoeducation.[64] This is described in greater detail in the later discussion.

In any chronic illness, an understanding of the psychosocial context of the child's life is critical to managing illness-related behavior and achieving adherence to management regimens that are often painful or uncomfortable and often in conflict with expectable developmental processes. For T1DM, the maintenance of treatment regimens is clearly related to medical outcomes. Short-term consequences of inadequate monitoring of blood glucose, changes in diet or exercise, or problems in insulin administration can potentially lead to seizures, unconsciousness, and death. Poor glycemic control can eventually cause blindness, renal failure, stroke, and myocardial infarction. The seriousness of these outcomes generates a great deal of understandable anxiety in parents and providers, anxiety that often does not yield improvements in treatment adherence, and which may, in fact, lead to conflict, resistance, and additional difficulty.

Understanding family and developmental factors in all pediatric illness and the need for family-based interventions is increasingly being addressed.[65] An understanding of illness-related behaviors in the child or adolescent and of the stress and emotional responses experienced by parents are critical if health care providers are to be effective in achieving helping the patients manage their illnesses effectively. In all serious illnesses in childhood and adolescence, parents can be expected to experience varying degrees of stress and frustration, which may lead to anxiety, depression, alterations in the marital relationship, and difficulties in the relationship with the child. When an illness causes ongoing disability, parents may need to grieve a real loss. These responses in parents are often associated with outcomes in the child, both morbidity (quality of life, psychosocial adjustment, physical complications) and mortality.

Adjustment to the illness and establishment of effective patterns of management of the illness are critical with T1DM. Adherence to treatment regimens and maintenance of metabolic control, while difficult for some to achieve during childhood, often becomes much more difficult with the transition to adolescence.[66] Problematic family interactional factors such as high levels of conflict and low cohesion are associated with poorer adherence to treatment regimens, poorer metabolic control, and worse health outcomes.[67,68]

The Effect of T1DM on Parents and Families

The diagnosis of T1DM in a child or adolescent is often an acute stressor in the lives of parents. They must quickly absorb a substantial amount of new and disturbing information. The physical demands of care are significant, involving blood glucose monitoring, insulin administration, attempts to regulate diet and activity, and time-consuming office visits and calls. Ongoing needs of the ill child's siblings, other family members, and work must be dealt with, and feelings of inadequacy or helplessness are understandable. Many parents experience subthreshold symptoms of distress and mood disturbance after the diagnosis.[40] A significant minority continues, weeks and months later, to experience anxiety and depression.[69] One study observed 22% of mothers of children with T1DM to have clinically significant levels of depression.[70] A study of pediatric parenting stress, as defined by the Pediatric Inventory for Parents, assessing the parents' communication with others, emotional functioning (eg, sleep, mood), the stress of performing the medical regimen, and effects on role functioning (eg, ability to work, care for other children) found that those who experienced a lower sense of self-efficacy in managing the child's medical care and greater parenting stress were more likely to report clinically significant symptoms of anxiety or depression.[71]

The experience of having a child with T1DM is a challenge for the parents' marriage, with consequences for the child's medical and psychosocial outcome. Mothers typically take on most child care, management of the illness, and communication with providers. In the study on parenting stress mentioned earlier, anxiety and depression were greater for mothers than fathers. The presence of each spouse participating in the child's care was a protective factor.[71] Higher levels of mother-reported spousal support have been found to be associated with less conflict with an adolescent with T1DM and with greater adherence to treatment.[70] Single-parent families clearly have greater difficulty with management of the illness than parents living together.[72]

Parents' emotional responses and coping styles interact with those of children and adolescents in a reciprocal or transactional manner. Maternal depression is associated with the quality of life and depressive symptoms in children with T1DM.[73] At the same time, maladaptive emotions and behavior on the part of the child add greatly to the stress on a parent.

Effects of the Child's Age or Developmental Level

Developmental considerations of the child or adolescent with IDDM include the child's age at diagnosis, the complexity of disease management, the ability to consent for treatment, and the trajectory through puberty. In many patients, diabetic control during the critical years of adolescence and early adulthood is determined by control established in late childhood.[74] The challenges to psychological adjustment and family interaction vary with the age or developmental level of the child. The cognitive capacity of the child, stability of attachment to parents, need for autonomy and other developmental needs, and medical issues associated with the patient's age all play a role. As children develop, they should gradually become the primary guardians of personal health and primary partners in medical decision making, assuming responsibility from their parents.[75] Developmentally, this involves a significant range of responsibility for self-care, ultimately resulting in responsibility for appropriate food choices, blood glucose monitoring, knowledge of HbA_{1c}, and appropriate insulin dose adjustment predictions to account the wide array of influencing variables.

It is not unusual for preschoolers to have become very ill and experienced an intense life-threatening condition that initially shapes their perception of what it means to have diabetes. Not surprisingly, this perception is also influenced by parental beliefs, expectations, and ability to effectively communicate with the child. Although the preschoolers have little responsibility in managing their diabetic care, they can begin to communicate subjective perceptions of what it feels to be hyper- or hypoglycemic. The greater risk of hypoglycemic episodes in preschool children often results in anxiety on the part of parents. Needle-related pain and distress may be a particular challenge with younger children, but children's ability and willingness to use needles are not age related.[76] Separation from parents, if hospitalization is necessary, can be a great cause of anxiety.

In latency, the child can begin to develop an understanding of the principles of diabetes, management techniques, and decision making related to considerations of consent. It is clear that "informed consent" has only limited direct application in children and adolescents. Only patients who have appropriate decisional capacity and legal empowerment can give their informed consent to medical care. In all other situations, parents or other surrogates provide "informed permission" for diagnosis and treatment of children with the assent of the child when appropriate. If physicians recognize the importance of assent, they empower children to the extent of their capacity.[75,77]

Assent should include at least the following elements[75]:

1. Helping the child achieve a developmentally appropriate awareness of the nature of his or her condition.
2. Telling each child what he or she can expect with tests and treatment.
3. Making a clinical assessment of the patient's understanding of the situation and the factors influencing how he or she is responding.
4. Soliciting an expression of the patient's willingness to accept the proposed care.

A child's refusal to assent to treatment may represent misunderstandings, fears, and concerns, which if initially respected by the clinician, may provide an opportunity for the exploration of refusal and a strengthening of the therapeutic relationship.

Although coercion or force may ultimately be necessary for medical reasons, it should be the last resort, keeping in mind the negative consequences of possible increased aversion to medical procedures.

A developmentally appropriate understanding of the nature of diabetes for childhood assent can often be expressed by latency-age children in simple meaningful terms. Describing "hypos" and "hypers" related to "sugar levels," their direct relation well-being, associated somatic feeling of each condition, and the relationship of food/insulin can usually be understood and expressed by these children. Children need to be helped to have some understanding that the benefit of treatment outweighs the problems of discomfort and inconvenience.

A child's expectation of tests and treatment is usually developed over time, as he or she begins to appreciate the regularity of injections. Appreciation of duration of treatment is more abstract however, and children may reference duration to the number of finger sticks throughout the day, rather than the lifetime.

In addition to simply asking the child to explain in his or her own words, making use of natural play can also indicate understanding of the situation and the factors influencing how he or she is responding. Demonstrations on dolls or asking the child how he or she would advise another boy or girl with diabetes is often perceived as fun and can often yield surprisingly insightful interpretations.

Although there has been little research about children's beliefs and goals or their ability to comanage a serious chronic condition, some studies have revealed that some children possess the knowledge, skill, and maturity to make personal decisions about their health care. It has been found that from around 4 years of age, children start to understand the principles and take responsible moral decisions about managing their diabetes. And yet, other research has indicated that instead of age or ability, experience is the salient factor in a child's intellectual and moral competence.[76,77]

In school-aged children with T1DM, parents still have to take very active responsibility for management.[78] Behaviors that are normal for the developmental stage, such as oppositional interactions, emotional liability, and increasing need for independence, can interfere with management. In addition to the life of the child in the family, challenges also arise with respect to school and peer relationships. The needs to regulate or at least monitor dietary intake and physical activity conflict with the child's need to be active with friends, to participate in sports, and to join activities involving food. A particular difficulty and point of conflict is misbehavior at mealtimes, such as playing with food, talking rather than eating, or refusal to eat, which generates anxiety in the parent who is concerned about the need for consistent intake. Such behavior tends to elicit ineffective, overreactive discipline from parents.[79] Patton and colleagues[80] observed that more parental activity, directing or commanding the child to eat, was associated with less eating as the meal progressed. This was not categorically different from mealtime interactions in healthy controls, but it was associated with poorer glycemic control in children with T1DM. An intervention, using principles similar to those of Parent Management Training,[81] effectively improved mealtime conflict by teaching parents to use short, direct commands that are associated with contingent positive attention.[82]

The transition to adolescence is a time when conflict with the family often increases and adherence to treatment regimens often deteriorates.[83] The same hormones that cause growth spurts in a child can also wreak havoc on his or her efforts to keep blood sugar level under control. As growth hormone increases during the early and middle adolescent years, the body becomes less sensitive to insulin. As a result, high glucose levels are common in late adolescents. When an adolescent reaches his or her full growth, these insulin-inhibiting hormones tend to decrease.[84,85] The increased adolescent physical demands of sports, dance, gymnastics, and many other strenuous activities can also change insulin requirements.

Increased autonomy in the formation of personal identity is an important developmental task of adolescence. This developmental task may be more complicated for adolescents with T1DM because at this time in their lives, metabolic control and treatment adherence often deteriorate and less parental involvement in diabetes care has been associated with poorer diabetes outcomes. Adolescents perceive support from family members primarily in the form of tangible support, such as reminding, helping, and even performing many of the self-management tasks.[86] Parent-child conflict is common and may take the form of parental worry and intrusive behaviors or blaming. Late adolescents often feel that their parents have identified them more in terms of the diabetes than their personality. Misunderstanding of the hormonal changes of development may lead to parental accusations of irresponsible diabetes management. Adolescents are most sensitive to being misunderstood and often either blatantly disregard appropriated diabetes management in response or create factitious blood sugar levels to satisfy the parents.

Issues common in adolescence, including the need for separation and a sense of autonomy; the adolescent's sense of invulnerability and propensity to risk taking; concerns about self-image, sexual identity, and peer group affiliation all complicate relationships with parents and management of the illness. At a time when peers are regarded increasingly as capable of managing certain aspects of their life and enjoy increasingly independent function, the adolescents with T1DM experience continuing vigilance on the part of their parents regarding their dietary intake, physical activity, and consistency with blood glucose monitoring and insulin administration.

Clinical practice consensus guidelines for "Diabetes in adolescence" were developed by the International Society for Pediatric and Adolescent Diabetes and published in 2008.[87] Providers who are sensitive to these issues, hoping to be responsive to the adolescent's need for a degree of mastery and autonomy may attempt a "loose" rather than a "tight" level of control of the illness. Parents and providers often need to be active in monitoring and managing treatment. Although adolescents have greater cognitive capacity and diabetes-related problem-solving skills than younger children, they were found to avoid using such skills in social situations in which they conflicted with acceptance by peers.[88] Active monitoring by parents is associated with better control of the illness.[89] Parents, providers, and adolescents need to find a sustainable balance between monitoring of the treatment regimen and allowing the adolescent to feel increasingly competent and independent.

There are clearly some protective factors. Those with more stable family communication and social support and with more positive self-perceptions experience less stress related to their illness and better glycemic control.[90,91]

INTERVENTIONS

Many children and adolescents have some degree of difficulty in maintaining good glycemic control, and a subset of adolescents has serious problems. These chronically poorly controlled patients are likely to experience multiple risk factors, including other family psychopathology, low levels of parental support and monitoring, irregular contact with care providers, lower socioeconomic status, and minority or single-parent homes.[61,92]

As noted earlier, children and adolescents may experience coexisting psychiatric disorders, such as anxiety, depressive disorders, and eating disorders. Other disorders that are fairly common in children and adolescents and not specifically related to diabetes, such as attention-deficit hyperactivity disorder or learning disabilities, may greatly complicate management. If such comorbid disorders are present, the first priority must be to treat them according to appropriate practice parameters. Family conflict may require family psychotherapy, and treatment of depression, anxiety, or other disorders in parents, either related to the child's diabetes or preexisting, may be indicated. Parents may be reluctant to seek help for themselves when they are preoccupied with a child's illness, but they must be helped to see the need to be functioning well if they are to be helpful to their child and families.

Several interventions, including educational programs, cognitive behavioral therapy, coping-skills training, and family-based interventions, specific to the difficulties experienced by families with a diabetic child have been studied. In a recent article, several interventions from different theoretical perspectives showed promise with respect to psychosocial outcomes and health service use, but without definitive effects on metabolic control.[93] A randomized controlled trial of an educational approach, Parent-Adolescent Teamwork, showed significantly decreased family conflict, but no significant effect on glycemic control.[63] A recent review of family-centered interventions indicated promising results with both family conflict and improved HbA_{1c} levels.[94]

The specific and important issue of needle-related distress has been the subject of successful interventions. Distraction, cognitive behavioral treatment (CBT), and hypnosis have shown promising results. CBT is "well established" for procedure-related pain.[95] Operant learning procedures with positive reinforcement including tokens, tangible rewards, or privileges are considered "probably efficacious," with increased adherence to blood glucose monitoring.[96]

MST is an intensive family-centered treatment modality that was originally developed to treat delinquent adolescents and has been extended to psychiatrically ill children and adolescents.[97] It has been adapted to treat chronically poorly controlled adolescents with T1DM.[98–100] The intensive home-based psychotherapeutic approach includes a wide menu of interventions appropriate to the individual patient and family. Family interventions included parent training regarding monitoring and improving communication. Individual interventions, such as CBT, for a depressed adolescent were used as needed. Treatment included collaboration with schools; involvement of peers, community, and extended family; and problem solving around barriers to keeping medical appointments and communicating with providers. A trend was seen regarding improvement of HbA_{1c} levels, with a decrease of 0.8% in the families completing treatment. Although the mean did not decrease to a level considered acceptable, this degree of improvement is associated with improved medical outcomes. The frequency of blood glucose monitoring increased and the number of hospital admissions for diabetic ketoacidosis decreased.

SUMMARY

In summary, the psychosocial adjustment and behavior of patients with T1DM is critical to their medical outcomes and quality of life, and family support, monitoring, and communication are essential levels of consideration. The illness is a significant and ongoing stressor for parents, and it confounds and complicates many aspects of normal child and adolescent development. Several careful studies have delineated important moderators and mediators of outcomes, and promising interventions have been developed and continue to be studied. Pediatricians, family physicians, nurse practitioners, child and adolescent psychiatrists, and other medical and mental health providers need to understand and address psychosocial adaptation to the illness if they are to improve the outcomes of their patients and their families. Protective factors such as family communication skills, spousal support, and enhancement of positive self-perception should be identified and promoted to minimize short- and long-term complications.

REFERENCES

1. Duncan G, Li S, Zhou X. Prevalence and trends of a metabolic syndrome phenotype among U.S. adolescents, 1999–2000. Diabetes Care 2004;27(10): 2438–43.
2. Duncan G. Prevalence of diabetes and impaired fasting glucose levels among US adolescents: National Health and Nutrition Examination Survey, 1999–2002. Arch Pediatr Adolesc Med 2006;160(5):523–8.
3. Nelson R, Bremer A. Insulin resistance and metabolic syndrome in the pediatric population. Metab Syndr Relat Disord 2009. [Epub ahead of print].
4. Hedley A, Ogden C, Johnson C, et al. Prevalence of overweight and obesity among US children, adolescents, and adults, 1999–2002. JAMA 2004; 291(23):2847–50.
5. Ogden C, Carroll M, Curtin L, et al. Prevalence of overweight and obesity in the United States, 1999–2004. JAMA 2006;295(13):1549–55.
6. Cohen D. Atypical antipsychotics and new onset diabetes mellitus. An overview of the literature. Pharmacopsychiatry 2004;37(1):1–11.
7. Cohen D, Huinink S. Atypical antipsychotic-induced diabetes mellitus in child and adolescent psychiatry. CNS Drugs 2007;21(12):1035–8.
8. Jerrell J, McIntyre R. Adverse events in children and adolescents treated with antipsychotic medications. Hum Psychopharmacol 2008;23(4):283–90.
9. McIntyre R, Jerrell J. Metabolic and cardiovascular adverse events associated with antipsychotic treatment in children and adolescents. Arch Pediatr Adolesc Med 2008;162(10):929–35.
10. Rosenbauer J, Herzig P, von Kries R, et al. Temporal, seasonal, and geographical incidence patterns of type I diabetes mellitus in children under 5 years of age in Germany. Diabetologia 1999;42(9):1055–9.
11. Bell R, Mayer-Davis E, Beyer J, et al. Diabetes in non-Hispanic white youth: prevalence, incidence, and clinical characteristics: the SEARCH for Diabetes in Youth Study. Diabetes Care 2009;32(Suppl 2):S102–11.
12. Felner E, Klitz W, Ham M, et al. Genetic interaction among three genomic regions creates distinct contributions to early- and late-onset type 1 diabetes mellitus. Pediatr Diabetes 2005;6(4):213–20.
13. Tillil H, Köbberling J. Age-corrected empirical genetic risk estimates for first-degree relatives of IDDM patients. Diabetes 1987;36(1):93–9.
14. Berhe T, Postellon D, Wilson B, et al. Feasibility and safety of insulin pump therapy in children aged 2 to 7 years with type 1 diabetes: a retrospective study. Pediatrics 2006;117(6):2132–7.
15. Nimri R, Weintrob N, Benzaquen H, et al. Insulin pump therapy in youth with type 1 diabetes: a retrospective paired study. Pediatrics 2006;117(6):2126–31.
16. Desrocher M, Rovet J. Neurocognitive correlates of type 1 diabetes mellitus in childhood. Child Neuropsychol 2004;10(1):36–52.
17. Hershey T, Perantie D, Warren S, et al. Frequency and timing of severe hypoglycemia affects spatial memory in children with type 1 diabetes. Diabetes Care 2005;28(10):2372–7.

18. Perantie D, Lim A, Wu J, et al. Effects of prior hypoglycemia and hyperglycemia on cognition in children with type 1 diabetes mellitus. Pediatr Diabetes 2008; 9(2):87–95.

19. Perantie D, Wu J, Koller J, et al. Regional brain volume differences associated with hyperglycemia and severe hypoglycemia in youth with type 1 diabetes. Diabetes Care 2007;30(9):2331–7.

20. Hershey T, Perantie D, Wu J, et al. Hippocampal volumes in youth with Type 1 diabetes. Diabetes 2010;59(1):236–41.

21. Rankins D, Wellard R, Cameron F, et al. The impact of acute hypoglycemia on neuropsychological and neurometabolite profiles in children with type 1 diabetes. Diabetes Care 2005;28(11):2771–3.

22. McDonnell C, Northam E, Donath S, et al. Hyperglycemia and externalizing behavior in children with type 1 diabetes. Diabetes Care 2007;30(9):2211–5.

23. Cameron F, Kean M, Wellard R, et al. Insights into the acute cerebral metabolic changes associated with childhood diabetes. Diabet Med 2005;22(5):648–53.

24. Blanz B, Rensch-Riemann B, Fritz-Sigmund D, et al. IDDM is a risk factor for adolescent psychiatric disorders. Diabetes Care 1993;16(12):1579–87.

25. Goldston D, Kelley A, Reboussin D, et al. Suicidal ideation and behavior and noncompliance with the medical regimen among diabetic adolescents. J Am Acad Child Adolesc Psychiatry 1997;36(11):1528–36.

26. Kovacs M, Goldston D, Obrosky D, et al. Psychiatric disorders in youths with IDDM: rates and risk factors. Diabetes Care 1997;20(1):36–44.

27. Garton A, Zubrick S, Silburn S. The Western Australian child health survey: a pilot study. Aust N Z J Psychiatry 1995;29(1):48–57.

28. Costello E. Developments in child psychiatric epidemiology. J Am Acad Child Adolesc Psychiatry 1989;28(6):836–41.

29. Bird H. Epidemiology of childhood disorders in a cross-cultural context. J Child Psychol Psychiatry 1996;37(1):35–49.

30. Northam E, Matthews L, Anderson P, et al. Psychiatric morbidity and health outcome in Type 1 diabetes–perspectives from a prospective longitudinal study. Diabet Med 2005;22(2):152–7.

31. Sawyer M, Arney F, Baghurst P, et al. The mental health of young people in Australia: key findings from the child and adolescent component of the national survey of mental health and well-being. Aust N Z J Psychiatry 2001;35(6):806–14.

32. Garrison M, Katon W, Richardson L. The impact of psychiatric comorbidities on readmissions for diabetes in youth. Diabetes Care 2005;28(9):2150–4.

33. Grey M, Boland E, Yu C, et al. Personal and family factors associated with quality of life in adolescents with diabetes. Diabetes Care 1998;21(6):909–14.

34. Smith M, Mauseth R, Palmer J, et al. Glycosylated hemoglobin and psychological adjustment in adolescents with diabetes. Adolescence 1991;26(101):31–40.

35. Kovacs M, Ho V, Pollock M. Criterion and predictive validity of the diagnosis of adjustment disorder: a prospective study of youths with new-onset insulin-dependent diabetes mellitus. Am J Psychiatry 1995;152(4):523–8.

36. Northam E, Todd S, Cameron F. Interventions to promote optimal health outcomes in children with Type 1 diabetes–are they effective? Diabet Med 2006;23(2):113–21.

37. Grey M, Cameron M, Lipman T, et al. Psychosocial status of children with diabetes in the first 2 years after diagnosis. Diabetes Care 1995;18(10):1330–6.

38. Kovacs M, Mukerji P, Iyengar S, et al. Psychiatric disorder and metabolic control among youths with IDDM. A longitudinal study. Diabetes Care 1996;19(4): 318–23.

39. Northam E, Anderson P, Adler R, et al. Psychosocial and family functioning in children with insulin-dependent diabetes at diagnosis and one year later. J Pediatr Psychol 1996;21(5):699–717.
40. Kovacs M, Feinberg T, Paulauskas S, et al. Initial coping responses and psychosocial characteristics of children with insulin-dependent diabetes mellitus. J Pediatr 1985;106(5):827–34.
41. Kovacs M, Goldston D, Obrosky D, et al. Prevalence and predictors of pervasive noncompliance with medical treatment among youths with insulin-dependent diabetes mellitus. J Am Acad Child Adolesc Psychiatry 1992;31(6):1112–9.
42. Liss D, Waller D, Kennard B, et al. Psychiatric illness and family support in children and adolescents with diabetic ketoacidosis: a controlled study. J Am Acad Child Adolesc Psychiatry 1998;37(5):536–44.
43. Jacobson A. The psychological care of patients with insulin-dependent diabetes mellitus. N Engl J Med 1996;334(19):1249–53.
44. Lustman P, Griffith L, Clouse R, et al. Psychiatric illness in diabetes mellitus. Relationship to symptoms and glucose control. J Nerv Ment Dis 1986;174(12):736–42.
45. Roy M, Roy A, Affouf M. Depression is a risk factor for poor glycemic control and retinopathy in African-Americans with type 1 diabetes. Psychosom Med 2007;69(6):537–42.
46. Massengale J. Depression and the adolescent with type 1 diabetes: the covert comorbidity. Issues Ment Health Nurs 2005;26(2):137–48.
47. Kanner S, Hamrin V, Grey M. Depression in adolescents with diabetes. J Child Adolesc Psychiatr Nurs 2003;16(1):15–24.
48. Kaminer Y, Robbins D. Insulin misuse: a review of an overlooked psychiatric problem. Psychosomatics 1989;30(1):19–24.
49. Cassidy E, O'Halloran D, Barry S. Insulin as a substance of misuse in a patient with insulin dependent diabetes mellitus. BMJ 1999;319(7222):1417–8.
50. McEwen B, Magariños A, Reagan L. Studies of hormone action in the hippocampal formation: possible relevance to depression and diabetes. J Psychosom Res 2002;53(4):883–90.
51. Goodnick P, Henry J, Buki V. Treatment of depression in patients with diabetes mellitus. J Clin Psychiatry 1995;56(4):128–36.
52. Cox D, Gonder-Frederick L, Polonsky W, et al. A multicenter evaluation of blood glucose awareness training-II. Diabetes Care 1995;18(4):523–8.
53. Dahan A, McAfee S. A proposed role for the psychiatrist in the treatment of adolescents with type I diabetes. Psychiatr Q 2009;80(2):75–85.
54. Jones J, Lawson M, Daneman D, et al. Eating disorders in adolescent females with and without type 1 diabetes: cross sectional study. BMJ 2000;320(7249):1563–6.
55. Smith F, Latchford G, Hall R, et al. Do chronic medical conditions increase the risk of eating disorder? A cross-sectional investigation of eating pathology in adolescent females with scoliosis and diabetes. J Adolesc Health 2008;42(1):58–63.
56. Antisdel J, Chrisler J. Comparison of eating attitudes and behaviors among adolescent and young women with type 1 diabetes mellitus and phenylketonuria. J Dev Behav Pediatr 2000;21(2):81–6.
57. Steel J, Young R, Lloyd G, et al. Abnormal eating attitudes in young insulin-dependent diabetics. Br J Psychiatry 1989;155:515–21.
58. Fairburn C, Peveler R, Davies B, et al. Eating disorders in young adults with insulin dependent diabetes mellitus: a controlled study. BMJ 1991;303(6793):17–20.

59. Minuchin S, Baker L, Rosman B, et al. A conceptual model of psychosomatic illness in children. Family organization and family therapy. Arch Gen Psychiatry 1975;32(8):1031–8.
60. Minuchin S, Fishman H. The psychosomatic family in child psychiatry. J Am Acad Child Psychiatry 1979;18(1):76–90.
61. Ellis D, Naar-King S, Templin T, et al. Improving health outcomes among youth with poorly controlled type I diabetes: the role of treatment fidelity in a randomized clinical trial of multisystemic therapy. J Fam Psychol 2007;21(3):363–71.
62. Ellis D, Podolski C, Frey M, et al. The role of parental monitoring in adolescent health outcomes: impact on regimen adherence in youth with type 1 diabetes. J Pediatr Psychol 2007;32(8):907–17.
63. Anderson B, Brackett J, Ho J, et al. An office-based intervention to maintain parent-adolescent teamwork in diabetes management. Impact on parent involvement, family conflict, and subsequent glycemic control. Diabetes Care 1999;22(5):713–21.
64. Lochrie A, Wysocki T, Burnett J, et al. Youth and parent education about diabetes complications: health professional survey. Pediatr Diabetes 2009;10(1):59–66.
65. Fiese B. Introduction to the special issue: time for family-based interventions in pediatric psychology? J Pediatr Psychol 2005;30(8):629–30.
66. Johnson S, Tomer A, Cunningham W, et al. Adherence in childhood diabetes: results of a confirmatory factor analysis. Health Psychol 1990;9(4):493–501.
67. Anderson B, Holmbeck G, Iannotti R, et al. Dyadic measures of the parent-child relationship during the transition to adolescence and glycemic control in children with type 1 diabetes. Fam Syst Health 2009;27(2):141–52.
68. Cohen D, Lumley M, Naar-King S, et al. Child behavior problems and family functioning as predictors of adherence and glycemic control in economically disadvantaged children with type 1 diabetes: a prospective study. J Pediatr Psychol 2004;29(3):171–84.
69. Chaney J, Mullins L, Frank R, et al. Transactional patterns of child, mother, and father adjustment in insulin-dependent diabetes mellitus: a prospective study. J Pediatr Psychol 1997;22(2):229–44.
70. Lewandowski A, Drotar D. The relationship between parent-reported social support and adherence to medical treatment in families of adolescents with type 1 diabetes. J Pediatr Psychol 2007;32(4):427–36.
71. Streisand R, Mackey E, Elliot B, et al. Parental anxiety and depression associated with caring for a child newly diagnosed with type 1 diabetes: opportunities for education and counseling. Patient Educ Couns 2008;73(2):333–8.
72. Cameron F, Skinner T, de Beaufort C, et al. Are family factors universally related to metabolic outcomes in adolescents with Type 1 diabetes? Diabet Med 2008;25(4):463–8.
73. Jaser S, Whittemore R, Ambrosino J, et al. Mediators of depressive symptoms in children with type 1 diabetes and their mothers. J Pediatr Psychol 2008;33(5):509–19.
74. Cameron F, Smidts D, Hesketh K, et al. Early detection of emotional and behavioural problems in children with diabetes: the validity of the Child Health Questionnaire as a screening instrument. Diabet Med 2003;20(8):646–50.
75. Bioethics Co. Informed consent, parental permission, and assent in pediatric practice. Pediatrics 1995;95:314–6.
76. Alderson P, Sutcliffe K, Curtis K. Children as partners with adults in their medical care. Arch Dis Child 2006;91(4):300–3.

77. Alderson P, Sutcliffe K, Curtis K. Children's competence to consent to medical treatment. Hastings Cent Rep 2006;36(6):25–34.
78. Palmer D, Berg C, Wiebe D, et al. The role of autonomy and pubertal status in understanding age differences in maternal involvement in diabetes responsibility across adolescence. J Pediatr Psychol 2004;29(1):35–46.
79. Wilson A, DeCourcey W, Freeman K. The impact of managing school-aged children's diabetes: the role of child behavior problems and parental discipline strategies. J Clin Psychol Med Settings 2009;16(3):216–22.
80. Patton S, Piazza-Waggoner C, Modi A, et al. Family functioning at meals relates to adherence in young children with type 1 diabetes. J Paediatr Child Health 2009. [Epub ahead of print].
81. Kazdin A. Parent management training: evidence, outcomes, and issues. J Am Acad Child Adolesc Psychiatry 1997;36(10):1349–56.
82. Stark L, Jelalian E, Powers S, et al. Parent and child mealtime behavior in families of children with cystic fibrosis. J Pediatr 2000;136(2):195–200.
83. Drotar D, Ievers C. Age differences in parent and child responsibilities for management of cystic fibrosis and insulin-dependent diabetes mellitus. J Dev Behav Pediatr 1994;15(4):265–72.
84. Effect of intensive diabetes treatment on the development and progression of long-term complications in adolescents with insulin-dependent diabetes mellitus: Diabetes Control and Complications Trial. Diabetes Control and Complications Trial Research Group. J Pediatr 1994;125:177–88.
85. Amiel S, Sherwin R, Simonson D, et al. Impaired insulin action in puberty. A contributing factor to poor glycemic control in adolescents with diabetes. N Engl J Med 1986;315(4):215–9.
86. Weinger K, O'Donnell K, Ritholz M. Adolescent views of diabetes-related parent conflict and support: a focus group analysis. J Adolesc Health 2001;29(5):330–6.
87. Court J, Cameron F, Berg-Kelly K, et al. Diabetes in adolescence. Pediatr Diabetes 2008;9(3 Pt 1):255–62.
88. Thomas A, Peterson L, Goldstein D. Problem solving and diabetes regimen adherence by children and adolescents with IDDM in social pressure situations: a reflection of normal development. J Pediatr Psychol 1997;22(4):541–61.
89. Horton D, Berg C, Butner J, et al. The role of parental monitoring in metabolic control: effect on adherence and externalizing behaviors during adolescence. J Pediatr Psychol 2009;34(9):1008–18.
90. Dashiff C, Hardeman T, McLain R. Parent-adolescent communication and diabetes: an integrative review. J Adv Nurs 2008;62(2):140–62.
91. Malik J, Koot H. Explaining the adjustment of adolescents with type 1 diabetes: role of diabetes-specific and psychosocial factors. Diabetes Care 2009;32(5):774–9.
92. Ellis D, Yopp J, Templin T, et al. Family mediators and moderators of treatment outcomes among youths with poorly controlled type 1 diabetes: results from a randomized controlled trial. J Pediatr Psychol 2007;32(2):194–205.
93. Couch R, Jetha M, Dryden D, et al. Diabetes education for children with type 1 diabetes mellitus and their families. Evid Rep Technol Assess (Full Rep) 2008;(166):1–144.
94. McBroom L, Enriquez M. Review of family-centered interventions to enhance the health outcomes of children with type 1 diabetes. Diabetes Educ 2009;35(3):428–38.
95. Powers S. Empirically supported treatments in pediatric psychology: procedure-related pain. J Pediatr Psychol 1999;24(2):131–45.

96. Lemanek K, Kamps J, Chung N. Empirically supported treatments in pediatric psychology: regimen adherence. J Pediatr Psychol 2001;26(5):253–75.

97. Henggeler S, Rowland M, Randall J, et al. Home-based multisystemic therapy as an alternative to the hospitalization of youths in psychiatric crisis: clinical outcomes. J Am Acad Child Adolesc Psychiatry 1999;38(11):1331–9.

98. Ellis D, Frey M, Naar-King S, et al. The effects of multisystemic therapy on diabetes stress among adolescents with chronically poorly controlled type 1 diabetes: findings from a randomized, controlled trial. Pediatrics 2005;116(6): e826–32.

99. Ellis D, Frey M, Naar-King S, et al. Use of multisystemic therapy to improve regimen adherence among adolescents with type 1 diabetes in chronic poor metabolic control: a randomized controlled trial. Diabetes Care 2005;28(7): 1604–10.

100. Ellis D, Templin T, Naar-King S, et al. Multisystemic therapy for adolescents with poorly controlled type I diabetes: stability of treatment effects in a randomized controlled trial. J Consult Clin Psychol 2007;75(1):168–74.

Pediatric Obesity: A Review for the Child Psychiatrist

Ann E. Maloney, MD[a,b,c],*

KEYWORDS

- Epidemic • Pediatric obesity • Psychiatric consultation
- Psychopharmacologic treatment • Physical activity

Pediatric obesity is an epidemic. Although the problem has been the focus of family physicians, pediatricians, and public health workers, few of them feel comfortable counseling patients and their families about changing behaviors. Child mental health providers may be asked to work alongside primary care physicians and other specialists who treat youngsters with obesity.

Child psychiatrists can assist families and other members of the multidisciplinary team in their attempts to control childhood and adolescent obesity, but expert consultation requires a thorough understanding of the crisis. This review of pediatric obesity assesses the epidemic's background, delineates the challenges of clinical care, and evaluates the therapeutic recommendations for this population of patients and their families.

DEFINITION AND CHARACTERIZATION OF OBESITY

Body mass index (BMI, calculated as weight in kilograms divided by the square of height in meters) is the standard measurement for determining an individual's weight-to-height relationship. This ratio is an indicator of the degree of body fat. Levels of child and adolescent BMI typically are measured as the sex-specific BMI for the age percentile (2–20 years old), which makes allowances for differences in body fat by gender and

A version of this article was previously published in the *Child and Adolescent Psychiatric Clinics of North America, 19:2.*

This work is supported by grants from the Maine Medical Center Research Institute (MMCRI). Work completed at Maine Medical Center Research Institute, 81 Research Drive, Scarborough, ME 04074-7205, USA.

[a] Center for Clinical and Translational Research, Maine Medical Center Research Institute, 81 Research Drive, Scarborough, ME 04074-7205, USA

[b] Tufts University Medical Center, Maine Medical Center, Portland, ME, USA

[c] Child & Adolescent Psychiatry, University of Vermont College of Medicine, Maine Medical Center, Portland, ME, USA

* Corresponding author. University of Massachusetts Memorial Medical Center, Department of Psychiatry, 55 Lake Avenue North, Worcester, MA 01655.

E-mail address: malona1@mmc.org

age. A child and adolescent BMI calculator can be found at http://www.cdc.gov/growthcharts. Pediatric obesity experts define child and adolescent obesity as a BMI greater than or equal to the 95th percentile, and overweight as a BMI greater than or equal to the 85th percentile.[1]

Obesity is a threat to the health of children. The condition is associated with genetic patterns, medical conditions, medications, and environmental factors. Fat cells were once believed to be inert storage depots of energy, but it is now understood that obesity is an inflammatory condition. Adipocytes play a significant role in endocrine signaling, and secreted adipokines have downstream effects on several organs. Biochemical mediators that regulate appetite and food intake include ghrelin, insulin, orexin, PYY-3-36, cholecystokinin, and adiponectin.

Adolescents are at slightly greater risk for obesity than younger children. The mechanisms of increased risk for weight gain seem to be multifactorial, but there seem to be 3 critical periods for the development of obesity that are normally characterized by marked developmental increases in BMI: infancy, the period of adiposity rebound between 5 and 7 years of age, and adolescence.[2]

SCOPE OF THE PROBLEM

Child and adolescent obesity rates in the United States are a public health issue, and evidence suggests that the current younger generation of Americans may have shorter life expectancies than their parents.[3] Rates of overweight and obesity among adolescents vary by gender, socioeconomic status, and ethnic background, and prevalence is further increased if factors of minority status, rural living, and lower socioeconomic status are considered.[4]

Child and adolescent overweight and obesity rates for girls and boys have greatly increased in the past 30 years. The National Health and Nutrition Examination Survey (NHANES) data suggest that 17.1% of children and adolescents between the ages of 2 and 19 years are at or above the 95th percentile of sex-specific BMI for age on growth charts.[4] Between NHANES I (1971–1974) and NHANES IV (2003–2006), the prevalence of obesity increased 12.4% for the 2- to 5-year-old group of children, 17% for the 6- to 11-year-old group, and 17.6% for the 12- to 19-year-old group. Among adolescents between the ages of 12 and 19 years, Mexican American boys and non-Hispanic black girls had the highest rates of obesity prevalence at 22.1% and 27.7%, respectively.[5] Obesity and socioeconomic status are linked, and lower levels of parent education are associated with multiple metabolic risks in adolescence.[6]

Goals published in the *Healthy People 2010* document include objective 19-3: "reduce to 5% the proportion of children and adolescents who are obese." Youths who are obese preschoolers are likely to be obese as adolescents, and this pattern is linked to adult-onset diabetes, hypertension, hyperlipidemia, asthma, and sleep apnea. The Centers for Disease Control and Prevention (CDC) compile obesity surveillance data for low-income, preschool-aged children participating in federally funded health and nutrition programs. The CDC examined trends between 1998 and 2008 and found that obesity prevalence among low-income, preschool-aged children increased steadily from 12.4% in 1998 to 14.5% in 2003. Since then, the rates have plateaued at a prevalence of 14.6% in 2008.[7] A follow-up study of more than 500 children who were overweight found that, after 40 years, 47% of the children were still overweight as adults. The severity of overweight in puberty was highly associated with weight-related morbidity and mortality in adulthood.[8]

A social network of 12,067 people was assessed repeatedly from 1971 to 2003 as part of the Framingham Heart Study.[9] The BMI was available for all subjects. The investigators reported social factors that seem to determine obesity in adults. They found that a person's chances of becoming obese increased by 57% (95% confidence interval [CI], 6–123) if he or she had a friend who became obese. This pattern was identified in pairs of adult siblings and in spouses. Neumark-Sztainer and colleagues[10] found that weight-specific socioenvironmental, personal, and behavioral variables were strong and consistent predictors of overweight status, binge eating, and extreme weight-control behaviors in teens. Social support from parents, peers, and teachers was associated with changes in physical activity over time for a population of inactive adolescent girls.

COST OF CHILD OBESITY

An attempt to quantify health care expenditures and health service use associated with childhood overweight and obesity found that this population had significantly higher health expenditures and service use rates than children of normal weight.[11] These figures included hospitalizations for comorbidities of obesity, outpatient and emergency department use, and prescription drug costs. Based on these results, researchers projected that costs of approximately $14.1 billion per annum are associated with increased pediatric BMI. These estimates are much higher if the adult population is included. Overall obesity-related direct heath care costs may be at least $90 billion per year and include coverage for a high number of people who were overweight or obese during youth and experienced the consequences in adulthood.[12] In Maine, adult obesity in an insured population has been estimated to cost $2.56 billion per year in avoidable medical and workers' compensation costs and lost productivity each year.[13] Although obesity prevention is not a suggested way to reduce overall health care costs, it is a cost-effective way to increase survival rates and quality of life.

Because children and adolescents who are obese and overweight are likely to carry their BMI status into adulthood,[14] the government has an incentive to support obesity prevention and treatment. At least one-half of obesity-related health care expenditures are financed by Medicare and Medicaid.[15] Schools and communities also deplete resources, and these stakeholders have a role in the reversal of this epidemic (**Fig. 1**).

MEDICAL AND PSYCHOSOCIAL CONSEQUENCES

Child and adolescent obesity can have medical and psychological consequences. Illnesses previously considered adult diseases are now occurring in youth. Short-term medical consequences include gastroesophageal reflux disease, obstructive sleep apnea (OSA), perioperative and postoperative complications, increased risk for injury, asthma, gallstones, sleep, dental caries, skeletal health, orthopedic injuries, and constipation. Long-term complications include coronary heart disease (CHD), hypertension, metabolic syndrome, diabetes mellitus, dyslipidemia, nonalcoholic fatty liver disease (NAFLD), and increased risk for certain cancers.[16,17]

Excess adiposity during the developing years is a morbidity and mortality risk factor, but it is not known whether total body fat or its distribution is responsible. One hypothesis is that intra-abdominal adipose tissue in childhood, independent from total body fat, increases the risk for disease in adults.

Mental Health Concerns

The psychological consequences of obesity include low self-esteem, victimization by peers, depression, anxiety, and increased risk for eating disorders. Fatigue is associated with obesity and overweight, but it can masquerade as a neurovegetative sign of a depressive disorder.[18,19] Obesity is associated with treatments for mental health

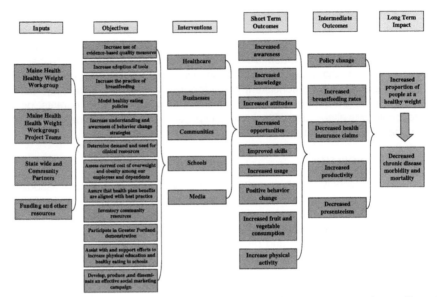

Fig. 1. The logic model for pediatric obesity shows the importance of coordinated approaches involving government, communities, health care providers, and individuals. (*Courtesy of* MaineHealth, Portland, ME; with permission.)

conditions, such as weight gain resulting from treatment with atypical antipsychotics. Overall mortality is increased for children with weight extremes, and youths with extreme perceptions of body size are at increased risk for suicidal ideation and suicide attempts.[20]

The Pediatric Quality of Life Inventory is an instrument designed to measure health-related quality of life for children and adolescents.[18] It is designed as a child self-report and parent proxy report to measure fatigue in pediatric patients.[18] Pediatric patients with obesity experienced fatigue comparable with pediatric patients receiving cancer treatment. Sedation from medication treatment, trauma symptoms, depression, and other mental illnesses can manifest as low energy levels. Current recommendations (http://www.mypyramid.gov/kids) are that youths participate in 1 hour of activity on most days, but it is challenging for the most obese to participate in activity when fatigue is a major symptom.

Early-onset obesity is associated with cognitive impairments. The *Journal of Pediatrics* reported that toddlers with early-onset morbid obesity had an average IQ of 78, whereas the control group of siblings had an average IQ of 106. Magnetic resonance imaging of infants who were early-onset morbidly obese revealed white matter lesions typically found in the brain of adults with Alzheimer disease or in children with untreated phenylketonuria.[19]

The stigma associated with youth overweight and obesity is pervasive in Western society, and it may come from peers, educators, or parents. Diet and body image are a national preoccupation, and anxiety about body image is a major concern for girls and boys in our culture. Youth obesity is associated with peer bullying, and peer victimization is associated with child-reported depression, anxiety, loneliness, and reduced physical activity.

Some studies show little or no association between child and adolescent obesity and poor emotional health.[21] Others report different results, particularly for minorities and women who may be more likely to have low self-esteem and engage in high-risk behaviors, although this effect may be decreased if body image is controlled for.[22]

Using data from a British birth cohort study, researchers examined the educational, social, socioeconomic, and psychological outcomes for individuals who were obese at age 10 and 30 years. Childhood obesity was associated with negative outcomes in adulthood for men and women, and persistent obesity in women was significantly associated with adverse employment and relationship status.[23] Obesity that begins in childhood or adolescence may be responsible for body image disturbances later in life, particularly in women.

Certain populations accumulate risk along with their weight. For example, obese Hispanic and white women have significantly lower levels of self-esteem by early adolescence and higher rates of sadness, loneliness, and nervousness. They are also more likely to engage in high-risk behaviors, such as smoking or drinking alcohol.[22] Vulnerable children who are exposed to abuse are more likely to be obese as adults.[24]

Comorbid Medical Conditions

Skeletal health

It was once believed that a husky weight status was good for bone, but it has been found that the developing skeleton suffers with rising adiposity.[25] Age-adjusted total body mineral content and bone area relative to body weight are lower in children who are overweight and obese than in children of lower adiposity. During the period of peak bone accrual, the teen years, obesity may have a long-term effect on osteoporosis for this population. Obesity may be a risk factor in pediatric trauma cases and may increase the incidence of extremity fractures that require surgical intervention.[26]

Childhood overweight and obesity are associated with several orthopedic complications, including Blount disease, acute fractures, slipped capital femoral epiphysis, and spinal complications.[16] A chart review of patients enrolled in pediatric clinics who were overweight and obese found that that these patients were more likely to report symptoms of decreased mobility and musculoskeletal discomfort, such as knee pain.[27]

Alimentary disorders

Caries and obesity coexist in children of low socioeconomic status.[28] Public health measures to improve dietary education, availability of appropriate foodstuffs, and access to dental care could decrease the risk of both diseases.

Obesity is a major predictor of gastroesophageal reflux disease among children between the ages of 7 and 16 years. This risk increases with corresponding increases in BMI.

Obesity is responsible for most gallstones in children with no other underlying medical problems.[29] It raises the risk of developing gallstones to 4 times that experienced by individuals of normal weight.

Among children and adolescents with constipation, there is a significantly higher prevalence of obesity than among controls, and this disorder may result from diet, activity level, or other influences.[30] The increased rate is not related to the presence of fecal incontinence or encopresis among children who are constipated. Children who are obese are also more likely to experience recurrent abdominal pain than children of normal weight.

Asthma

A study of 14,654 junior high school students found that increased BMI was one of the risk factors for asthma, and that higher BMI scores were correlated with an increased prevalence of asthma in this population.[31] Obese children with asthma experience more symptoms of asthma and recover more slowly from an acute-onset attack.

Sleep

Cardiovascular and metabolic processes are affected by sleep-wake cycles. Sleep-wake cycles are partly under the direct control of the master circadian pacemaker located in the suprachiasmatic nucleus. Basic functions, such as heart rate and levels of leptin (involved in appetite control), show circadian variation.[32]

Adolescents who are obese have a greater likelihood of experiencing sleep disorders such as OSA. This disorder can cause sleep deprivation and disrupted metabolism, which can further increase BMI and exacerbate other obesity-related conditions. Sleep deprivation is linked to impaired mood and poor school performance. A study of almost 300 children and adolescents found that sleep-disordered breathing, such as OSA, contributed to significantly lower levels of physical health and greater complaints of body pain. Even mild sleep-disordered breathing created measurable decreases in health-related quality of life.[33] OSA is a predictor of nocturnal hypertension in children, and hypertension is a direct complication of obesity and a serious risk factor for cardiovascular disease.

Persistent short sleep duration (<10 hours) during early childhood significantly increases the risk of excess weight.[34] Studies have focused on the importance of sleep duration and sleep hygiene in the creation of obesity and overweight in youth. A prospective cohort study of more than 1100 children who were followed from infancy found that persistent sleep duration of less than 10 hours per night had a significant effect on the risk of developing excess weight.[34] Similar support for the role of shorter sleep duration in developing obesity was found in a study of third- and sixth-graders.[35]

Hypertension

The long-term consequences of childhood obesity include primary hypertension. Children who are obese have 3 times the risk of hypertension compared with peers of normal weight.[36] Charts with norms for children are available at the National Institutes of Health (NIH) Web site (http://www.nhlbi.nih.gov/guidelines/hypertension/child_tbl.htm). The link between obesity and hypertension may be mediated in part by sympathetic nervous system hyperactivity (ie, increased levels of plasma catecholamines) and by neural manifestations such as increased peripheral sympathetic nerve traffic.[36]

In a study of 546 children and adolescents who were obese and between the ages of 4 and 17 years, television viewing was independently associated with hypertension, even after controlling for BMI. Television viewing was also positively associated with increasing BMI.[37] Converting sedentary screen time to active screen time is an ongoing area of research.[38] Limiting screen time is important for other reasons besides blood pressure. For each additional hour of television viewing, youths consume an additional 167 kcal/d (95% CI 136–198 kcal/d; $P<.001$), and they consume the foods commonly advertised on television.[39]

CHD

A retrospective study of 276,835 school children found a strong association between increased BMI in childhood (7–13 years old) and future fatal and nonfatal CHD. The risk of CHD increases with BMI and with the age of the child.[40] Other studies have shown no association between early childhood, increased BMI, and later CHD.

One study was designed to measure prescriptions for diabetes, hypertension, and dyslipidemia among children and adolescents. Using a cross-sectional study design, a pharmacy benefits manager database was used to provide descriptive statistics of insured US children and adolescents between the ages of 6 and 18 years. From 2004 to June 30, 2007, these medications increased 15.2% from 3.3 per 1000 youths in

2004 to 3.8 per 1000 youths in 2007. Older teens (16–18 years old) had the highest prevalence overall, but the greatest rate of increase was found among those 6 to 11 years old: 18.7% for girls and 17.3% for boys.[41]

Diabetes

Increased BMI is a major risk factor for developing type 2 diabetes.[42] The endocrine disruption caused by obesity can result in insulin resistance. The prevalence of new diagnoses of diabetes in children 0 to 19 years old increased from 4% before 1992 to 16% in 1994. Adolescents 10 to 19 years old accounted for 33% of the diabetes diagnoses in 1994.[43] Rates for new cases of diabetes in 2002 and 2003 are shown in **Fig. 2**. Children with type 2 diabetes may show no or few symptoms and remain undiagnosed for long periods, increasing the risk of developing later cardiovascular diseases.

Fatty liver disease

NAFLD is becoming a more common pediatric diagnosis as the obesity epidemic continues. The exact pathophysiology of NAFLD is unknown, but the result is an accumulation of fat in the liver, causing scarring and potential liver failure. The prevalence of NAFLD among children is difficult to measure because people have no signs, symptoms, or complications. However, reviews of pediatric autopsy results show that approximately 10% of children and adolescents 2 to 19 years old may have this condition.[44] Prevalence may be higher among boys than among girls, and it is significantly associated with visceral fat mass, insulin resistance, and type 2 diabetes. The prevalence of NAFLD among hospitalized children and young adults increased between 1986 and 2006, which correlates with the obesity epidemic.[45]

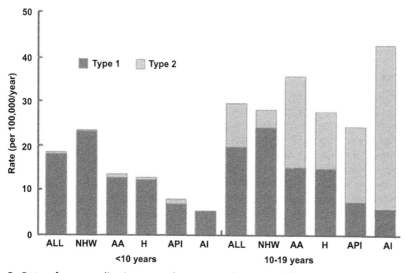

Fig. 2. Rate of new pediatric cases of type 1 and type 2 diabetes according to age or ethnicity. (*From* National Diabetes Statistics, 2007; National Diabetes Information Clearing-house, a service of the National Institute of Diabetes and Digestive and Kidney Diseases (NIDDK), NIH. Available at: http://diabetes.niddk.nih.gov/DM/PUBS/statistics/#d_allages.)

Cancer

Evidence is mounting in support of a relationship between obesity and many adult cancers, and childhood obesity may provide an additional risk factor for developing cancer. Researchers of a prospective cohort study of more than 900,000 adults estimated that 14% of cancer deaths in men and 20% of cancer deaths in women could be attributed to current rates of overweight and obesity in the United States.[46] The National Cancer Institute strongly supports obesity prevention and treatment research.

Perioperative and Postoperative Complications

Children who are overweight and obese presenting for tonsillectomy and adenoidectomy have a higher incidence of perioperative complications and are more likely to be admitted and to stay longer than children of normal weight.[47] Children who are obese undergoing elective surgical procedures have more preexisting comorbid medical conditions and an increased incidence of perioperative adverse respiratory events.

PREDISPOSING FACTORS
Perinatal Environment

Metabolic pathways that are altered during prenatal and perinatal development can increase an individual's risk for developing obesity later in life. Rodent studies show that protein or calorie restriction during the prenatal or suckling period promotes increased levels of hyperphagia, risk for obesity, glucose intolerance, and hypertension in adult rodents.[48] Barker and Martyn[49] posits that prenatal undernutrition may create a "metabolically thrifty" phenotype due to a predicted lifetime environment in which caloric intake is low. A person with this phenotype may be predisposed to obesity when mismatched with an obesogenic environment.[16,49]

The metabolic changes that predispose children to obesity can be manipulated by many factors, including postnatal leptin exposure, prenatal zinc restriction, and preconception maternal nutrition. Maternal diabetes, maternal obesity, and maternal smoking also are associated with an increased risk for their offspring developing obesity. Like prenatal undernutrition, infant overfeeding can increase the likelihood of childhood and adolescent obesity.

Genetics

Twin studies have shown a genetic link, but at a population level, the increase in obesity rates is too rapid to be explained entirely by a genetic shift. Approximately 5% of childhood obesity cases are directly related to genetic defects that cause impaired functioning. Genetic defects have been implicated in many obesity syndromes, including Prader-Willi, Bardet-Biedl, Cohen, Ayazi, and macrosomia, obesity, macrocephaly, and ocular abnormalities (MOMO). However, most obesity cases involve genetic risk, rather than genetic determination, which is influenced by environmental factors. As many as 41 genetic polymorphisms associated with obesity in the right environment have been determined,[50] and each may have partial and additive effects.

Breastfeeding

Decades of epidemiologic research have established that breastfeeding is associated with a reduction in the risk for later overweight and obesity.[51] Drawing from attachment theory and temperament styles taught in psychiatry, it is possible that breastfeeding encourages the infant's self-regulation.[51] One study showed a beneficial association between breastfeeding in early life and bone mass in 8-year-old children born at term, particularly those breastfed for 3 months or longer.[52]

Idiopathic Factors

Most cases of child obesity are not directly caused by coexisting medical conditions. The most common endogenous causes of child and adolescent obesity account for less than 10% of cases, including hormonal effects, hypothyroidism, hypercortisolism, primary hyperinsulinism, pseudohypoparathyroidism, acquired hypothalamic disorders, familial lipodystrophy, and Prader-Willi, Laurence-Moon/Bardet-Biedl, Alström, Börjeson-Forssman-Lehmann, Cohen, Turner, Beckwith-Wiedemann, Sotos, Weaver, and Ruvalcaba syndromes.

Dietary Factors

Caloric intake and dietary habits affect individual weight, but most of what is presented regarding these factors and BMI in the literature is based on inference.[53] Many Americans eat a poor-quality diet, falling short of many of the recommended daily allowances for calcium, dietary fiber, whole grains, and fruits and vegetables, but studies show that the effect of each of these factors on BMI is mixed.[53]

Schools are a major part of the lives of millions of youths, but they have had little effect on reducing or preventing pediatric obesity. Most children do not consume diets that meet the recommended dietary guidelines, nor do they achieve adequate levels of daily physical activity. Fast food consumption has risen steeply in the past 2 decades. Economic conditions and scarcity of fresh produce are drivers of this problem, especially in rural communities.

Sugar-sweetened beverages, such as soda, are under scrutiny as contributors to the obesity epidemic. Youths are increasing their total calorie intake with these products, which are being substituted for more nutritious foods. As a result, children and adolescents are likely to have inadequate intakes of calcium, folate, and iron. Decreasing the intake of these beverages may be the most effective way to reduce energy consumption, and some states are considering additional taxes on sugar-sweetened beverages. Increased fat intake may play a role in current obesity levels. Studies of dietary habits have shown mixed results, but there is some evidence to support the relationship between missing breakfast, snacking, and eating at fast-food establishments and increased BMI levels among youths.[54]

Physical Activity

Less than 3% of youths meet *Healthy People 2010* objective 22.7, which calls for bouts of continuous vigorous physical activity.[55] Nonexercise activity thermogenesis (NEAT) has been described as the crouching tiger behind the hidden dragon of obesity.[56] NEAT is the energy expenditure of all physical activities other than volitional sportslike exercise. Levine and colleagues[56] argue that our chair-enticing environment should be reengineered so that work, school, and home environments render active living the option of choice. Research into the built environment (eg, parks, recreation, trails) and safe routes to school to encourage walking and biking are areas of considerable policy attention.

The No Child Left Behind Act (2002) had an unintended consequence, because schools cut physical education to devote time to new testing requirements, de-emphasizing subjects other than reading and mathematics. The decision to cut physical education programs has been supported by tighter budgets in a time of economic crisis. These cuts are ill-conceived, because physical fitness correlates with better academic test scores, and physical activity offers many physical, emotional, and social benefits.

Television and electronic screen time can affect body weight through substitution of physical activity, increased caloric intake during screen time, and reduced resting metabolism.[57] Lower levels of activity and increased television viewing are each independently associated with obesity,[58] and seated video game use in particular has been linked to obesity.[59] Active games, such as Dance Dance Revolution and Wii Sports, may be helpful in decreasing sedentary screen time.[38]

Conceptual Diagnostic Classification

Obesity is currently classified as a medical condition (coded as 278.00 Obesity, unspecified) by the International Classification of Diseases (ICD) and is not considered a psychiatric disorder by the Diagnostic and Statistical Manual of Mental Disorders, Fourth Edition, Text Revision (DSM-IV-TR). However, binge eating disorder and eating disorders not otherwise specified are recognized by the DSM-IV-TR. Excess weight is a possible warning sign for this diagnosis but is not considered a classification criterion. Binge eating disorder, night eating syndrome, and sleep-related eating disorder are often associated with overweight in adolescents.[60] Youths with binge eating, restricting, extreme weight-control measures, or purging behavior should be thoroughly evaluated for eating disorders.[61]

ASSESSMENT, PREVENTION, AND TREATMENT

Imbalance of energy intake and energy expenditure is the core problem of overweight youths, but correcting this simple discrepancy requires complex inputs to achieve re-equilibration. Emotions and behavior can be changed, but they require well-timed reinforcement and ongoing individualized care. A parent-child approach, in which parents are directly engaged in supporting their child's behavioral modification, has been successfully used in treatment interventions. Interventions with mandatory parental participation have achieved the greatest and most persistent weight changes.[62]

Free, comprehensive, and detailed information is available online (http://pediatrics. aappublications.org/cgi/reprint/120/Supplement_4/S254). An overview of pediatric obesity and a family handout are available from the American Academy of Child and Adolescent Psychiatry (http://www.aacap.org/cs/root/facts_for_families/facts_for_ families).

Medical Assessment and Intervention

The American Medical Association convened a panel to address the prevention and treatment of pediatric obesity (**Fig. 3**).[61] The Expert Committee recommends that primary care providers address the issue of weight with all children at least once each year. Practitioners are urged to assess key dietary habits (eg, consumption of sweetened beverages), physical activity habits, readiness to change lifestyle habits, and family history of obesity and obesity-related illnesses. Laboratory testing recommendations are tailored to the degree of obesity and comorbid illnesses.

The main framework from the Expert Committee is a stepped approach, which is a 4-stage plan for treatment of childhood obesity. This comprehensive approach to weight management includes prevention, structured weight management, comprehensive multidisciplinary intervention, and tertiary care intervention.[53] This framework outlines the standard of care for youths who are obese and provides developmentally sensitive interventions.

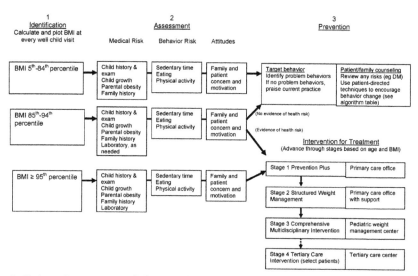

Fig. 3. Universal assessment of obesity risk and steps to prevention and treatment. DM, diabetes mellitus. (*From* Barlow SE, The Expert Committee. Expert committee recommendations regarding the prevention, assessment, and treatment of child and adolescent overweight and obesity: summary report. Pediatrics 2007;120(Suppl):S164–92; with permission. Available at: http://pediatrics.aappublications.org/content/vol120/Supplement_4/images/large/zpe1120743790001.jpeg.)

Recommendations for treating obesity include advising families to limit consumption of sweetened beverages and fast food, to limit sedentary screen time, to engage in physical activity for at least 60 minutes per day, and to eat nutritious and balanced meals every day. Sharing well-prepared meals with family members helps to instill healthier eating habits. The main summary message that has been adopted by our colleagues in pediatrics is 5-2-1-0, which stands for 5 servings of fresh fruits and vegetables (minimum) per day, 2 hours or less of screen time, 1 hour of physical activity, and zero sugar-sweetened beverages.

Primary care has developed tool kits and cue cards to communicate with parents of preschoolers about obesity. Physicians have been reluctant to use these tools, particularly because of time constraints.[63] Messages such as 5-2-1-0 help practitioners keep a mnemonic in mind when talking with families and therefore facilitate the process. Flip charts and tool kits also assist in organizing the data and the messages to families. The Maine Youth Overweight Collaborative is an award-winning program (http://www.mcph.org/Major_Activities/keepmehealthy.htm) that has shifted clinic behavior and increased the number of providers documenting BMI percentile.[64]

Approaches to Prevention and Treatment

Many different treatments have been studied, but mostly for short periods (3–6 months). Medications, lifestyle changes, physical activity, surgery, and diets have been modified. Laboratory and research settings have been used, along with community care. Many programs have success in the short-term, but maintaining lower weight is elusive. Epstein and colleagues,[65] in a 25-year review of rigorous trials, showed that family treatment works, especially for younger children and girls.

Simultaneously treating parents and children can improve relationships in the family and is beneficial because obesity tends to run in families. However, parents of children who are obese are not always ready to make a change when the provider calls for action. This tendency poses a challenge for physicians, because the milieu of a child is most often the family, and most studies support the use of family-based treatment. Children living in 2 homes because of custody arrangements can complicate treatment.

Maintenance interventions to augment the effects of initial weight-loss programs have been studied.[66] Children were assigned to the control group, 4 months of behavioral skills maintenance (BSM), or social facilitation maintenance (SFM) treatment. Children receiving BSM or SFM maintained relative weight significantly better than children assigned to the control group. The group with social problems in SFM treatment had the best outcomes compared with those of the control group.

Prevention efforts must begin earlier to avoid the consequences of the obesity epidemic. Primary care physicians often see young children, but visits are scheduled less frequently as children become older. Child psychiatrists may see children more often than their primary care counterparts, depending on the age of the child and the severity of the psychiatric disorder, and they are therefore positioned to help identify at-risk children who may benefit from diagnosis and treatment and from assistance with early lifestyle changes. In this epidemic, all providers who see children regularly should at least measure them for BMI percentile, chart this information, and share it with the family.

Because child psychiatrists are familiar with cognitive-behavioral therapies, motivational interviewing, brief negotiation, and other addiction treatments, they may be more comfortable applying these methods in practice. They see illnesses as chronic matters and know the importance of staying aligned with families for the "long haul." Primary care physicians feel ill equipped to address the problems of obesity. Some believe they do not have the time in the clinic, and others are resentful about what they perceive as insufficient patient or parent motivation. Moreover, physicians report negative attitudes about obesity that may affect patient care. Child psychiatrists understand countertransference and time pressures, and they can relate to feelings of being "out of the scope of practice." However, this epidemic calls for action from many stakeholders.

Treatment Theories

There are many parallels between obesity and addictive behaviors. Because of common neurobiologic pathways in the brain, addiction and obesity have shared certain methods of research and treatment. Theory of planned behavior, theory of reasoned action, and social cognitive learning theory are the basis for considering treatments that may be effective. For instance, motivational enhancement and cognitive-behavioral strategies used in addiction treatment constitute the cornerstone of treatments for pediatric obesity. Cognitive-behavioral therapy combined with family-based intervention has proved the most effective,[67] especially for children who are morbidly obese and have life-threatening medical conditions. One program was organized in a series of treatment modules: (1) starting treatment: preadmission phase; (2) establishing and maintaining weight loss; (3) encouraging acceptance, addressing realistic expectations to body weight, and addressing body image concerns; and (4) long-term weight maintenance. The program included family intervention and physical activity intervention.

Weight and Medications

Body composition can be affected by certain medications, such as insulin, sulfonylureas, thiazolidinediones, antidepressants, steroids, anticonvulsants, pizotifen, and hormonal contraception agents. The effects of medications are evaluated during the intake process by child psychiatrists, who must try to protect patients from adverse drug effects.

There have been significant increases in the use of second-generation antipsychotics (SGAs) for adolescents from 1996 to 2001.[68] Older and newer antipsychotics are associated with rapid weight gain and with other adverse effects, such as dyslipidemia. The magnitude of body-weight gain was found to be higher with the SGAs, and youths are affected to a greater extent than adults. Clozapine and olanzapine produce the greatest weight gain, ziprasidone and aripiprazole produce less weight gain, and quetiapine and risperidone cause intermediate effects. Appetite stimulation is probably a key cause of weight gain, but genetic polymorphisms can modify the weight response during treatment with SGAs. Nizatidine, amantadine, reboxetine, topiramate, sibutramine, and metformin been used in preventing or reversing SGA weight gain with some success, but side effects exist for these agents as well. Metformin has been the most studied.[69] Correll and Carlson[70] stress monitoring and lifestyle modification, and clearly more studies are needed in this vulnerable population, as reviewed by Shin and colleagues.[71]

Few agents are approved for obesity, and there have been many safety concerns. Rimonabant (Acomplia), which blocks the endocannabinoid system, showed promise, but it was not approved by the US Food and Drug Administration (FDA) because suicidal ideation was identified during clinical trials. The combination of fenfluramine and phentermine produced primary pulmonary hypertension and harmed many patients, and it serves as a warning to put safety first in the treatment of obesity.

Sibutramine (Meridia) acts on the brain to inhibit deactivation of norepinephrine, serotonin, and dopamine, and it decreases appetite. Orlistat (Xenical) or over-the-counter Alli blocks fat absorption by inhibiting reversibly pancreatic lipase. Metformin has been used in clinical trails but is not FDA-approved for this indication. Psychostimulants are not approved for pediatric obesity.

Bariatric Approaches

Although there are risks associated with surgical interventions such as laparoscopic adjustable gastric banding (Lap-Band) and Roux-en-Y gastric bypass, there is some indication that these interventions may provide a weight-loss option and improved quality of life for eligible older children. Early results suggest that these methods, along with lifestyle changes, may provide sustained weight loss, but more studies are needed to determine longer-term outcomes. Teaching hospitals, such as Stanford, began offering this therapy in 2004, and the NIH has a large trial underway to provide efficacy and safety data about this procedure. In one study of 41 adolescents, 18 had a Lap-Band for at least 3 years, the mean BMI had decreased to 29 ($\pm$6) kg/m^2 (range, 23–47 kg/m^2), and it was maintained at 5 years.[72] In that case series, 83% were no longer obese.

School, Community, and Governmental Interventions

To combat pediatric obesity, sweeping actions must be taken by all levels of government, the food industry, the media, the health care industry, and educational institutions. School-based health improvement programs are overwhelmingly supported by parents, and some changes in schools are beginning to happen. For example, the Arkansas Act 1220 of 2003 mandated the removal of food and beverage vending machines from elementary schools and required schools to provide parents with information about BMI, nutrition, and physical activity as it relates to health. Early evaluation data show that BMI levels have not increased since the start of the program in 2004.[73]

Direct food marketing to children by television advertisements has been identified as a significant promoter of the obesity epidemic. One-half of all advertisements during children's programming are for food items, most of which have no or low nutritional value.[74] Many are endorsed by children's favorite characters, making them even more appealing. Because self-regulation by the food and beverage industries failed to change advertising patterns, researchers have called for legislative regulation of advertising to children. Public support exists for addressing the obesity epidemic through school-, community-, and media-based programs.

In the future, there are likely to be social marketing Web sites, cell-phone diets, text messaging, and other forms of mobile communication used in ambulatory strategies. Preliminary data for adults suggest that Internet-delivered, theoretically sound, evidence-based treatments can be accessed remotely.[75] Using text messaging in the treatment of pediatric obesity and certain eating disorders has already been piloted.[76]

SUMMARY

Because specialty treatment centers for pediatric obesity are not available for most youths, child psychiatrists can, as physicians, provide sensible and balanced nutrition and physical-activity advice in our practice. Using the 5-2-1-0 message and referring families to the Web site (http://www.mypyramid.gov), culturally relevant care can be delivered to children and families, and improvements in the child's environment can be advocated. By using consistent messaging with our primary-care colleagues and assisting them with comorbid mental-health concerns, child psychiatrists can be part of the effort to control pediatric obesity. Regular documentation and sensitive discussion of BMI values are helpful measures that can be implemented now. Referral to specialty stage 3 or stage 4 teams, which consist of registered dieticians, exercise specialists, and mental-health professionals, will likely increase as they become more widespread.

ACKNOWLEDGMENTS

The author wishes to thank Elizabeth Horton, Kristina Medinger, and Clifford Rosen; editorial assistance from Ann Morris is kindly acknowledged.

REFERENCES

1. Barlow SE, Dietz WH. Obesity evaluation and treatment: expert committee recommendations. The Maternal and Child Health Bureau, Health Resources and Services Administration and the Department of Health and Human Services. Pediatrics 1998;102(3):E29.
2. Dietz WH. Critical periods in childhood for the development of obesity. Am J Clin Nutr 1994;59(5):955–9.
3. Finkelstein EA, Brown DS, Wrage LA, et al. Individual and aggregate years-of-life-lost associated with overweight and obesity. Obesity (Silver Spring) 2010;18(2):333–9.
4. Goodman E. Letting the "Gini" out of the bottle: social causation and the obesity epidemic. J Pediatr 2003;142(3):228–30.
5. Ogden CL, Carroll MD, Curtin LR, et al. Prevalence of overweight and obesity in the United States, 1999–2004. JAMA 2006;295(13):1549–55.

6. Goodman E, McEwen BS, Huang B, et al. Social inequalities in biomarkers of cardiovascular risk in adolescence. Psychosom Med 2005;67(1):9–15.

7. Centers for Disease Control and Prevention (CDC). Obesity prevalence among low-income, preschool-aged children—United States, 1998–2008. MMWR Morb Mortal Wkly Rep 2009;58(28):769–73.

8. Mossberg HO. 40-year follow-up of overweight children. Lancet 1989;2(8661): 491–3.

9. Christakis NA, Fowler JH. The spread of obesity in a large social network over 32 years. N Engl J Med 2007;357(4):370–9.

10. Neumark-Sztainer DR, Wall MM, Haines JI, et al. Shared risk and protective factors for overweight and disordered eating in adolescents. Am J Prev Med 2007;33(5):359–69.

11. Trasande L, Liu Y, Fryer G, et al. Effects of childhood obesity on hospital care and costs, 1999–2005. Health Aff (Millwood) 2009;28(4):w751–60.

12. Daviglus ML. Health care costs in old age are related to overweight and obesity earlier in life. Health Aff (Millwood) 2005;24(Suppl 2). W5R97–100.

13. Chenoweth D. 2004. 2004. Anthem: press release. Available at: http://www.anthem.com/wps/portal/ahpfooter?content_path=shared/noapplication/f0/s0/t0/pw_ad087829.htm&label=Press%20Release. Accessed December 22, 2009.

14. Iughetti L, De Simone M, Verrotti A, et al. Thirty-year persistence of obesity after presentation to a pediatric obesity clinic. Ann Hum Biol 2008;35(4):439–48.

15. Finkelstein EA, Trogdon JG, Cohen JW, et al. Annual medical spending attributable to obesity: payer- and service-specific estimates. Health Aff (Millwood) 2009;28(5):w822–31.

16. Lee YS. Consequences of childhood obesity. Ann Acad Med Singapore 2009; 38(1):75–7.

17. Maffeis C, Tato L. Long-term effects of childhood obesity on morbidity and mortality. Horm Res 2001;55(Suppl 1):42–5.

18. Varni JW, Limbers CA, Bryant WP, et al. The PedsQL Multidimensional Fatigue Scale in pediatric obesity: feasibility, reliability and validity. Int J Pediatr Obes 2009;10:1–9.

19. Miller J, Kranzler J, Liu Y, et al. Neurocognitive findings in Prader-Willi syndrome and early-onset morbid obesity. J Pediatr 2006;149(2):192–8.

20. Eaton DK, Lowry R, Brener ND, et al. Associations of body mass index and perceived weight with suicide ideation and suicide attempts among US high school students. Arch Pediatr Adolesc Med 2005;159(6):513–9.

21. Swallen KC, Reither EN, Haas SA, et al. Overweight, obesity, and health-related quality of life among adolescents: the National Longitudinal Study of Adolescent Health. Pediatrics 2005;115(2):340–7.

22. Strauss RS. Childhood obesity and self-esteem. Pediatrics 2000;105(1):e15.

23. Viner RM, Cole TJ. Adult socioeconomic, educational, social, and psychological outcomes of childhood obesity: a national birth cohort study. BMJ 2005; 330(7504):1354.

24. Alvarez J, Pavao J, Baumrind N, et al. The relationship between child abuse and adult obesity among California women. Am J Prev Med 2007;33(1):28–33.

25. Goulding A, Taylor RW, Jones IE, et al. Overweight and obese children have low bone mass and area for their weight. Int J Obes Relat Metab Disord 2000;24(5):627–32.

26. Rana AR, Michalsky MP, Teich S, et al. Childhood obesity: a risk factor for injuries observed at a level-1 trauma center. J Pediatr Surg 2009;44(8):1601–5.

27. Taylor ED, Theim KR, Mirch MC, et al. Orthopedic complications of overweight in children and adolescents. Pediatrics 2006;117(6):2167–74.

28. Marshall TA, Eichenberger-Gilmore JM, Broffitt BA, et al. Dental caries and childhood obesity: roles of diet and socioeconomic status. Community Dent Oral Epidemiol 2007;35(6):449–58.

29. Baker S, Barlow S, Cochran W, et al. Overweight children and adolescents: a clinical report of the North American Society for Pediatric Gastroenterology, Hepatology and Nutrition. J Pediatr Gastroenterol Nutr 2005;40(5):533–43.

30. Pashankar DS, Loening-Baucke V. Increased prevalence of obesity in children with functional constipation evaluated in an academic medical center. Pediatrics 2005;116(3):e377–80.

31. Chu YT, Chen WY, Wang TN, et al. Extreme BMI predicts higher asthma prevalence and is associated with lung function impairment in school-aged children. Pediatr Pulmonol 2009;44(5):472–9.

32. Martin EY, Molly SB. Potential role for peripheral circadian clock dyssynchrony in the pathogenesis of cardiovascular dysfunction. Sleep Med 2007;8(6):656–67.

33. Rosen CL, Palermo TM, Larkin EK, et al. Health-related quality of life and sleep-disordered breathing in children. Sleep 2002;25(6):657–66.

34. Touchette E, Petit D, Tremblay RE, et al. Associations between sleep duration patterns and overweight/obesity at age 6. Sleep 2008;31(11):1507–14.

35. Lumeng JC, Somashekar D, Appugliese D, et al. Shorter sleep duration is associated with increased risk for being overweight at ages 9 to 12 years. Pediatrics 2007;120(5):1020–9.

36. Sorof J, Daniels S. Obesity hypertension in children: a problem of epidemic proportions. Hypertension 2002;40(4):441–7.

37. Pardee PE, Norman GJ, Lustig RH, et al. Television viewing and hypertension in obese children. Am J Prev Med 2007;33(6):439–43.

38. Maloney AE, Bethea TC, Kelsey KS, et al. A pilot of a video game (DDR) to promote physical activity and decrease sedentary screen time. Obesity (Silver Spring) 2008;16(9):2074–80.

39. Wiecha JL, Peterson KE, Ludwig DS, et al. When children eat what they watch: impact of television viewing on dietary intake in youth. Arch Pediatr Aldolesc Med 2006;160:436–42.

40. Baker JL, Olsen LW, Sorensen TI. Childhood body-mass index and the risk of coronary heart disease in adulthood. N Engl J Med 2007;357(23):2329–37.

41. Liberman JN, Berger JE, Lewis M. Prevalence of antihypertensive, antidiabetic, and dyslipidemic prescription medication use among children and adolescents. Arch Pediatr Adolesc Med 2009;163(4):357–64.

42. Goran MI, Ball GDC, Cruz ML. Obesity and risk of type 2 diabetes and cardiovascular disease in children and adolescents. J Clin Endocrinol Metab 2003;88(4):1417–27.

43. Pinhas-Hamiel O, Dolan LM, Daniels SR, et al. Increased incidence of non-insulin-dependent diabetes mellitus among adolescents. J Pediatr 1996;128(5 Pt 1):608–15.

44. Schwimmer JB, Deutsch R, Kahen T, et al. Prevalence of fatty liver in children and adolescents. Pediatrics 2006;118(4):1388–93.

45. Koebnick C, Getahun D, Reynolds K, et al. Trends in nonalcoholic fatty liver disease-related hospitalizations in US children, adolescents, and young adults. J Pediatr Gastroenterol Nutr 2009;48(5):597–603.

46. Calle EE, Rodriguez C, Walker-Thurmond K, et al. Overweight, obesity, and mortality from cancer in a prospectively studied cohort of U.S. adults. N Engl J Med 2003;348(17):1625–38.

47. Nafiu OO, Green GE, Walton S, et al. Obesity and risk of peri-operative complications in children presenting for adenotonsillectomy. Int J Pediatr Otorhinolaryngol 2009;73(1):89–95.

48. Orozco-Solis R, Lopes de Souza S, Barbosa Matos RJ, et al. Perinatal undernutrition-induced obesity is independent of the developmental programming of feeding. Physiol Behav 2009;96(3):481–92.

49. Barker DJ, Martyn CN. The maternal and fetal origins of cardiovascular disease. J Epidemiol Community Health 1992;46(1):8–11.

50. Poirier P, Giles TD, Bray GA, et al. Obesity and cardiovascular disease: pathophysiology, evaluation, and effect of weight loss. Arterioscler Thromb Vasc Biol 2006;26(5):968–76.

51. Bartok CJ, Ventura AK. Mechanisms underlying the association between breast-feeding and obesity. Int J Pediatr Obes 2009;4(4):196–204.

52. Jones G, Riley M, Dwyer T. Breastfeeding in early life and bone mass in prepubertal children: a longitudinal study. Osteoporos Int 2000;11(2):146–52.

53. Spear BA, Barlow SE, Ervin C, et al. Recommendations for treatment of child and adolescent overweight and obesity. Pediatrics 2007;120(Suppl 4):S254–88.

54. Taveras E, Berkey C, Rifas-Shiman S, et al. Association of consumption of fried food away from home with body mass index and diet quality in older children and adolescents. Pediatrics 2005;116(4):e518–24.

55. Pate RR, Freedson PS, Sallis JF, et al. Compliance with physical activity guidelines: prevalence in a population of children and youth. Ann Epidemiol 2002; 12(5):303–8.

56. Levine JA, Vander Weg MW, Hill JO, et al. Non-exercise activity thermogenesis: the crouching tiger hidden dragon of societal weight gain. Arterioscler Thromb Vasc Biol 2006;26(4):729–36.

57. Robinson TN. Television viewing and childhood obesity. Pediatr Clin North Am 2001;48(4):1017–25.

58. Singh GK, Kogan MD, Van Dyck PC, et al. Racial/ethnic, socioeconomic, and behavioral determinants of childhood and adolescent obesity in the United States: analyzing independent and joint associations. Ann Epidemiol 2008; 18(9):682–95.

59. Vandewater EA, Shim MS, Caplovitz AG. Linking obesity and activity level with children's television and video game use. J Adolesc 2004;27(1):71–85.

60. Powers PS, Bruty H. Pharmacotherapy for eating disorders and obesity. Child Adolesc Psychiatr Clin N Am 2009;18(1):175–87.

61. Barlow SE. Expert committee recommendations regarding the prevention, assessment, and treatment of child and adolescent overweight and obesity: summary report. Pediatrics 2007;120(Suppl 4):S164–92.

62. Jelalian E, Saelens BE. Empirically supported treatments in pediatric psychology: pediatric obesity. J Pediatr Psychol 1999;24(3):223–48.

63. Woolford SJ, Clark SJ, Ahmed S, et al. Feasibility and acceptability of a 1-page tool to help physicians assess and discuss obesity with parents of preschoolers. Clin Pediatr (Phila) 2009;48(9):954–9.

64. Polacsek M, Orr J, Letourneau L, et al. Impact of a primary care intervention on physician practice and patient and family behavior: Keep ME Healthy—The Maine Youth Overweight Collaborative. Pediatrics 2009;123(Suppl 5): S258–66.

65. Epstein LH, Paluch RA, Roemmich JN, et al. Family-based obesity treatment, then and now: twenty-five years of pediatric obesity treatment. Health Psychol 2007;26(4):381–91.

66. Wilfley DE, Stein RI, Saelens BE, et al. Efficacy of maintenance treatment approaches for childhood overweight: a randomized controlled trial. JAMA 2007;298(14):1661–73.
67. Fennig S, Fennig S. Can we treat morbid obese children in a behavioral inpatient program? Pediatr Endocrinol Rev 2006;3(Suppl 4):590–6.
68. Patel NC, Crismon ML, Hoagwood K, et al. Trends in the use of typical and atypical antipsychotics in children and adolescents. J Am Acad Child Adolesc Psychiatry 2005;44(6):548–56.
69. Shin L, Bregman H, Breeze JL, et al. Metformin for weight control in pediatric patients on atypical antipsychotic medication. J Child Adolesc Psychopharmacol 2009;19(3):275–9.
70. Correll CU, Carlson HE. Endocrine and metabolic adverse effects of psychotropic medications in children and adolescents. J Am Acad Child Adolesc Psychiatry 2006;45(7):771–91.
71. Shin L, Bregman H, Frazier J, et al. An overview of obesity in children with psychiatric disorders taking atypical antipsychotics. Harv Rev Psychiatry 2008;16(2):69–79.
72. Fielding GA, Duncombe JE. Laparoscopic adjustable gastric banding in severely obese adolescents. Surg Obes Relat Dis 2005;1(4):399–405 [discussion: 405–397].
73. Raczynski JM, Thompson JW, Phillips MM, et al. Arkansas Act 1220 of 2003 to reduce childhood obesity: its implementation and impact on child and adolescent body mass index. J Public Health Policy 2009;30(Suppl 1):S124–40.
74. Stitt C, Kunkel D. Food advertising during children's television programming on broadcast and cable channels. Health Commun 2008;23(6):573–84.
75. Tate DF, Jackvony EH, Wing RR. Effects of Internet behavioral counseling on weight loss in adults at risk for type 2 diabetes: a randomized trial. JAMA 2003;289(14):1833–6.
76. Shapiro JR, Bauer S, Hamer RM, et al. Use of text messaging for monitoring sugar-sweetened beverages, physical activity, and screen time in children: a pilot study. J Nutr Educ Behav 2008;40(6):385–91.

Psychiatric Concerns in Pediatric Epilepsy

I. Simona Bujoreanu, PhD*, Patricia Ibeziako, MD,
David Ray DeMaso, MD

KEYWORDS

- Epilepsy • Seizures • Children • Psychiatric • Psychosocial
- Cognitive functioning

Pediatric epilepsy is a common, chronic, and challenging physical illness for children and their families. Approximately 45,000 children younger than 15 years develop a new seizure each year, with a median age of onset between ages 5 and 6 years.[1,2] By 20 years of age, 1% of the US population can be expected to have developed epilepsy.[1] In 7 of every 10 cases, there is no known cause, leading to a diagnosis of *idiopathic* epilepsy.[1] A *secondary* or *symptomatic* epilepsy diagnosis is given when there is a known cause for the seizures (eg, anoxic damage, physical trauma, infection, or tumor).[3] Finally, *cryptogenic* or *probably symptomatic* epilepsy implies that an underlying cause for epilepsy exists but cannot be identified.[4]

Childhood epilepsy can place substantial cognitive and psychosocial burdens on young patients and their families. Research on the psychiatric concerns of pediatric epilepsy has grown exponentially over the years (eg, PubMed search on 11/14/2009 found 134 articles published by 1980, 1182 articles between 1981–2000, and 2013 articles from 2001–2009). Focusing primarily on literature from the last 2 decades, this article provides a medical overview along with reviews of cognitive functioning, psychosocial adjustment, and psychiatric management of children and adolescents with pediatric epilepsy. A thorough understanding of these interrelated domains can enable providers to promote resiliency and adaptation in the patients and families facing pediatric epilepsy.

MEDICAL OVERVIEW

Seizures are changes in motor function, sensation, and/or consciousness that are the consequences of abnormal synchronized electrical discharges in the brain.[5] In 2001, the Commission on Epidemiology of the International League Against Epilepsy (ILAE)[6] published a diagnostic scheme based on the following 5 axes: (1) behavior during the

A version of this article was previously published in the *Child and Adolescent Psychiatric Clinics of North America, 19:2.*

Department of Psychiatry, Children's Hospital Boston, Harvard Medical School, 300 Longwood Avenue, Boston, MA 02115, USA

* Corresponding author.

E-mail address: simona.bujoreanu@childrens.harvard.edu

doi:10.1016/j.pcl.2011.06.001
0031-3955/11/$ – see front matter © 2011 Elsevier Inc. All rights reserved.
pediatric.theclinics.com

seizure, (2) types of seizures, (3) detailing specific syndromes, (4) causes, and (5) resultant impairments.[7] **Box 1** provides an overview of the ILAE diagnostic schema; for a detailed review of seizure types the reader is referred to Friedman and Sharieff.[8]

Approximately 70% of children with epilepsy become seizure free on antiepileptic drugs (AEDs) within a few years of diagnosis and subsequently can safely discontinue their medications without recurrence of seizures.[2] Seizure remission is associated with a defined cause of seizure, absence of an epilepsy syndrome, onset before 10 years of age, a low seizure frequency, and early treatment response.[9] In a prospective study of childhood-onset epilepsy, only about 10% of the sample met the criteria for intractable epilepsy (defined as having failed 2 or more AEDs and having had 1 or more seizures per month during a period of 18 months).[10]

There is a multifactorial approach to treatment, which is based on patient's age; type of seizure; risks of recurrence and potential for injury; psychosocial implications; other predisposing medical issues; or effects of treatment, such as toxicity, expense, and cognitive and emotional well-being correlates.[8] Generally, AED monotherapy is

---

Box 1
Overview of ILAE diagnostic scheme

Axis I: ictal phenomenology

Description of the seizure event

Axis II: seizure type

Self-limited

    Generalized: begins deep in the brain and reaches all parts at the same time (eg, tonic-clonic, clonic, absence, spasms, neocortical temporal, myoclonic seizures)

    Focal: begins in one region of the cortex (eg, focal sensory or motor seizures)

        Simple: consciousness is preserved

        Complex: consciousness is impaired

Continuous

    Generalized status epilepticus

    Focal status epilepticus

Reflect: ictal events participated by sensory stimuli (visual, thinking, music, eating, reading, startle, hot water)

Axis III: syndrome

Complex of signs and symptoms that define a unique epilepsy condition (eg, febrile seizures, alcohol withdrawal, progressive myoclonic epilepsy, childhood absence, Lennox-Gastaut syndrome, familial temporal lobe, limbic or neocortical epilepsies, or reflex epilepsies)

Axis IV: cause

Symptomatic: resulting from structural brain lesions (secondary epilepsy)

Probably symptomatic: believed to be symptomatic but no cause identified (cryptogenic)

Idiopathic: primary epilepsy with no identifiable structural brain lesion, presumed to be genetic

Axis V: impairment

Description of disability caused by the epileptic condition

Data from Poduri A, Manicone PE. Seizures. In: Zaoutis LB, Chiang VW, editors. Comprehensive pediatric hospital medicine. Philadelphia: Mosby; 2007. p. 791–800.

more efficacious and results in fewer and less-significant side effects. Polytherapy generally occurs after the failure of more than 1 individual AED trial.[11] For those children with disabling uncontrolled epilepsy and localized regions of seizure activity, surgery has become a treatment option. Temporal or extratemporal resections or corpus callosotomies have been found to significantly decrease seizures in 50% to 90% of such children.[12]

Additional treatment options have been considered for the 20% to 30% of those who do not respond to AEDs, who are not surgical candidates, and/or who have failed surgery.[13] Vagal nerve stimulation, an approved therapy down to age 12 years, has been found to lead to improvement in patients' health-related quality of life.[14] Similar positive effects have also been found with a ketogenic diet in which 80% of the total daily caloric intake is fat.[11,15]

COGNITIVE FUNCTIONING

Pediatric epilepsy is often associated with significant cognitive comorbidity. Cognitive functioning varies in youngsters with epilepsy because of varying interactions between the underlying cause of epilepsy (eg, physiologic disturbance, genetic defect), direct effects of seizure activity on brain structure and function, and/or the medications used to treat seizures.[16,17] The interactions between these factors help explain the difficulty in obtaining a single unified picture of the neuropsychological strengths and vulnerabilities for the pediatric epilepsy population as a whole.

Similar to previous pediatric population studies, Berg and colleagues[16] found that 73.6% of children had normal intellectual functioning, whereas 26.4% fell in a range of cognitive functioning suggestive of subnormal abilities. They found that the level of cognitive functioning was strongly associated with the underlying cause and type of epilepsy (ie, remote symptomatic cause), age at onset (worse outcome if child was younger than 5 years at the time of diagnosis), and medication status (worse outcome if child was still taking medication 5 years postdiagnosis). Furthermore, each of these factors was independently associated with a moderate increase in the risk of falling in the below-normal cognitive range, with a higher degree of impairment for children who experienced more than 1 factor.

Different neuropsychological profiles have emerged depending on the type of epilepsy, the specific focus of the seizures, or the type of treatment. The rate of co-occurring attention-deficit/hyperactivity disorder (ADHD) is increased more than that expected by chance, likely as a result of the bidirectional relationship between those diagnoses.[18] The rate of executive functioning struggles seems increased as evidenced by deficits in processing speed, working memory, planning, organization, and/or mental flexibility. Visual spatial functions and concept formation/abstract reasoning are also affected, as are language abilities and motor skills.[11]

Efforts to define cognitive functioning in children with idiopathic absence seizures, complex partial seizures, and generalized tonic-clonic seizures found an overall low average IQ as well as lower verbal skills, visual memory, and visual attention skills in these patients.[19] Hemisphere-specific disruptions of cognitive skills have been found in temporal lobe epilepsy, with left-sided lesions showing lower performance on verbal memory tasks and right-sided lesions having decreased visual memory functioning.[19] Children with cryptogenic localized epilepsy were found to display reduced psychomotor speed, poor alertness, slower central information-processing speed, and poorer visual long-term memory.[20] Additional details on the neuropsychological profiles of children with epileptic syndromes may be obtained from the works of Mac-Allister and Schaffer[4] and Hamiwka and Wirrell.[21]

Effect of AEDs

Worsening scores in arithmetic abilities for children on topiramate and greater improvement for the maze task for children treated with carbamazepine have been found.[22] In another study, no differences were found in the cognitive scores for children who were newly diagnosed with partial seizures and treated with either oxcarbazepine or carbamazepine/valproate during a 6-month treatment period.[23] In a comparison study, the discontinuation of phenobarbital improved the total IQ score in the case group compared with the control group, mostly in nonverbal performance skills, with verbal skills remaining almost unchanged.[24] More information on studies that are focused on the cognitive side effects of AEDs in children can be obtained from Loring and Meador[25] and Aldenkamp and colleagues.[26]

Academic achievement

Children with epilepsy are more likely to experience school problems, with lower academic achievement. The type of epilepsy (eg, localized and symptomatic generalized epilepsies) has been found to be the dominant factor that explains educational underachievement.[27] Specific neuropsychological vulnerabilities in verbal skills, memory, and executive functioning are strongly related to reading, math, and writing problems. However, it is worth noting that studies show that, in addition to specific cognitive deficits, academic struggles are also moderated by demographic and psychosocial variables. For instance, family environment characterized by support and organization significantly moderated the effect of cognitive deficits on writing and reading in children with epilepsy.[28]

PSYCHOSOCIAL ADJUSTMENT
Emotional Functioning

Children with epilepsy seem to be at risk for emotional and behavioral problems. However, there has been significant variation across studies exploring the rate of psychopathology in children. Similar to the factors affecting epilepsy prognosis and cognitive functioning, seizure frequency/control, type of epilepsy, age of onset, illness duration, and AED medications also likely contribute to the differences found between studies.[29] In addition, differences in the methodology used across studies to assess emotional functioning may also contribute to the varying prevalence rates of emotional and behavioral difficulties in the pediatric epilepsy population.

The Isle of Wight study found that 28% of children with epilepsy had psychiatric disorders.[30] Ott and colleagues[31] found that children with complex partial seizures or partial generalized with absence seizures had comparable rates of anxiety and affective struggles (16%), disruptive behaviors (23%), and psychiatric comorbidity (20%). The investigators concluded that, whether by parent report or by diagnostic interview, children with epilepsy are 3 to 6 times more likely to develop psychopathology than the general population.

Nonepileptic (or nonelectrical) seizures (NESs) are estimated to occur in 17% to 30% of patients referred to comprehensive epilepsy centers (a slightly lower frequency is reported in children) and are paroxysmal events with clinical similarity to epileptic seizures, in the absence of concurrent electrographic ictal pattern.[32] Because a high proportion of patients with NESs have concurrent epilepsy that can be difficult to distinguish from epileptic events, NESs should be suspected when events (1) are refractory to medication changes, (2) have atypical clinical features, (3) are exacerbated by stress, and (4) are not associated with incontinence or a postictal period.[33] Psychosocial stressors are associated with NESs, and common underlying psychiatric diagnoses include mood and/or anxiety disorders (especially separation anxiety, social anxiety, and school phobia).[34] NESs are common in children, and the gold standard of diagnosis is ictal video electroencephalogram (EEG) recording. Early diagnosis is essential for the institution of appropriate psychotherapeutic interventions, and it allows a reduction in the morbidity of unnecessary AED therapy. Video-EEG evidence also helps parents comprehend the emotional, nonepileptic nature of the events.[33]

In a comparison with healthy children, youngsters with epilepsy had significantly more anxiety/affective disorders (63%) and disruptive disorders (26.1%) as well as suicidal ideation (20%).[35] In the same study, only a few patients (5.2%) had depression as a single-standing diagnosis because most cases of depression were comorbid with anxiety disorders (3.5%) or disruptive disorders (28%). When using categorical and dimensional measures of psychopathology in children diagnosed with epilepsy in the preceding 6 months, Dunn and colleagues[36] found that the risk for a psychiatric diagnosis was 3 to 4 times higher for attention-deficit hyperactivity, oppositional defiant, conduct, and dysthymic disorders than that for healthy comparison children.

Multiple studies show that suicide is more common in people with epilepsy.[37] A history of psychiatric disease increases the risk of suicide in a person with epilepsy, but the risk of suicide in people with epilepsy is increased also in the absence of a psychiatric history. The relationship between seizures and depression or suicidal behavior may be bidirectional, and major depression and attempted suicide increase the risk of developing seizures.[37]

In children with epilepsy with comorbid nonverbal cognitive problems, psychosocial problems (including internalizing and externalizing problems) were much more frequent than among controls.[38] Although far less frequent, thought disorders in pediatric epilepsy seem to occur at a higher rate when compared with community-based population estimates.[39]

The question of cause-effect relationship between epilepsy and psychiatric difficulty remains an area of inquiry. Behavioral problems have been identified as early as 6 months before the child's first recognized seizure, with nearly 32% of the newly diagnosed children having a preexisting baseline of psychiatric symptomatology within the clinical or the at-risk ranges.[40] A developmental perspective in explaining the psychological and behavioral difficulties of children with epilepsy suggests a model whereby the cognitive and language difficulties found in pediatric epilepsy adversely affect a child's ability to follow normal emotional and social skill developmental tracks.[31]

In a meta-analysis examining the types and severity of psychopathology in children with epilepsy, the magnitude of differences revealed small to medium effect sizes when compared with children with other chronic physical illnesses (eg, asthma, diabetes, cardiac disease, and migraine), suggesting that the psychopathology in pediatric epilepsy may be attributed partly to the chronicity of the physical disease as opposed to an illness-specific effect of epilepsy. Furthermore, within the larger population of children with other physical illnesses affecting the central nervous system, the rates for anxiety and depression were similar to those in the pediatric epilepsy population.[41]

Epilepsy during adolescence poses a period of vulnerability that can hinder the development of psychosocial independence,[42] and treatment relies on AEDs, which must be taken daily.[43] Nonadherence is common and problematic because of lack of education about epilepsy (ie, why take medications in the absence of seizures), desire to avoid adverse medication side effects, difficulties in controlling seizures, forgetfulness, disorganization, and/or oppositionality. Negative outcomes of nonadherence include seizure recurrence, missing school, absence from social events, emergency department visits, and/or hospitalization.[42] Studies have shown that treatment nonadherence is as high as 50% in chronic pediatric illnesses.[44] Caregiver involvement in their children's epilepsy management, which is greater than what has been found in other chronic physical illnesses, has implications with regard to monitoring treatment adherence.[42] A meta-analysis of psychological interventions developed to increase adherence has revealed that applied behavioral interventions (eg, problem solving, parent training) and multicomponent interventions incorporating educational treatment models, social support, social skills training, or family therapy seemed to be relatively potent in promoting adherence among chronically physically ill youth.[44]

Despite the common desire of adolescents with epilepsy to drive, seizures pose the risk of a crash, which may result in property damage, injuries, and even deaths. Today, every state in the United States permits people with controlled seizures to drive with required seizure-free periods ranging from about 3 to 12 months.[45] Many patients with epilepsy frequently do not inform their physicians about seizure occurrence, fearing loss of driving privileges and other social consequences[45]; therefore, it is recommended that physicians engage adolescents directly in discussions about their health condition, including the safety issues related to driving.

Family Functioning

Physical illness in a child is a significant source of stress for families.[46] Given its chronic nature, childhood epilepsy presents ongoing demands on the family's ability to adapt and function.[29] Parents of children with epilepsy have reported feeling more emotionally overwhelmed and fearful than parents of children with special health care needs.[47] Parents have been found to experience posttraumatic stress symptoms and major depressive disorder,[48] to express anxiety and decreased quality of life,[49] or to express increased stress levels, especially if comorbid depression and learning difficulties were present in the child.[50]

The increased parenting stress caused by having a child with epilepsy has been found to adversely affect parent-child interaction, leading to behavioral and emotional problems.[51] A meta-analysis of the research on the psychosocial adjustment of children with epilepsy reveals that behavioral and emotional disturbances are related to parental criticism and parental psychological control, whereas parental acceptance was associated with lower levels of externalizing behavior problems.[41] These findings of parental negative perceptions and stigma in relationship with adjustment to childhood epilepsy have offered mixed results; overall, having epilepsy and mental health problems may possibly lead to an increase in the stigma load for these children.[29]

Long-term consequences of epilepsy may be a result of any or all of the childhood psychological struggles, effects on cognitive functioning, and/or family adjustment and stressors. Considering the elevated prevalence of psychopathology in adults with epilepsy (about 65%),[52] the less-than-desirable outcome of children with generalized epilepsy 20 years postdiagnosis,[53] and the poor quality of life for seizure-free or off-medication adults 30 years from the diagnosis,[54] successfully identifying and treating emergent psychopathology in the pediatric population warrants early identification and early preventive interventions.

Psychiatric Management

Establish a collaborative health care approach

A pattern of delayed recognition and diagnosis of epilepsy has been observed with a variety of interrelated reasons including parental delay in seeking treatment, health care providers not recognizing a presentation as epilepsy, and/or health care providers initiating inappropriate treatment.[55] Unrecognized seizures can have adverse physical and psychosocial consequences. According to a survey of pediatricians and child neurologists, most of them were unaware of the greater need for mental health referrals in children with epilepsy, identified limited resources in their own expertise about the mental health system, and recognized their lack of collaboration with mental health providers.[56] This becomes evident because more than 60% of children with epilepsy do not receive needed mental health services despite diagnosable psychiatric disorders.[31] In this context, it is critical for the child mental health clinicians to establish an integrated health care approach characterized by communication and collaboration with a child's family, primary care clinician, and specialty care clinician (eg, child neurologist). This will allow the mental health clinician not only to convey important psychiatric considerations to the physical health clinicians but also to be alert to important changes in the course and physical treatment of the child's epilepsy.

The care of patients with pediatric epilepsy does involve workforce shortages, which create significant challenges for the patient, family, and primary care clinicians in obtaining specialty care. There are approximately 8000 child psychiatrists,[57] 1200 child neurologists,[58] and 500 developmental behavioral pediatricians in the United States.[59] This means that primary care clinicians often need to undertake the tasks of both medical and psychiatric care of childhood epilepsy without the ability to collaborate with child-trained psychiatrists or neurologists who specialize in the developmental, psychosocial, or biologic aspects of these patients.

Because not every youngster with epilepsy needs mental health and educational assessment or intervention, primary care clinicians are increasingly adopting standardized screening tools and/or queries to identify only the youngsters who are most in need of mental health intervention.[60] In this context, child mental health clinicians with strong interests in chronic pediatric physical illnesses have tremendous opportunities to collaboratively work with primary care clinicians to develop innovative and integrative health care approaches for children and their families.

Evaluate academic functioning

The use of neuropsychological evaluations for the pediatric epilepsy population has been a topic of debate. Arguments for and against this intervention have been discussed: the need for early identification of learning or mental health problems, ability to learn in school, or successful negotiation of social peer interaction versus an indiscriminate use of time-consuming and expensive evaluations, the potential inappropriate labeling of children as "learning disabled," or the risk of attached stigma. Overall, the conclusion is that the option of a neuropsychological evaluation should be at least considered by mental health clinicians in the course of their evaluation and management of children with epilepsy.[61]

Children identified as "students in need of services" can benefit from services ranging from simple classroom accommodations to specialized instruction. Communication among home, school, and medical providers is an essential step in ensuring that an integrated health care approach that increases a child's chance for success is implemented. The mental health clinician needs to be alert to parental stress levels when negotiating with the educational system because research has noted increased parent struggles when their children present with learning disabilities co-occurring with epilepsy.[50] To communicate effectively, school personnel and parents must be educated about neurocognitive effects that a particular child may experience. In addition, knowledge of state and federal laws regarding the education of children with special needs will aid in the parents' ability to navigate through the education system and to best advocate for their child.

As part of this process, the child mental health clinician must provide psychoeducation and guidance to parents regarding the neuropsychological correlates of their child's epilepsy, from a thorough evaluation of potential cognitive weaknesses to explaining the role of neuropsychologists and educational advocates in the community or the school.

Consider psychotherapy

Psychotherapy is an important treatment that should be considered for emotional and behavioral problems in children with epilepsy. The treatment, which should include the child and family, targets the enhancement of coping mechanisms that promote continued psychological development and adaptation to illness.[62] Effective psychotherapy can help patients understand the meaning of and responses to their illness, improve treatment adherence, and enhance psychosocial functioning.[62] As with other physical illnesses, there continues to be a paucity of empirical evidence that supports the efficacy of any psychotherapeutic modality in children with epilepsy.

In a review of the existing successful intervention programs designed to provide support to children and families facing epilepsy, identified treatment goals were delineated, such as: reducing children's concerns and fears; problem behaviors; minimizing associated stress; increasing epilepsy knowledge and decision-making skills; improving attitudes toward epilepsy; and improving epilepsy management, independence, coping skills, and efficient communication.[63] These interventions were delivered in through a variety of modalities including individual meetings, parent groups, phone interviews/conferences, video conferencing, and summer camps. Both individual and group cognitive behavioral intervention strategies, including relaxation and biofeedback, predominated as the treatment approach.[63]

Overall, these evidence-based psychological interventions have shown improved psychological adjustment and some evidence that seizure severity and frequency may be reduced.[63] Although these therapeutic efforts provide support for the use of psychological interventions in childhood epilepsy, methodologically sound randomized clinical trials are still needed before taking for granted the implications of their effectiveness. Nonetheless, despite numerous methodological weaknesses in existing studies, there is a sufficiently strong evidence base to support the integration of psychotherapy treatment as part of comprehensive pediatric care in physically ill children and adolescents.[62]

Manage psychopharmacologic treatment

It is beyond the scope of this article to review the pharmacologic treatment of the different types of epilepsy in childhood. The prescribing mental health clinician should be familiar with the medications being used in the treatment of seizures in each individual child and their common associated neuropsychiatric effects (**Table 1**).

The US Food and Drug Administration (FDA) has issued an update after the completion of its analysis concerning the risk of suicidality (suicidal behavior or ideation) that was observed during clinical trials of various AEDs compared with placebo in the treatment of epilepsy, psychiatric disorders, and other conditions.[64] The pooled analysis of 199 clinical trials involving 11 AEDs (carbamazepine, divalproex sodium, felbamate, gabapentin, lamotrigine, levetiracetam, oxcarbazepine, pregabalin, tiagabine, topiramate, zonisamide) used as monotherapy or as adjuvant therapy showed that patients receiving an AED had a 0.43% risk of suicidal behavior/ideation compared with 0.24% risk in patients receiving placebo. Increased risk was observed as early as 1 week after the initiation of AED and continued through the duration of trials (most trials lasted up to 24 weeks); risk did not vary significantly by age (age range, 5–100 years).

Table 1
Common AEDs and neuropsychiatric effects

Generic Name	Trade Name	Neuropsychiatric Side Effects
Phenobarbital	Luminal	Drowsiness, somnolence, central nervous system depression, paradoxic excitement, hyperkinetic activity, cognitive impairment, defects in general comprehension, short-term memory deficits, decreased attention span, ataxia, suicidal thinking and behavior
Phenytoin	Dilantin	Slurred speech, dizziness, drowsiness, lethargy, coma, ataxia, dyskinesias, mood changes, suicidal thinking and behavior
Carbamazepine	Tegretol	Sedation, dizziness, drowsiness, somnolence, fatigue, slurred speech, ataxia, confusion, suicidal thinking and behavior
Oxcarbazepine	Trileptal	Headache, dizziness, somnolence (incidence in children up to 34.8%), fatigue, ataxia or gait disturbances (children: up to 23.2%), tremor, insomnia, cognitive symptoms (children: up to 5.8%; psychomotor slowing, difficulty concentrating, speech/language problems), anxiety, nervousness, emotional lability, suicidal thinking and behavior
Levetiracetam	Keppra	Behavioral symptoms such as aggression, anger, apathy, depersonalization, depression, emotional lability, hostility, hyperkinesias, irritability, (incidence in children 38%); somnolence (children 23%); headache, hostility (children 12%); nervousness (children 10%); dizziness (children 7%); personality disorder; pain (children 6%); agitation (children 6%); emotional lability (children 6%); depression (children 3%); amnesia; anxiety, confusion (children 2%); psychotic symptoms; suicidal thinking and behavior
Valproic acid	Depakote	Drowsiness, somnolence, irritability, confusion, restlessness, nervousness, hyperactivity, malaise, headache, ataxia, dizziness, abnormal dreams, amnesia, anxiety, abnormal coordination, depression, personality disorder, hyperammonemic encephalopathy, suicidal thinking and behavior
Lamotrigine	Lamictal	Agitation, anxiety, ataxia, depression, difficulty concentrating, dizziness, emotional lability, headache, incoordination, insomnia, irritability, nervousness, sedation, somnolence, speech disorder, suicidal thinking and behavior
Gabapentin[a]	Neurontin	Somnolence, dizziness, ataxia, fatigue, depression, nervousness, suicidal thinking and behavior; neuropsychiatric adverse events in children 3–12 y of age: emotional lability (behavioral problems): 6% incidence; hostility (including aggressive behaviors): 5.2%; hyperkinesia (hyperactivity, restlessness): 4.7%; thought disorder (problems with concentration and school performance): 1.7%. Note: most of these pediatric neuropsychiatric adverse events are mild to moderate in terms of intensity but discontinuation of gabapentin may be required; children with mental retardation and attention-deficit disorders may be at increased risk for behavioral side effects.
Topiramate	Topamax	Ataxia, difficulty in concentrating, dizziness, memory difficulties, fatigue, nervousness, somnolence, psychomotor slowing, speech/language problems, confusion, depression, mood problems, anxiety, cognitive problems; fever, irritability, and sleep disturbances (reported in children), suicidal thinking and behavior. Note: somnolence and fatigue are the most common neuropsychiatric adverse effects in children

[a] Abrupt withdrawal may precipitate status epilepticus or increase in seizures; decrease dose gradually over at least 1 week.

Depressive disorders

Selective serotonin reuptake inhibitors (SSRIs) seem to be a good therapeutic option in patients with co-occurring depressive disorders and epilepsy, considering their efficacy in remitting depressive symptoms, having few adverse effects, and maintaining satisfactory seizure control.[65] Although older tricyclic and monoamine oxidase inhibitor antidepressants have a dose-dependent potential to decrease seizure threshold, second-generation antidepressants, particularly the SSRIs, do not lower seizure threshold and may even have an anticonvulsant effect.[66]

Bupropion immediate release (IR) has higher rates of seizures compared with other second-generation antidepressants, and EEG abnormalities have been reported in some patients on bupropion IR therapy.[67] Seizures are especially prominent at single doses greater than 150 mg or daily doses greater than 450 mg, and the estimated seizure incidence was found to increase tenfold at dosages of more than 450 mg/d.[68] There is an increased risk of seizures in patients who take extra doses of bupropion IR on an "as needed" basis.[69] In addition, about 21% of patients admitted with intentional bupropion IR overdose present with seizures.[70]

Anxiety disorders

Gamma-aminobutyric acid (GABA), the predominant inhibitory neurotransmitter of the central nervous system, is involved in the pathophysiology of a wide variety of disorders, including anxiety. Many of the anticonvulsant agents target this neurotransmitter and therefore potentially have a beneficial effect for anxiety in patients with or without comorbid epilepsy.

The SSRIs are the first line of treatment for patients with comorbid anxiety and seizures.[71] The selective norepinephrine reuptake inhibitor, venlafaxine, has also shown to have some benefit.[71]

Gabapentin has been demonstrated to have anxiolytic action. Its exact mechanism of action is not understood, although modes of action involving calcium channels and some GABAergic and glutamatergic systems have been hypothesized.[72] Pregabalin, an adjunctive medication used for partial epilepsy, acts at presynaptic calcium channels, modulating neurotransmitter release in the central nervous system, a property it shares with gabapentin. The clinical development of pregabalin during the past decade has included its use in the treatment of neuropathic pain and generalized anxiety disorder in addition to epilepsy.[73] Tiagabine hydrochloride acts as a selective GABA reuptake inhibitor and is used in epilepsy treatment; it may also be useful in the treatment of acute anxiety and generalized anxiety disorder.[74] However, there remains a paucity of studies involving children; most data cited earlier are from adult studies.

Attention-deficit/hyperactivity disorder

Stimulants are the first line of treatment in patients with comorbid ADHD and epilepsy. With regard to the efficacy of methylphenidate in alleviating ADHD symptoms in children with dual diagnosis of epilepsy, multiple studies have shown improvement in symptoms in more than 70% of children.[75]

There is no definitive evidence supporting the possibility that methylphenidate aggravates or induces epilepsy. Methylphenidate affects the presynaptic uptake of noradrenaline and dopamine but has no effect on neurotransmitters such as GABA, glutamate, and aspartic acid or sodium or calcium channels, which have been associated with the pathophysiology of epilepsy.[76] There is also insufficient evidence in the literature to justify performing encephalography in an otherwise healthy child with ADHD before starting methylphenidate treatment. At present, EEG is considered only in children who are suspected of having clinical seizures or when absence or complex partial seizures are part of the differential diagnosis of an attention problem.

Atomoxetine is a potent specific norepinephrine reuptake inhibitor and has not been associated with an increased risk of seizures in patients treated for ADHD.[77] There has been a fair amount of clinical use of alpha2-agonists such as guanfacine and clonidine in children with comorbid ADHD and epilepsy.[78] There is 1 case report on the possible association of clonidine with new-onset seizures but there is insufficient evidence supporting the association of alpha2-agonists with increased seizures.[79]

Psychosis

Pediatric patients with epilepsy have an increased risk of suffering from psychotic symptoms, which are generally classified according to their temporal relationship with the seizure itself as ictal, postictal, and interictal psychosis. Ictal psychosis is most commonly associated with complex partial seizures, with most discharges having a focus on the limbic and isocortical components of the temporal lobe, although they may sometimes originate from the frontal lobe.[80] Postictal psychosis is, however, the most common form of psychosis found in people with epilepsy.[81]

The treatment of epilepsy in youngsters with concomitant psychotic symptoms is complicated further by the side effects of the antiepileptic and antipsychotic drugs and by the drug-drug interactions. For example, research has shown that some AEDs can precipitate psychosis, whereas all antipsychotic drugs have the propensity to cause paroxysmal EEG abnormalities and induce seizures.[80] Furthermore, antipsychotic drugs also have pharmacokinetic interactions with antiepileptic medications. Among the antipsychotic drugs, clozapine is the most epileptogenic, with seizures reported in 0.3% to 5% of people treated with therapeutic doses.[82]

Bipolar disorder

Anticonvulsant monotherapy is a reasonable approach for patients with comorbid epilepsy and bipolar spectrum disorder. Strict interpretation of the Diagnostic and Statistical Manual of Mental Disorders, fourth edition (DSM-IV) diagnostic criteria for bipolar disorder requires exclusions based on a co-occurring physical illness. This poses a diagnostic challenge in childhood epilepsy because there is an association of mood disorder symptoms with interictal and periictal states, which makes it difficult to identify comorbidity outside of the context of epilepsy.[83] Anticonvulsants may function in these patients by decreasing neuronal hyperexcitability and reducing the likelihood for affective instability and seizure activity.

Although controlled trials are necessary, in retrospective studies, carbamazepine, divalproex sodium, lamotrigine, and oxcarbazepine have demonstrated the most evident improvement as monotherapy in patients with co-occurring epilepsy and bipolar spectrum illness.[84] Carbamazepine, divalproex sodium, and lamotrigine are FDA-approved drugs for the treatment of bipolar disorder in adults but not in children, whereas oxcarbazepine is not FDA approved for the treatment of bipolar disorder in either adults or children. Small, open-label trials of divalproex sodium and carbamazepine support their efficacy in the treatment of youngsters with bipolar disorder, whereas oxcarbazepine has also been shown in case reports to be effective for the treatment of childhood bipolar disorder.[85]

SUMMARY

Medical science has made great strides in understanding the process of diagnosis and treatment of pediatric epilepsy, leading to significant improvements in the medical prognosis of this complex illness. Although the developing brain has great capacity for plasticity and resilience, understanding the biologic, psychiatric, and social aspects associated with pediatric epilepsy is critical. Research in the fields of child psychiatry and pediatric psychology has led to significant advancements in understanding the cognitive functioning and psychosocial adjustment of children with epilepsy. The care of the pediatric epilepsy population should, therefore, be the point of convergence between state-of-the-art medical treatments and cross-discipline treatments focusing on psychoeducation, therapeutic intervention, and school support, for the ultimate goal of promoting the development of independence, competence, and well-being at the maximum level for the child, in the initial phases of the illness and diagnosis and in the future.

REFERENCES

1. Epilepsy Foundation of America. Available at: http://www.epilepsyfoundation.org/. Accessed October 10, 2009.
2. Shinnar S, Pellock JM. Update on the epidemiology and prognosis of pediatric epilepsy. J Child Neurol 2002;17:S4–17.
3. World Health Organization. Available at: http://www.who.int/en/. Accessed November 1, 2009.
4. MacAllister WS, Schaffer SG. Neuropsychological deficits in childhood epilepsy syndromes. Neuropsychol Rev 2007;17(4):427–44.
5. Martini R. Neurological disease. In: Shaw RJ, DeMaso DR, editors. Textbook of pediatric psychosomatic medicine: mental health consultation with physically ill children. Washington, DC: American Psychiatric Press Inc; 2010. p. 387–403.
6. Commission on Epidemiology of the International League Against Epilepsy. Available at: http://www.ilae-epilepsy.org/. Accessed November 11, 2009.
7. Poduri A, Manicone PE. Seizures. In: Zaoutis LB, Chiang VW, editors. Comprehensive pediatric hospital medicine. Philadelphia: Mosby; 2007. p. 791–800.
8. Friedman MJ, Sharieff GQ. Seizures in children. Pediatr Clin North Am 2006; 53(2):257–77.
9. Nair GC, Bharucha NE. Prognosis of pediatric epilepsy. J Pediatr Neurosci 2008; 3:41–7.
10. Berg AT, Shinnar S, Levy SR, et al. Early development of intractable epilepsy in children: a prospective study. Neurology 2001;56(11):1445–52.
11. Williams J, Sharp GB. Epilepsy. In: Yeates KO, Ris MD, Taylor HG, editors. Pediatric neuropsychology: research, theory, and practice. New York: Guilford Press; 2000. p. 47–73.
12. Smith ML, Elliott IM, Lach L. Memory outcome after pediatric epilepsy surgery: objective and subjective perspectives. Child Neuropsychol 2006; 12(3):151–64.
13. Bagić A, Theodore WH, Boudreau EA, et al. Towards a non-invasive interictal application of hypothermia for treating seizures: a feasibility and pilot study. Acta Neurol Scand 2008;118(4):240–4.
14. Sherman EM, Connolly MB, Slick DJ, et al. Quality of life and seizure outcome after vagus nerve stimulation in children with intractable epilepsy. J Child Neurol 2008;23(9):991–8.
15. Kossoff EH, Pyzik PL, Rubenstein JE, et al. Combined ketogenic diet and vagus nerve stimulation: rational polytherapy? Epilepsia 2007;48(1):77–81.
16. Berg AT, Langfitt JT, Testa FM, et al. Residual cognitive effects of uncomplicated idiopathic and cryptogenic epilepsy. Epilepsy Behav 2008;13(4):614–9.

17. Henkin Y, Sadeh M, Kivity S, et al. Cognitive function in idiopathic generalized epilepsy of childhood. Dev Med Child Neurol 2005;47(2):126–32.
18. Hamoda HM, Guild DJ, Gumlak S, et al. Association between attention-deficit/ hyperactivity disorder and epilepsy in pediatric populations. Expert Rev Neurother 2009;9(12):1–8.
19. Williams J, Griebel ML, Dykman RA. Neuropsychological patterns in pediatric epilepsy. Seizure 1998;7(3):223–8.
20. van Mil SG, Reijs RP, van Hall MH, et al. Neuropsychological profile of children with cryptogenic localization related epilepsy. Child Neuropsychol 2008;14(4):291–302.
21. Hamiwka LD, Wirrell EC. Comorbidities in pediatric epilepsy: beyond 'just' treating the seizures. J Child Neurol 2009;24(6):734–42.
22. Kang H-C, Eun B-L, Lee CW, et al. The effects on cognitive function and behavioral problems of topiramate compared to carbamazepine as monotherapy for children with benign rolandic epilepsy. Epilepsia 2007;48(9):1716–23.
23. Donati F, Gobbi G, Campistol J, et al. Oxcarbazepine Cognitive Study Group. The cognitive effects of oxcarbazepine versus carbamazepine or valproate in newly diagnosed children with partial seizures. Seizure 2007;16(8):670–9.
24. Tonekaboni SH, Beyraghi N, Tahbaz HS, et al. Neurocognitive effects of phenobarbital discontinuation in epileptic children. Epilepsy Behav 2006;8(1):145–8.
25. Loring DW, Meador KJ. Cognitive side effects of antiepileptic drugs in children. Neurology 2004;62(6):872–7.
26. Aldenkamp AP, De Krom M, Reijs R. Newer antiepileptic drugs and cognitive issues. Epilepsia 2003;44(4):21–9.
27. Aldenkamp AP, Weber B, Overweg-Plandsoen WC, et al. Educational underachievement in children with epilepsy: a model to predict the effects of epilepsy on educational achievement. J Child Neurol 2005;20(3):175–80.
28. Fastenau PS, Shen J, Dunn DW, et al. Neuropsychological predictors of academic underachievement in pediatric epilepsy: moderating roles of demographic, seizure, and psychosocial variables. Epilepsia 2004;45(10):1261–72.
29. Austin JK, Caplan R. Behavioral and psychiatric comorbidities in pediatric epilepsy: toward an integrative model. Epilepsia 2007;48(9):1639–51.
30. Rutter M, Graham P, Yule W. A neuropsychiatric study in childhood. Philadelphia: JB Lippincott; 1970.
31. Ott D, Siddarth P, Gurbani S, et al. Behavioral disorders in pediatric epilepsy: unmet psychiatric need. Epilepsia 2003;44(4):591–7.
32. Thompson NC, Osorio I, Hunter EE. Nonepileptic seizures: reframing the diagnosis. Perspect Psychiatr Care 2005;41(2):71–8.
33. Paolicchi JM. The spectrum of nonepileptic events in children. Epilepsia 2002; 43(Suppl 3):60–4.
34. Bhatia MS, Sapra S. Pseudoseizures in children: a profile of 50 cases. Clin Pediatr 2005;44(7):617–21.
35. Caplan R, Siddarth P, Gurbani S, et al. Psychopathology and pediatric complex partial seizures: seizure-related, cognitive, and linguistic variables. Epilepsia 2005;45(10):1273–81.
36. Dunn DW, Austin JK, Perkins SM. Prevalence of psychopathology in childhood epilepsy: categorical and dimensional measures. Dev Med Child Neurol 2009; 51(5):364–72.
37. Bell GS, Sander JW. Suicide and epilepsy. Curr Opin Neurol 2009;22(2):174–8.
38. Høie B, Sommerfelt K, Waaler PE, et al. The combined burden of cognitive, executive function, and psychosocial problems in children with epilepsy: a population-based study. Dev Med Child Neurol 2008;50(7):530–6.

39. Caplan R, Siddarth P, Bailey CE, et al. Thought disorder: a developmental disability in pediatric epilepsy. Epilepsy Behav 2006;8(4):726–35.
40. Austin JK, Harezlak J, Dunn DW, et al. Behavior problems in children before first recognized seizures. Pediatrics 2001;107(1):115–22.
41. Rodenburg R, Stams GJ, Meijer AM, et al. Psychopathology in children with epilepsy: a meta-analysis. J Pediatr Psychol 2005;30(6):453–68.
42. Asato MR, Manjunath R, Sheth RD, et al. Adolescent and caregiver experiences with epilepsy. J Child Neurol 2009;24(5):562–71.
43. Snodgrass SR, Vedanarayanan VV, Parker CC, et al. Pediatric patients with undetectable anticonvulsant blood levels: comparison with compliant patients. J Child Neurol 2001;16(3):164–8.
44. Kahana S, Drotar S, Frazier T. Meta-analysis of psychological interventions to promote adherence to treatment in pediatric chronic health conditions. J Pediatr Psychol 2008;33(6):590–611.
45. Krumholz A. Driving issues in epilepsy: past, present, and future. Epilepsy Curr 2009;9(2):31–5.
46. Kazak AE, Kassam-Adams N, Schneider S, et al. An integrative model of pediatric medical traumatic stress. J Pediatr Psychol 2006;31(4):343–55.
47. Modi AC. The impact of a new pediatric epilepsy diagnosis on parents: parenting stress and activity patterns. Epilepsy Behav 2009;14(1):237–42.
48. Izeri PK, Ozten A, Aker AT. Posttraumatic stress disorder. Epilepsy Behav 2006;8: 250–5.
49. Williams J, Steel C, Sharp GB, et al. Parental anxiety and quality of life in children with epilepsy. Epilepsy Behav 2003;4(5):483–6.
50. Cushner-Weinstein S, Dassoulas K, Salpekar JA, et al. Parenting stress and childhood epilepsy: the impact of depression, learning, and seizure-related factors. Epilepsy Behav 2008;13(1):109–14.
51. Rodenburg R, Meijer AM, Deković M, et al. Family predictors of psychopathology in children with epilepsy. Epilepsia 2006;47(3):601–14.
52. Blumer D, Montouris G, Hermann B. Psychiatric morbidity in seizure patients on a neurodiagnostic monitoring unit. J Neuropsychiatry Clin Neurosci 1995;7(4): 445–56.
53. Camfield C, Camfield P. Twenty years after childhood-onset symptomatic generalized epilepsy the social outcome is usually dependency or death: a population-based study. Dev Med Child Neurol 2008;50(11):859–63.
54. Sillanpää M, Haataja L, Shinnar S. Perceived impact of childhood-onset epilepsy on quality of life as an adult. Epilepsia 2004;45(8):971–7.
55. Buelow JM, Shore CP. Childhood epilepsy: failures along the path to diagnosis and treatment. Epilepsy Behav 2006;9(3):440–7.
56. Smith K, Siddarth P, Zima B, et al. Unmet mental health needs in pediatric epilepsy: insights from providers. Epilepsy Behav 2007;11(3):401–8.
57. American Academy of Child and Adolescent Psychiatry: Child and Adolescent Psychiatrists Champion Child Healthcare Crisis Relief Act. Press release. Available at: http://www.aacap.org/cs/2007_press_releases/child_and_adolescent_ psychiatrists_champion_child_healthcare_crisis_relief_act. Accessed January 3, 2010.
58. Bale JF, Currey M, Firth S, et al. The child neurology workforce study: pediatrician access and satisfaction. J Pediatr 2009;154(4):602–6.
59. Gupta VB. The future of developmental behavioral pediatrics. J Dev Behav Pediatr 2005;26(3):254–5.

60. Goldstein J, Plioplys S, Zelko F, et al. Multidisciplinary approach to childhood epilepsy: exploring the scientific rationale and practical aspects of implementation. J Child Neurol 2004;19(5):362–78.

61. Buelow JM, McNelis A. Should every child with epilepsy undergo a neuropsychological evaluation? Epilepsy Behav 2002;3(31):210–3.

62. Szigethy E, Noll RB. Individual psychotherapy. In: Shaw RJ, DeMaso DR, editors. Textbook of pediatric psychosomatic medicine: mental health consultation with physically ill children. Washington, DC: American Psychiatric Press Inc; 2010. p. 423–38.

63. Wagner JL, Smith G. Psychosocial intervention in pediatric epilepsy: a critique of the literature. Epilepsy Behav 2006;8(1):39–49.

64. US Food and Drug Administration. Antiepileptic drugs and suicidality. Available at: http://www.fda.gov/downloads/Drugs/Drugsafety/PostmarketDrugSafetyInformation forPatientsandProviders/UCM192556.pdf. Accessed December 5, 2009.

65. Thome-Suoza MS, Kuczynski E, Valente KD. Sertraline and fluoxetine: safe treatments for children and adolescents with epilepsy and depression. Epilepsy Behav 2007;10:417–25.

66. Alper K, Schwartz KA, Kolts RL, et al. Seizure incidence in psychopharmacological clinical trials: an analysis of Food and Drug Administration (FDA) summary basis of approval reports. Biol Psychiatry 2007;62:345–54.

67. Shah GD, Hirsch LJ. Bitemporal epileptiform discharges induced by bupropion: a case report. Clin Neuropharmacol 2001;24:304–6.

68. Physicians' desk reference. 61st edition. Montvale (NJ): Thomson Healthcare, Inc; 2007. p. 1603–7.

69. Shepherd G. Adverse effects associated with extra doses of bupropion. Pharmacotherapy 2005;25:1378–82.

70. Spiller HA, Ramoska EA, Krenzelok EP, et al. Bupropion overdose: a 3-year multicenter retrospective analysis. Am J Emerg Med 1994;12:43–5.

71. Ipser JC, Stein DJ, Hawkridge S, et al. Pharmacotherapy for anxiety disorders in children and adolescents. Cochrane Database Syst Rev 2009;(3):CD005170.

72. Onder E, Tural U, Gokbakan M. Does gabapentin lead to early symptom improvement in obsessive-compulsive disorder? Eur Arch Psychiatry Clin Neurosci 2008; 258:319–23.

73. Hamandi K, Sander JW. Pregablin: a new antiepileptic drug for refractory epilepsy. Seizure 2006;15:73–8.

74. Schaller JL, Thomas J, Rawlings D. Low-dose tiagabine effectiveness in anxiety disorders. MedGenMed 2004;6(3):8.

75. Gucuyener K, Erdemoglu K, Senol S, et al. Use of methylphenidate for attention-deficit hyperactivity disorder in patients with epilepsy or electroencephalographic abnormalities. J Child Neurol 2003;18:109–12.

76. Kaufmann R, Goldberg-Stern H, Shuper A. Attention-deficit disorders and epilepsy in childhood: incidence, causative relations and treatment possibilities. J Child Neurol 2009;24:727–33.

77. Wernicke JF, Holdrige KC, Jin L, et al. Seizure risk in patients with attention deficit hyperactivity disorder treated with atomoxetine. Dev Med Child Neurol 2007;49: 498–502.

78. Torres AR, Whitney J, Gonzalez-Heydrich J. Attention-deficit/hyperactivity disorder in pediatric patients with epilepsy: review of pharmacological treatment. Epilepsy Behav 2008;12:217–33.

79. Feron FJ, Hendriksen JG, Nicolai J, et al. New-onset seizures: a possible association with clonidine? Pediatr Neurol 2008;38:147–9.

80. Farooq S, Sherin A. Interventions for psychotic symptoms concomitant with epilepsy. Cochrane Database Syst Rev 2008;(4):CD006118.
81. Toone BK. The psychoses of epilepsy. J Neurol Neurosurg Psychiatr 2000;69(1): 1–3.
82. Langosch JM, Trimble MR. Epilepsy, psychosis and clozapine. Hum Psychopharmacol 2002;17(2):115–9.
83. Kudo T, Ishida S, Kubota H, et al. Manic episode in epilepsy and bipolar 1 disorder: a comparative analysis of 13 patients. Epilepsia 2001;160:430–7.
84. Salpekar JA, Conry JA, Doss W, et al. Clinical experience with anticonvulsant medication in pediatric epilepsy and comorbid bipolar spectrum disorder. Epilepsy Behav 2006;9(2):327–34.
85. Lopez-Larson M, Frazier JA. Empirical evidence for the use of lithium and anticonvulsants in children with psychiatric disorders. Harv Rev Psychiatry 2006; 14:285–304.

Psychiatric Considerations in Children and Adolescents with HIV/AIDS

Tami D. Benton, MD

KEYWORDS

- Human immunodeficiency virus • Children • Adolescents
- Psychiatric disorders

The psychosocial impact of human immunodeficiency virus (HIV) disease has been recognized since the beginning of the epidemic for affected adults, but there has been less focus on the impact of HIV on young people. Among HIV-positive (HIV+) adults, high levels of distress, psychiatric symptoms, and their associations with worse health outcomes were recognized early in the epidemic. Subsequently, many studies have focused on understanding the prevalence of psychiatric symptoms among HIV+ adults and on identifying effective treatments for these symptoms. Fewer studies have examined these symptoms and their treatments among HIV+ children and adolescents. This article reviews what is known about psychiatric syndromes among HIV+ youths, their treatments, and other psychosocial factors of concern to the psychiatrist when treating children and adolescents with HIV disease.

EPIDEMIOLOGY

Despite tremendous progress in our understanding of the HIV virus, its mode of transmission, and treatments to prevent its progression, HIV disease continues to be pandemic. Worldwide, an estimated 4.8 million people became newly infected in 2003 and more than 20 million people have died since the first cases of acquired immune deficiency syndrome (AIDS) were identified in 1981.[1] An estimated 1,106,400 persons in the United States were living with HIV infection, with 21% undiagnosed and unaware of their infection at the end of 2006.[2] In 2007, the estimated number of persons diagnosed with AIDS in the United States was approximately 37,041.

A version of this article was previously published in the *Child and Adolescent Psychiatric Clinics of North America, 19:2.*
Department of Child and Adolescent Psychiatry, The Children's Hospital of Philadelphia, 3440 Market Street, Suite 410, Philadelphia, PA 19104, USA
E-mail address: bentont@email.chop.edu

Most new HIV infections still occur among men who have sex with men (MSM). The Centers for Disease Control and Prevention (CDC) estimated that approximately 56,300 people were newly infected with HIV in 2006, with over half of these new infections occurred in gay and bisexual men. Black/African American men and women were strongly affected, and were estimated to have an incidence rate that was 7 times as high as that among whites.[3] At the end of 2007, the estimated number of persons, adults and children, living with HIV/AIDS in the United States with confidential name-based HIV/AIDS infection reporting was 571,378. The estimated number of deaths of persons with AIDS in the United States through 2007 was 583,298.

Highly active antiretroviral therapies (HAART) and prenatal detection of HIV-infected women has caused the rates of congenitally acquired HIV to decline dramatically in developed countries, though rates remain high in less developed nations. Only 9300 cases of AIDS in children younger than 13 years were reported in the United States at the end of 2002, and only 59 cases of congenitally acquired cases were reported to the CDC in 2003.[4] Since the advent of HAART, children acquiring HIV through vertical transmission are living longer and are now young adults, living with a chronic condition. Many of these young adults are attending college, are working, and are now beginning to have their own children.[5]

Although new case rates for congenitally acquired HIV are low, many young people are acquiring HIV disease. Of new HIV infections reported to the CDC, adolescents account for 50% as well as 25% of new sexually transmitted diseases reported annually to the CDC.[4] Infection rates among adolescents in the United States are increasing. The most common modes of transmission among adolescents and young adults was male to male sexual transmission, accounting for 42% of all cases; high-risk heterosexual contact accounted for 31%, and injection drug use 21%. The highest rates of new infections were among African Americans, and 19% were among Hispanics. HIV infection is a growing problem among adolescents, especially minority adolescents, emphasizing the importance of prevention efforts focused on the adolescent population.

ETIOLOGY OF HIV/AIDS INFECTION AMONG YOUTH

Infected mothers transmit HIV during pregnancy or delivery, or through breast milk. Person to person transmission occurs through blood contacts such as transfusions or needle sharing; or through sexual contact with an infected partner. Transmission through blood products is rare in the United States but prevalent in some other countries. Perinatal transmission of HIV has been significantly reduced by the implementation of voluntary routine prenatal screening for HIV implemented by the CDC in 2001,[6] and the use of reverse transcriptase inhibitors in HIV+ pregnant women during the prepartum and intrapartum periods and during breast feeding. Recent revisions to the CDC's recommendations include voluntary testing in all health care settings for individuals aged 13 to 64 years. It is further recommended that individuals at risk for acquiring HIV disease and their sex partners be tested annually.[6]

Once exposure to HIV has occurred, the virus infects helper T cells and replicates in the peripheral blood and lymphoid organs. The immune system responds by generating cytotoxic T lymphocytes (CTLs) that recognize and kill viral particles. The initial invasion and viremia may be experienced as a mild flu-like syndrome initially, but then the reduced viremia, resulting from the CTLs, produces a phase of clinical latency, an asymptomatic phase that can last for years. Unfortunately, the immune system eventually deteriorates with increased viremia, the development of symptoms, and eventually AIDS. AIDS is diagnosed when the CD4+CD3− count falls below 200 cells/mL or when one AIDS-defining condition occurs.

Early detection of HIV viral infection is critical to effective treatment. New technologies that allow earlier, quicker, and more accurate detection have been developed. For acquired HIV, rapid diagnostic tests using saliva can provide screening results in as little as 20 minutes. However, serum samples are still required to confirm the presence of HIV infection. These tests generally detect the virus or its antibody, 2 to 12 weeks after the initial infection, and include enzyme-linked immunosorbent assay (ELISA) or enzyme immunoassay, Western blot, p24 antigen capture assay, HIV-1 DNA polymerase chain reaction (PCR), and HIV-1 RNA assay.[7] HIV antibody detection, however, cannot be used to make a diagnosis of HIV disease in infants when vertical acquisition of HIV is suspected. Virologic testing to identify antibodies to the virus and its components, using DNA and RNA PCR, are made within the first 48 hours of birth, at 1 to 2 months, and again at 3 to 6 months to distinguish the infant antibodies from maternal antibodies, which should decline over time. Definitions for defining AIDS in the pediatric population are similar to those for adults, with some exceptions (**Table 1**).[8] Another classification system has been developed to include infants exposed to HIV whose status remains to be determined. The Baylor International Pediatric AIDS Initiative Education Resources provides a comprehensive description of these conditions.[9]

NEUROLOGIC EFFECTS OF HIV INFECTION

HIV primarily infects microglia of the central nervous system and macrophages. Its neurotoxic effects are thought to result primarily from the virus's ability to induce inflammatory factors that result in neuronal cell damage and death. In the adult population, the late effects of the neuronal cell damage presents as HIV-associated dementia (HAD). In children and adolescents, 2 types of encephalopathies may be seen: (1) a progressive encephalopathy characterized by acquired microcephaly, loss of previously acquired skills, and corticospinal tract abnormalities, and (2) a static encephalopathy presenting with cognitive and motor delays, but without a loss of acquired skills or neurologic deficits.[10] How the neurologic findings of a child or adolescent manifests clinically are related to many factors including length of infection, severity of deficits, rate of decline, and mode of transmission; for example, HIV encephalopathy is most commonly seen in those children and adolescents who were infected through vertical transmission.[11] High rates of severe, progressive encephalopathy were commonly seen with pediatric HIV disease at the beginning of the epidemic (50%–90%); however, improved antiretroviral therapy reduces viral load, thus reducing the numbers of infected cells in the central nervous system

Table 1 Revised human immunodeficiency virus pediatric classification system: immune categories based on age-specific CD4+ T-lymphocyte count and percentage			
Immune Categories	Less Than 12 Months No./μL (%)	1–5 Years No./μL (%)	6–12 Years No./μL (%)
Category 1: no suppression	>1500 (>25%)	>1000 (>25%)	>500 (>25%)
Category 2: moderate suppression	750–1499 (15%–24%)	500–999 (15%–24%)	200–499 (15%–24%)
Severe suppression	<750 (<15%)	<500 (<15%)	<200 (15%)

Data from CDC. Revised classification system for human immunodeficiency virus infection in children less than 13 years of age. MMWR 1994;43(RR-12):1–10.

(CNS) and slowing the progression of CNS disease.[11] Current rates of HIV encephalopathy presenting with brain atrophy, cognitive delays, and motor deficits are much less common and estimated to be present in 13% to 23% of infected children.[11] Findings associated with encephalopathy are increased calcifications of the basal ganglia, brain atrophy, enlarged ventricles, and enlarged cortical sulci.[12] Recent studies further suggest that higher viral loads are associated with severity of cerebral atrophy and are not associated with the presence of intracerebral calcifications.[13] Magnetic resonance imaging (MRI) studies have been recommended for children with progressive neurocognitive dysfunction, who do not exhibit symptoms of an AIDS-defining illness.[14] MRI screening may detect mass lesions associated with lymphomas or toxoplasmosis, and cerebrovascular complications that are more commonly seen in HIV-infected adolescents.[15]

Cognitive findings in HIV-infected children are generally characterized by impairments in expressive and receptive language skills, with expressive language commonly impacted more than receptive language, as well as frequent impairments in visuomotor skills and spatial learning.[16]

HAD, which has been well described in adults, has not been described in adolescents. HAD, a subcortical dementia, presents with progressive cognitive decline, behavioral abnormalities, and motor dysfunction. The frontal-cortical thinning found in HAD has been associated with declining attention, executive functioning, and working memory.[17] Although not well described in adolescents, case studies describing the presence of dementia in adolescents suggest that this syndrome may become a more frequent observation in the future as adolescents live longer with this chronic disease.[18] For adolescents who are HIV+, a significant risk factor for the development of CNS disease is strongly related to adherence to HAART, which requires multiple daily dosing of multiple medications. Poor adherence to antiretroviral treatments with consequent suboptimal medication levels can lead to viral drug resistance, higher viral loads, and increased risk for CNS disease. For school-aged children and adolescents, cognitive impairments, particularly undetected cognitive deterioration, can lead to academic failure, impaired occupational functioning, and impaired capacity to adhere to treatment recommendations. At present, neurodevelopmental assessment and testing are recommended every 6 months for children younger than 2 years; once a year for children aged 2 to 8 years who are asymptomatic, and more often if symptomatic; and every 2 years for asymptomatic, stable children 8 years and older.[19]

Among adolescents who acquire HIV through transfusions, needle sharing, or sexual contact, the use of antiretroviral therapies have increased the length of time lived with HIV. Long-term survivors are more likely to have problems with attention, memory, and other cognitive processes. Adolescents who develop AIDS may show late neurocognitive changes with progressive bradykinesia, spasticity, and hallucinations.[20]

PSYCHIATRIC SYNDROMES IN CHILDREN AND ADOLESCENTS WITH HIV DISEASE

The recognition of psychiatric syndromes in HIV-uninfected adolescents and in HIV+ adolescents, and the use of available interventions when recognized are extremely important. A large body of evidence supports the associations between adolescents with mental health conditions and the greater risk for HIV transmission. Psychiatrically ill adolescents are more likely to be sexually active at an early age, to engage more often in unprotected intercourse, to have multiple sexual partners,[21,22] to have histories of sexually transmitted diseases, and to use drugs or alcohol when having sex, and are less likely to use a condom.[5]

Recognizing psychiatric symptoms and other behavioral problems presenting in the context of HIV disease results from many complex and interacting factors, and it is important that the clinician understand how these factors might affect the child's or adolescent's presentation of emotional distress. The direct or indirect effects of the virus on the CNS, genetic factors, prenatal exposure to substances, opportunistic infections, adequacy of medical care, family and peer relationships, and other environmental factors affect the presentation of these symptoms. Another factor affecting the presentation of behavioral problems is that the majority of youngsters exposed to HIV face environmental stressors associated with living in demographically distressed areas affected by poverty, family stress, and alcohol and substance abuse.[5]

Families living with HIV also face several unique challenges. Mothers with HIV frequently become aware of their own illness during their pregnancies and must come to accept the diagnosis of a chronic and ultimately fatal illness for themselves, while caring for their newborn infants. Parents living with HIV must adhere to demanding treatment regimens while parenting infected children, parenting their children who are not HIV+ (affected children), soliciting family and social support for their families in the face of stigma, facing decisions about disclosure of their HIV status, and planning for their own deaths and the future care for their children. Children living with HIV-infected parents must also face the burden of living with chronically ill parents, many of whom struggle with addictions or mental health conditions, who will eventually succumb to this ultimately fatal illness.

For children and adolescents living with HIV disease, many factors associated with their illness threaten their emotional well being: coping with the pain of their physical illness, worries about their physical health or prognosis, frequent disruptions of social and academic activities due to hospitalizations and medical appointments, social stigma and isolation, fears related to disclosure, losses, and concerns about their own body image related to wasting, lipodystrophy, or dermatologic conditions associated with their illness. For younger children, feelings of guilt for having done something wrong to deserve HIV are common. Feelings of depression, social withdrawal, loneliness, anger, and confusion are not uncommon among youths struggling to cope with HIV disease.

Prevalence rates of psychiatric disorders among HIV+ adolescents have varied widely due to differing study methodologies and study designs. Clinical reports suggest high rates of mental health problems in perinatally infected adolescents.[23] Few well-controlled studies have examined prevalence rates of psychiatric disorders among adolescents who have vertically or behaviorally acquired HIV disease.[24–26]

In one study, Scharko[24] reviewed published studies of the prevalence of psychiatric disorders among HIV-infected youth, finding only 8 studies that examined psychiatric disorders using *Diagnostic and Statistical Manual* (fourth edition; DSM-IV) criteria. These investigators found high prevalence rates of psychiatric disorders: 28.6% with attention-deficit/hyperactivity disorder (ADHD), 24.3% with anxiety disorders, and 25% with depression. Generalizability of this study is limited as data collected across studies had varying populations and sample sizes were small; modes of infection, diagnostic methods, age range of samples, and use of control groups varied. A controlled study of behavioral problems in perinatally infected children found high rates of behavioral problems, but they did not differ from those of a control group of children who were perinatally exposed but not infected with HIV, suggesting that HIV infection was not a contributor to the development of behavior problems.[27] Another study found high rates of psychiatric hospitalizations among perinatally infected children and adolescents when compared with non-HIV–infected peers, with the primary admitting diagnosis being depression, ADHD, and oppositional defiance disorder (ODD).[23] One small study of HIV-infected youth aged 6 to 15 years described high rates of depression (47%) and attentional problems (29%). These investigators suggested that depression might be associated with encephalopathy and worsening immune function.[28]

In one of the few studies using a structured interview to obtain psychiatric diagnosis, Pao and Lyon[25] used the SCID (Structured Clinical Interview for DSM-IV axis I Disorders) to evaluate 34 HIV+ adolescents attending an urban clinic, for current and lifetime rates of psychiatric disorders. The investigators found very high prevalence rates of lifetime psychiatric diagnosis. In this sample, 68% had a diagnosis of depression, 59% substance abuse, and 29% conduct disorder. It was further found that the majority of these youths had psychiatric disorders preceding their diagnosis, and that approximately half of them had a current affective disorder. These rates of disorders are significantly higher than those found among the general adolescent population whose rates of psychiatric disorders range between 10% and 22%. These data suggest that HIV+ adolescents have higher rates of depression, substance abuse, and conduct disorders.[29] In another study using the Diagnostic Interview Schedule for Children (DISC-IV) to determine the presence of psychiatric disorders in 47 perinatally infected youths aged 9 to 16 years, 55% of youths evaluated met criteria for a psychiatric disorder, with anxiety disorders being most prevalent (40%), followed by ADHD (21%) and disruptive behavior disorders (24%).

Recent well-controlled studies of psychiatric diagnosis among perinatally acquired HIV+ youth suggests rates of psychiatric disorders ranging from 48%[30] to 61%.[26] These studies together support high rates of psychiatric illnesses among adolescents who have acquired their HIV infections both behaviorally and perinatally, further emphasizing the importance of the biopsychosocial approach in the evaluation and treatment of HIV-infected youth.[31]

TREATMENT

Recommendations for pharmacologic treatment of psychiatric disorders in HIV-infected youth are largely empirical.[5] Data obtained from adults suggest that medications commonly used to treat psychiatric symptoms in nonmedically ill individuals, including psychostimulants, antidepressants, and antipsychotic medications, are useful for the treatments of those disorders in the medically ill, including those who are HIV+.[32]

However, when choosing to use psychotropic medications, careful consideration and caution should be used when prescribing these medications in HIV+ youths who are using HAART. Many psychotropic medications, as well as antiretroviral ones, are widely metabolized by the cytochrome P450 system, especially the subgroups 3A4 and 2D6, and have a high potential for drug-drug interactions (Table 2). For medications that are metabolized by the liver, enzyme systems may be inhibited or stimulated by these medications, thus increasing or decreasing levels of one or both. Although the clinical significance of many of these interactions is unclear, certain classes of antiretrovirals are known to pose the greatest risk for changes in drug levels that are significant in HIV+ individuals. The protease inhibitors, specifically ritonavir, has the greatest impact on the inhibition of 3A4, and to a lesser extent on 2D6; Efavirenz has been shown to induce CYP3A4, which potentially decreases plasma levels of coadministered medications principally metabolized by this pathway.[33]

Before considering psychotropic medication use for HIV+ children receiving antiretroviral therapies, factors beyond the presenting behavioral complaints must be evaluated and considered. Developmental, environmental, social, and family factors may

Drug Name	Interactions With HAART
Table 2	
Common interactions of antiretroviral therapies and psychotropic medications	
Citalopram	Lopinavir/r, ritonavir increase citalopram levels
Fluoxetine and fluvoxamine	Increase levels of amprenavir, delavirdine, efavirenz, indinavir, lopinavir/r, nelfinavir, ritonavir, saquinavir
	Nevirapine decreases flluoxetine levels
Paroxetine	Lopinavir/r, ritonavir increase paroxetine levels
Sertraline	Lopinavir/r, ritonavir increase sertraline levels

influence the behavioral presentation, and must be considered. A comprehensive assessment including information from the child or adolescent, as well as collateral information from schools, primary care providers, specialists, counselors, family members, and others involved in caregiving should be compiled. A thorough family psychiatric history and histories of stressors is extremely important in reaching diagnostic conclusions.

Another consideration when prescribing for youths relates to the absence of evidence guiding psychotropic administration and dosing in this population. When choosing medications and dosing, the clinician must consider the child's weight, body mass index and Tanner stage, status of medical illness, potential drug interactions, and side effects of medications. When evidence of neurologic disease is present, the potential for medication side effects is even greater. It is important to start with low doses of medication, and to titrate slowly to minimize adverse effects that might decrease adherence.

MOOD DISORDERS: DEPRESSION AND BIPOLAR DISORDER

The prevalence of depressive disorders increases in frequency from childhood to adolescence for HIV-negative (HIV−) and HIV+ populations.[29] The presentation of depression in adolescents who are HIV+ is similar to adult populations. As in adults, depressed mood and irritability of at least 2 weeks' duration are criteria. Complicating this diagnosis of depression in the HIV+ child or adolescent, however, is the overlap between the vegetative symptoms of depression and the symptoms of the medical illness, or side effects of HIV treatments. Symptoms such as anorexia, fatigue, or other somatic complaints may be related to depression or HIV disease. When establishing the diagnosis, evaluation for worsening of medical status, poor adherence with resulting drug resistance, recent stressors with resulting adjustment disorder, or other psychological factors should be considered.

Although antidepressants of all classes have been prescribed to HIV+ children and adolescents based on the adult literature, selective serotonin reuptake inhibitors (SSRIs) are the most commonly prescribed antidepressant medications, though no evidence currently exists to support differences in efficacies. However, only fluoxetine has been approved for the treatment of depression in children older than 8 years, and has the greatest empirical support.[34] Amitriptyline is approved for depression in patients older than 12 years. Tricyclic antidepressants (TCAs) have been used empirically to help with pain syndromes, insomnia, and anxiety, but their sedating side effects and potential for toxicity in overdose limits their usefulness.[35] Fluoxetine, and its metabolite norfluoxetine, may inhibit CYP 3A3 and 3A4, contraindicating its use with macrolide antibiotics, azole antifungal medication, and several other medications.[36] Citalopram and mirtazepine are commonly used because they have fewer drug interactions and more favorable side effect profiles. In addition, mirtazepine has been helpful in promoting weight gain and sleep. Careful monitoring for the emergence of suicidal ideation is warranted with the use of the medications during treatment.

The presence of bipolar disorder in prepubertal youth and adolescents, and its clinical presentation, has been supported by a large evidence base, although no studies have examined the prevalence of these disorders in HIV+ youth.[37] The presence of grandiosity, elevated and expansive mood, racing thoughts, decreased need for sleep, and hypersexuality can also present in the pediatric population, and can occur with other childhood psychiatric disorders such as ADHD and substance abuse.[38] Treatment recommendations for children and adolescents with bipolar disorder are similar to those recommended for adults,[39] with the caveats that drug interactions, hepatotoxicity, and side effect profiles must be considered in the presence of HIV disease.

ATTENTION-DEFICIT/HYPERACTIVITY DISORDER

Several studies suggest high rates of ADHD in HIV-infected youths,[24,40] though few studies have examined the use of psychotropic medications in this group. The efficacy of psychostimulants for the treatment of ADHD in nonmedically ill populations is well validated, and is the pharmacotherapeutic treatment of choice for this disorder. Although commonly prescribed in HIV+ children, few studies exist that examine dosage or efficacy in the HIV+ population.

Empirical data suggest initiating treatment at the same dosages as those in the nonmedically ill population, and titrating those dosages as recommended. Stimulant medications have few drug-drug interactions, making them relatively safe in combination with antiretrovirals; however, it is important to observe for side effects.

ANXIETY DISORDERS

Anxiety disorders appear to be common among HIV+ youths, frequently comorbid with other psychiatric disorders. Social and specific phobias, separation anxiety disorders, agoraphobia, generalized anxiety, panic, and obsessive compulsive disorders have been reported, but the prevalence rates of specific anxiety disorders are unclear.[26] When present in HIV+ youth and significant enough to interfere with normative function, cognitive and behavioral therapies are indicated. The use of SSRIs and TCAs have demonstrated some efficacy in cases of anxiety disorders that fail to respond to behavioral strategies.

POSTTRAUMATIC STRESS DISORDER

The epidemiology of HIV in United States women increases the risk of exposure to trauma for youth living with HIV. The majority of perinatally exposed youths live in inner cities where stress, poverty, and trauma are prevalent.[41] Trauma related to traumatic events and trauma related to medical procedures place HIV+ youth at risk for posttraumatic stress disorder (PTSD) and/or traumatic stress.[42] The evidence further suggests that trauma exposure may adversely affect adherence to treatment recommendations among HIV+ youth.[43]

In one study examining the prevalence of PTSD and posttraumatic stress symptoms (PTSS) in a sample of HIV+ youth, 30 adolescents and young adults with HIV/AIDS were evaluated using a trauma symptoms checklist keyed to DSM-IV PTSD symptoms. The investigators found high rates of PTSD (13.3%) and PTSS (20%) in response to receiving a diagnosis of HIV infection. Even higher rates of PTSD and PTSS (23.3% and 23.3%) were observed when examining other traumatic events experienced by this same group of adolescents.[43]

Treatment studies for adolescents with PTSD suggest that cognitive behavioral therapies focused on PTSD symptomatology are more effective than other therapies in the management of symptoms and that medications can be helpful, although support for medication use in adolescents are weak.[44]

For children and adolescents experiencing anxiety related to procedures, benzodiazepines used in low doses, such as lorazepam, in conjunction with distraction techniques and psychotherapy have been helpful. Clonazepam has been used as an adjunct to psychotherapy for children and adolescents experiencing more pervasive and prolonged anxiety. Benzodiazepines may cause sedation and behavioral disinhibition, especially in patients with CNS disease, and should be monitored closely.[45]

Antihistamines have been used to sedate anxious children, but are not recommended for the treatment of anxiety. In addition, the anticholinergic properties of antihistamines can precipitate or worsen delirium.[45]

DELIRIUM AND DEMENTIA

The evidence suggests that delirium in the pediatric population presents with the same clinical picture as that of adults, and that the DSM-IV diagnostic criteria are applicable across the lifespan. Impairments in attention, responsiveness, levels of consciousness, orientation, confusion, affective lability, and sleep disturbance are present in pediatric patients with delirium, although paranoia, perceptual disturbances, and memory impairment are less common in younger children. The most common etiologies involve medical conditions.[46]

Treatment recommendations for pediatric delirium have been based on those found in the adult literature, and consist of developmentally appropriate strategies to maintain orientation and to provide environmental cues that will be reassuring for the child. Low doses of atypical antipsychotic agents have been used empirically, although one case report suggests that the atypical agent risperidone failed to adequately address symptoms of delirium in an adolescent with HAD.[18]

While the presence of HIV-associated dementia has been well described among adults with HIV disease, this late-appearing neuropsychiatric presentation has not been well described in the pediatric population.[47] HIV-related progressive and static encephalopathies have been observed and described among perinatally infected youth.[10] One case report of an adolescent presenting with delirium and HAD suggests that our conventional thinking about the presentation of HIV-associated dementia among youths may be changing as adolescents with perinatally acquired HIV and adolescents with behaviorally acquired HIV are living longer with this chronic illness.[24]

OTHER PSYCHOSOCIAL FACTORS THAT MAY BE A FOCUS OF CLINICAL INTERVENTION
Adherence

Current treatments for HIV/AIDS use antiretroviral medications. Four classes of medications, each with different mechanisms of action, are used in combination with a protease inhibitor to prevent the entry, replication, and cell destruction caused by HIV: nucleoside analogue reverse transcriptase inhibitors (NRTIs), nonnucleoside reverse transcriptase inhibitors (NNRTIs), fusion inhibitors, and protease inhibitors. These medications require multiple day dosing, have unpleasant side effects, require caution when used with other medications, and have potential for multiple drug interactions. To gain optimal benefit from these medications, compliance must be near

100%.[48] Poor or inconsistent adherence can result in increasing viral loads, progression to AIDS, and the development of resistance to current therapies. The Reach study[49] demonstrated the important relationships between psychiatric illness and adherence. These investigators examined longitudinal adherence to antiretroviral treatments among HIV+ adolescents for 1 year. Depression was associated with poor adherence to antiretroviral medications. At the initial study visit, 69% of the adolescents were adherent to medications by self-report, with only 50% being adherent at 12 months. Those with later stage disease were less adherent. Failure to maintain adherence was significantly associated with depression. Williams[50] examined predictors of adherence, demographics, and psychosocial characteristics of a large cohort of HIV+ children and adolescents (vertically transmitted) and their caregiver participants in the Pediatric AIDS Clinical Trials Group. Among this cohort of 2088 children and adolescents, factors associated with increases in nonadherence included increasing age in years, female gender, detectable viral load, recent stressful life events, grade retention, and a diagnosis of depression or anxiety. These findings were similar to those of Murphy and colleagues,[49] whose cohort were adolescents who were not congenitally infected.

Disclosure

The issues related to the disclosure of a child's or adolescent's HIV status are complex, and as a result, many caregivers and medical care providers are ambivalent about disclosing to children. This ambivalence is fueled by very realistic concerns about the stigma associated with HIV disease and the potential consequences of disclosure on the child and family. This is especially true given that disclosure of a child's HIV status may reveal parental HIV status as well, thus affecting the whole family.

The American Academy of Pediatrics has endorsed the disclosure of HIV to older children and adolescents and has developed guidelines to help families and clinicians cope with this difficult issue.[51] Studies examining the impact of disclosure have been conflicting. Some studies report higher esteem, promotion of trust, improved adherence, and better health and well being.[52] Other studies suggest that learning of one's HIV status may increase distress and contribute to the development of depression, anxiety, and behavioral problems.[53] Disclosure optimally should occur in a planned and structured setting with parents or other caregivers and health care providers. The information should be provided in a developmentally, socioculturally, sensitive manner. It is also important that parents and providers be prepared for the potential postdisclosure reactions, which may be immediate or delayed and can range from no apparent emotion to severe distress. Most children and adolescents eventually go on to adjust to living with their illness.[54]

It is clearly critical that adolescents be informed of their HIV status before they become sexually active, to maximize their own health behaviors and to decrease risk of transmission to others. Fear of rejection by peers if HIV status were known can prevent adolescents from disclosing, adhering to treatment recommendations, or from engaging in safe sex practices so as not to raise suspicions. It is crucial that adolescents understand their illness, when to disclose to supportive individuals, and how to elicit support when needed to cope with the demands of their illness.

SUMMARY

Youths infected with HIV are living longer. While most are doing well, many struggle with the burden of their illness and the demands of living with this chronic condition. The focus of our efforts must be prevention of new HIV infections. The recognition and treatment of psychiatric conditions for adolescents who are HIV− and for those who are HIV+ are an important component of this effort.

Psychiatric conditions are increasingly recognized among HIV+ youths who were born with their HIV disease and among those who acquire their disease. Furthermore, psychiatric conditions have been identified as a risk factor for acquisition of HIV disease, transmission of HIV, and poor outcomes for those who are infected by decreasing the likelihood of adherence to treatment. Child psychiatrists and other mental health professionals can play important roles in the prevention of HIV infection for adolescents receiving psychiatric treatment by the identification and treatment of psychiatric conditions that may predispose adolescents to risk, evaluating the adolescents' sexual practices and risky behaviors that place them at risk, and intervening when appropriate.[5]

When evaluating psychiatric disorders in HIV+ youth a comprehensive biopsychosocial assessment, using multiple informants involved in the child's or adolescent's care including caregivers, schools, and other agencies, should be used to understand the context in which the symptoms occur. A comprehensive assessment includes the identification of any stressors or events that might contribute to adjustment difficulties such as loss of family or friends, or changes in health status. An assessment of cognitive status, and adherence to antiretroviral treatments and safe health practices, should be included as well.

Although many child and adolescent psychiatrists express discomfort about asking or discussing sexual behaviors with high-risk teenagers who are HIV− or HIV+, clinicians can use direct questioning to ask adolescents about their sexual behaviors, the role of sexual relationships, the use of condoms, the context in which sexual activities occur, sexual attitudes and behaviors of their peer groups, and the quality of these relationships. A comprehensive assessment of sexual behavior and discussion with an adolescent in therapy provides a forum for open discussions about their sexual practices. Initiating these discussions with the adolescent within a therapeutic context demonstrates the importance of his or her concerns and the therapist's concerns about the adolescent's safety. Adolescents may use this process to gain awareness of unsafe sexual behaviors and to increase their motivation for change.[55]

Although few treatment studies have focused specifically on treatments for psychiatric conditions among medically ill children and adolescents, and even fewer have focused on HIV+ children and adolescents, the few studies available suggest that interventions currently used for non-HIV+ children and adolescents may be effective. Special considerations and attention must be given to the side effect profiles of psychotropic medications, potential for interactions with other medications, and ease of administration for youths who may already be using antiretroviral therapies.

HIV remains a significant health risk for adolescents, and psychiatric illness may predispose adolescents to risk, perpetuate the burden of illness for those infected, and increase the risk for further transmission. Psychiatrists can play an important role in curbing this epidemic by identification and treatment of adolescents at risk, as well as improving the quality of life for those already struggling with this illness.

REFERENCES

1. UNAIDS. 2004 report of the global AIDS epidemic. Available at: http://www.unaids.org/bangkok2004/GAR2004_html/GAR2004_00_en.htm. Accessed December 12, 2009.
2. Center for Disease Control. HIV prevalence estimates—United States, 2006. MMWR Morb Mortal Wkly Rep 2008;57(39):1073–6.

3. Hall HI, Ruiguang S, Rhodes P, et al. Estimation of HIV incidence in the United States. JAMA 2008;300:520–9.

4. US Department of Health and Human Services. HIV/AIDS surveillance report 2003. 2003;15:1–40.

5. Donenberg G, Pao M. Youths and HIV/AIDS: psychiatry's role in the changing epidemic. J Am Acad Child Adolesc Psychiatry 2005;44(8):728–47.

6. Branson BM, Handsfield HH, Lampe MA, et al. Revised recommendations for HIV testing in adults, adolescents and pregnant women in health care settings. MMWR Recomm Rep 2006;55:1–17.

7. Fauci A. HIV disease: AIDS and related disorders. In: Braunwald E, editor. Harrison's principles of internal medicine. 15th edition. New York: McGraw-Hill; 2001. p. 1852–913.

8. Centers for Disease Control. Revised classification system for human immunodeficiency virus infection in children less than 13 years of age. MMWR 1995; 43(RR-12):1–10.

9. Kline MW. Pediatric HIV infection. Baylor international pediatric AIDS initiative. Available at: http://bayloraids.org/resources/pedaids/manifestations.html. Accessed December 12, 2009.

10. Belman A. HIV-1 associated CNS disease in infants and children. In: Price R, Perry S III, editors. Research publications: association for research in nervous and mental disease, vol. 72. New York: Raven Press; 1994. p. 289–310.

11. Tardieu M, Chenadec JL, Persoz A. The French pediatric HIV infection study and the SEROCO group. HIV-1 related encephalopathy in infants compared with children and adults. Neurology 2000;54:1089–95.

12. Brouwers P, DeCarli C, Tudor-Williams G, et al. Interrelations among patterns of change in neurocognitive, CT brain imaging and CD4 measures associated with anti-retroviral therapy in children with symptomatic HIV infection. Adv Neuroimmunol 1994;4:223–31.

13. Brouwers P, Civitello L, DeCarli C, et al. Cerebrospinal fluid viral load is related to cortical atrophy and not to intracerebral calcifications in children with symptomatic HIV disease. J Neurovirol 2000;6:390–7.

14. Pastalides AD, Wood LV, Atac GK, et al. Cerebrovascular disease in HIV-infected pediatric patients: neuroimaging findings. AJR AM J Roentgenol 2002;179:999–1003.

15. Civitello L. Neurologic aspects of HIV infection in infants and children: therapeutic approaches and outcome. Curr Neurol Neurosci Rep 2003;3:120–8.

16. Frank EG, Foley GM, Kuchuk A. Cognitive functioning in school-age children with HIV. Percept Mot Skills 2007;85:267–72.

17. Thompson PM, Dutton RA, Hayashi KM, et al. Thinning of the cerebral cortex visualized in HIV/AIDS reflects CD4 + T lymphocyte decline. Proc Natl Acad Sci U S A 2005;102(43):15647–52.

18. Scharko AM, Baker E, Kothari P, et al. Case study: delirium in an adolescent girl with human immunodeficiency virus-associated dementia. J Am Acad Child Adolesc Psychiatry 2006;45:104–8.

19. Wolters PL, Brouwers P. Neurobehavioral function and assessment of children and adolescents with HIV-1 infection. In: Zeichner SL, Read JS, editors. Textbook of pediatric care. Cambrige (UK): Cambridge University Press; 2005. p. 510–29.

20. Watkins JM, Cool VA, Usner JA, et al. Attention in HIV infected children: results from the Hemophilia Growth and Development Study. J Int Neuropsychol Soc 2000;6:443–54.

21. Brown LK, Danokovsy MB, Lourie JK. Adolescents with psychiatric disorders and the risk of HIV. J Am Acad Child Adolesc Psychiatry 1997;36:1609–17.

22. Tubman JG, Gil AG, Wagner EF, et al. Patterns of sexual risk behaviors and psychiatric disorders in a community sample of young adults. J Behav Med 2003;26:473–500.

23. Gaughan DM, Hughes MD, Oleske, et al. Psychiatric hospitalizations among children and youths with human immunodeficiency virus infection. Pediatrics 2004; 113:e544–51.

24. Scharko AM. DSM psychiatric disorders in the context of pediatric HIV/AIDS. AIDS Care 2006;18(5):441–5.

25. Pao M, Lyon M. Psychiatric diagnosis in adolescents seropositive for the human immunodeficiency virus. Arch Pediatr Adolesc Med 2000;154:240–4.

26. Mellins CA, Brackis-Cott E, Cheng-Shiun L, et al. Rates and types of psychiatric disorders in perinatally human immunodeficiency virus-infected youth and seroconverters. Journal of Child Psychology and Psychiatry 2009;50(9):1131–8.

27. Mellins CA, O'Driscoll P, Magder LS, et al. High rates of behavioral problems in perinatally infected HIV infected children are not linked to HIV disease. Pediatrics 2003;111:384–93.

28. Misdrahi D, Vila G, Funk-Brentano I, et al. DSM-IV mental disorders and neurological complications in children and adolescents with human immunodeficiency virus type 1 infection (HIV-1). Eur Psychiatry 2004;19:182–4.

29. Lewinsohn PM, Hops H, Roberts RE, et al. Adolescent psychopathology. I: prevalence and incidence of depression and other DSMIIIR disorders in high school students. J Abnorm Psychol 1993;102:133–44.

30. Wood SM, Shah SS, Steenhoff, et al. The Impact of AIDS diagnosis on long term neurocognitive and psychiatric outcomes of surviving adolescents with perinatally acquired HIV. AIDS 2009;23:1859–65.

31. Brown LK, Lourie KJ, Pao M. Children and adolescents living with HIV and AIDS: a review. J Child Psychol Psychiatry 2000;41(1):81–96.

32. Evans DL, Charney D, Lewis L, et al. Mood disorders in the medically ill: scientific review and recommendations. Biol Psychiatry 2005;58:175–89.

33. Thompson A, Silverman B, Dzeng L, et al. Psychotropic medications and HIV/AIDS. Clin Infect Dis 2006;42(1):1305–10.

34. Emslie GJ, Rush J, Weinberg WA, et al. A double-blind, randomized, placebo-controlled trial of fluoxetine in children and adolescents with depression. Arch Gen Psychiatry 1997;54(11):1031–310.

35. Geller B, Resising D, Leonard H, et al. Critical review of tricyclic antidepressant use in children and adolescents. J Am Acad Child Adolesc Psychiatry 1999; 38(5):513–6.

36. Rosenstein DR, Pao M, Cai J. Psychopharmacologic management in oncology. In: Abraham J, Allegra CJ, Gulley J, editors. Bethesda handbook of clinical oncology. 2nd edition. Philadelphia: Lippincott Williams and Wilkins; 2005. p. 521–8.

37. Geller B, Zimmerman B, Williams M, et al. Phenomenology of prepubertal and early adolescent bipolar disorder: examples of elated mood, grandiose behaviors, decreased need for sleep, racing thoughts and hypersexuality. J Child Adolesc Psychopharmacol 2002;12(1):3–9.

38. Joshi G, Wilens T. Comorbidity in pediatric bipolar disorder. Child Adolesc Psychiatr Clin N Am 2009;18(2):291–319.

39. Kowatch RA, DelBello MP. Pediatric bipolar disorder: emerging diagnostic and treatment approaches. Child Adolesc Psychiatr Clin N Am 2006;15:73–108.

40. Mellins CA, Brackis-Cott E, Dolezal C, et al. Psychiatric disorders in youth with perinatally acquired human immunodeficiency virus infection. Pediatr Infect Dis J 2006;25:432–7.

41. Havens JF, Mellins CA. Psychiatric Aspects of HIV/AIDS in childhood and adolescence. In: Rutter M, Taylor E, editors. Child and adolescent psychiatry. 5th edition. Oxford (UK): Blackwell; 2002. p. 1101–13.

42. Stuber M, Shemesh E. Post-traumatic stress and responses in children with life-threatening illnesses. Child Adolesc Psychiatr Clin N Am 2003;12(2):195–209.

43. Jerilynn Radcliffe, Fleisher CL, Hawkins LA, et al. Posttraumatic stress and trauma history in adolescents and young adults with HIV. J Adolesc Health 2006;38(2):110–1.

44. Treatment of children and adolescents. In: Cohen JA, Berliner L, March JS, et al, editors. Effective treatments for PTSD: practice guidelines from the International Society for Traumatic Stress Studies. New York: Guilford Press; 2000. p. 330–2 388, xii.

45. Pao M, Weiner L. Childhood and adolescence. In: Cohen M, Gorman J, editors. Textbook of AIDS psychiatry. New York: Oxford publishing Inc; 2009. p. 307–36.

46. Turkel SB, Tavaré JA. Delirium in children and adolescents. J Neuropsychiatry Clin Neurosci 2003;15:431–5.

47. McArthur J. HIV dementia: an evolving disease. J Neuroimmunol 2004;157:3–10.

48. Feingold AR, Rutstein RM, Meislich D, et al. Protease inhibitor therapy in HIV-infected children. AIDS Patient Care STDS 2000;14:589–93.

49. Murphy DA, Belzer M, Durako SJ, et al. Longitudinal antiretroviral adherence among adolescents infected with human immunodeficiency virus. Arch Pediatr Adolesc Med 2005;159:764–70.

50. Williams PL. Predictors of adherence to antiretroviral medication s in children and adolescents with HIV infection. Pediatrics 2006;118(6):1745–57.

51. American Academy of Pediatrics. Disclosure of illness status to children and adolescents with HIV infection. Pediatrics 1999;103:164–6.

52. Mellins CA, Brackis-Cott E, Dolezal C. Patterns of status disclosure to perinatally HIV infected children and subsequent mental health outcomes. Clin Child Psychol Psychiatry 2002;7:101–14.

53. Lester P, Chesney M, Cooke M, et al. When the time comes to talk about HIV: factors associated with diagnostic disclosure and emotional distress in HIV-infected children. J Acquir Immune Defic Syndr 2002;31:309–17.

54. Wiener L, Havens J, Ng W. Psychosocial problems in pediatric HIV infection. In: Shearer WT, editor. Medical management of AIDS in children. Philadelphia: W.B. Saunders; 2003. p. 119–28.

55. Brown LK, Lourie KJ. Motivational interviewing and the prevention of HIV among adolescents. In: Monti PM, Colby SM, O'Leary TA, editors. Adolescents, alcohol and substance abuse: reaching teens through brief interventions. New York: Guilford; 2001. p. 244–74.

Psychiatric Aspects of Pediatric Cancer

Brian P. Kurtz, MD[a,b], Annah N. Abrams, MD[b,c,d],*

KEYWORDS

- Cancer • Psychosocial issues • Psychiatry
- Pediatric • Coping

The diagnosis and treatment of children and adolescents with cancer has a tremendous and lasting effect on the patients, their families, and other individuals in their social network. It carries a host of psychological and behavioral ramifications, from questions of mortality to changes in levels of functioning in multiple domains. This review looks at the psychosocial and treatment-related issues that arise in children with cancer.

OVERVIEW OF CHILDHOOD CANCERS

Cancers of any kind during childhood are rare. Childhood cancer accounts for less than 2% of all cancers diagnosed each year. About 150 to 160 per 1,000,000 children, or around 12,000 children in total, will be diagnosed in any given year.[1,2] By comparison, asthma, the most common chronic illness of childhood, is prevalent in 8.5% of the child population (6.2 million children), and juvenile diabetes has an annual incidence rate 1.5 to 2 times greater than cancer (about 240 per 1,000,000).[3,4] The most common forms of childhood cancer are leukemias (28%), specifically acute lymphocytic leukemia (ALL)

A version of this article was previously published in the *Child and Adolescent Psychiatric Clinics of North America, 19:2.*

Please note that this review includes reference to investigations into uses of medications for indications other than those which have received FDA approval (such as use of antipsychotics to treat severe mood symptoms secondary to corticosteroid treatment and antidepressants to treat depressive symptoms occurring in the context of cancer or interferon treatment). Careful clinical judgment is encouraged when using medications for indications other than those approved by the FDA.

[a] Department of Psychiatry, Division of Pediatric Psychiatry, Tufts Medical Center and Floating Hospital for Children at Tufts Medical Center, 800 Washington Street #1007, Boston, MA 02111, USA

[b] Department of Psychiatry, Tufts University School of Medicine, 136 Harrison Avenue, Boston, MA 02111, USA

[c] Harvard Medical School, 25 Shattuck Street, Boston, MA 02115, USA

[d] Department of Pediatric Hematology Oncology, Massachusetts General Hospital, 55 Fruit Street, Yawkey 8B, Boston, MA 02114, USA

* Corresponding author. Departments of Child and Adolescent Psychiatry and Pediatric Hematology Oncology, Massachusetts General Hospital, 55 Fruit Street, Yawkey 8B, Boston, MA 02114.

E-mail address: aabrams@partners.org

Pediatr Clin N Am 58 (2011) 1003–1023
doi:10.1016/j.pcl.2011.06.009
0031-3955/11/$ – see front matter © 2011 Elsevier Inc. All rights reserved.

(21%), and central nervous system (CNS) tumors (18%), which together account for almost half of all malignancies. Other tumor types include germ cell tumors (7%), Hodgkin lymphoma (7%), non-Hodgkin lymphoma (6%), neuroblastoma (5%), acute myeloid leukemia (5%), Wilms tumor (4%), osteosarcoma (3%), rhabdomyosarcoma (3%), thyroid carcinoma (3%), melanoma (3%), retinoblastoma (2%), and Ewing sarcoma (1%).[5] Childhood cancer remains the leading cause of illness-related death in childhood, but significant advances in survival have been made in the past 35 years.[2] The overall 5-year survival rate for 0- to 19-year-olds diagnosed between 1975 and 1979 was 62.9%, compared with 81.5% in 2001.[1]

Much of this progress has come from the collaboration of pediatric oncology researchers and clinicians. The Children's Oncology Group (COG), supported by the National Cancer Institute, creates standardized treatment protocols for pediatric cancers and then analyzes the responses to care and disseminates this information to all pediatric cancer providers.[6]

To appreciate the experience of a child who has cancer it is helpful to have an understanding of the treatments involved. Treatment of pediatric cancer may involve chemotherapy, radiation, surgery, or stem cell/bone marrow transplant, or some combination of these modalities. In children with ALL, the most common type of childhood cancer, children receive chemotherapy for 2 to 3 years depending on their risk stratification. The stages of treatment of ALL are divided into induction, CNS-directed treatment and intensification, reinduction, and maintenance. Children initially receive chemotherapy treatment in an inpatient pediatric unit, and subsequently receive chemotherapy treatment in the outpatient setting.[7,8] In contrast, children with primary CNS malignancies, the second most common cancer of childhood, may have surgery only (eg, children with a pilocytic astrocytoma) or have surgery, radiation, and intensive chemotherapy (eg, children with medulloblastoma).[9,10]

PSYCHOLOGICAL ADJUSTMENT

As with any severe stressor, the way in which a child is affected by cancer and responds psychologically varies with age. It is useful to view adjustment to a cancer diagnosis and the subsequent treatments through a developmental lens, keeping in mind key markers for each age group.[11] Ultimately, some children with cancer may develop problems with mood or anxiety.

Preschool Age

During the preschool years (ages 2–6 years), children are egocentric (a perspective of being at the center of everything) and use associative logic, which means that any 2 unrelated things can be understood in terms of 1 causing the other. The combination of egocentricity and associative logic results in magical thinking and interweaving of reality and fantasy. The use of magical thinking may lead a child to believe that his cancer is a punishment for a bad thought or deed. An example of this might be a 4 year-old boy who thinks he has leukemia because he took his sister's toy or he ate too many cookies. As a result procedures and treatment side effects may feel like punishments, especially if the child is unable to localize the medical illness to a particular body part, as is the case in leukemia. These feelings are consistent with a perception of whole body vulnerability, that "my whole body is sick," even though only 1 organ system is involved. Whole body vulnerability is made more real for the child with cancer who endures intravenous lines, hair loss, and nausea and vomiting. For children with leukemia this vulnerability is heightened, as it is difficult to grasp the concept of a hematologic malignancy.

The concept of time develops gradually in this age range. Although parents may be focused on the seriousness of a diagnosis, the expected course of treatment, and probabilities of survival, the child will likely only comprehend what will affect him or her in the moment.

The dominant social sphere of the preschool child, and the area most affected by the illness, is family life. Children aged 3 to 6 years spend most of their time with their immediate family, and their contacts outside the home are usually limited to preschool and day care. Separations from family members and care providers can be anxiety provoking and challenging during the course of treatment.

School Age

School age is characterized by mastery of skills. There is the emergence of logical thinking (causal logic) and more appreciation for another's point of view. School and peer groups play an increasing role in a child's life. Therefore, disrupted functioning in school performance and peer relationships are common social sequelae, either from direct effects of cancer (time missed from school and friends) or a regressive loss of coping skills. Offering school tutors and age-appropriate activities (such as board games, video games, computers, puzzles, and arts and crafts) can help children to function closer to their premorbid level and may serve as a counterweight to the regressive pull of dependency, helplessness, and loss of control that often accompanies intensive medical treatment.

When school-age children are diagnosed with cancer, they are able to understand the simple functional explanations of their illness and often pride themselves in mastering the names or procedures and treatments they have received. Innovative programs targeting this developmental level include "My Story in Beads"[12] which allows children to mark off each procedure and treatment with a special bead on a string (Elyse Levin-Russman, MSW, LICSW, personal communication, January 2010). Children create a narrative about how their cancer was diagnosed and the treatment they are receiving, allowing them to be active participants in their care. Rules provide predictability in this age group, but a cancer diagnosis disrupts this way of thinking because there are no identifiable causes for most childhood cancers, unlike some adult cancers (eg, smoking leading to lung cancer). It can be frustrating to a child who plays by the rules and follows the doctors' orders to then face setbacks in treatment despite their best efforts. Helping this age group feel competent in the midst of medical complications can be challenging.

Adolescence

During normal adolescence, areas of growth include identity and independence, sexual development, and peer group involvement. Cognitively, adolescents are able to think abstractly and can understand the complexity of a chronic illness in the same way as adults. They can appreciate the meaning of a life-threatening or chronic illness, but often are not prepared to manage the changes in their lifestyle and activities that the treatment requires.[13]

The multiple demands of living with cancer (including enduring the diagnosis and treatments, physical discomfort, limitations, pain, effect on appearance, and fears about the present and future) threaten the adolescent's ability to exercise newly acquired independence. These demands occurs at the same time as the adolescent is striving to individuate from parents and trying to establish an independent identity. An adolescent's identity usually relies on the peer group to determine what is "in" and what is "out," and attractiveness within this group plays a significant role in determining one's self-esteem. Time away from school and other activities may strain friendships and create feelings of isolation at a time when feeling connected to peers is of utmost importance to the development of identity. Often the illness occurs at a time when other tensions between the adolescent and parent make relying on the parents uncomfortable or unacceptable. Logistical and emotional reasons thwart individuation; parents may need to bring the adolescent to appointments or stay at the bedside during a hospitalization, or may experience longing for closeness with the adolescent when faced with the issues of mortality raised by cancer. In the setting of this emotionally complex dilemma, some teens become sullen, aggressive, nonadherent, or withdrawn, whereas others are able to negotiate the discomfort of returning to a more dependent supportive relationship with parents.

A recent study examined the rates and types of distress experienced by teenagers 4 to 8 weeks after they were diagnosed with cancer.[14] The main areas included physical concerns (eg, mucositis), personal changes (eg, hair loss, fatigue, and weight changes) and treatment-related worries (eg, missing school and missing leisure activities).

Body image and sexuality are tremendously affected by cancer. In adolescence, an extraordinary amount of time is spent on one's appearance and presentation because it often determines one's self-esteem. For the adolescent with cancer, physical attractiveness takes on new meaning. Competence and interest in developing interpersonal and intimate relationships depend on having a positive sense of self and body image. Both of these are challenged during treatment because of feelings of being different and physical appearance changes such as hair loss caused by chemotherapy or weight gain caused by corticosteroids. As a result of low self-esteem and body image concerns expressed by adolescents with cancer, they avoid or are less likely to establish intimate relationships.[15] Future fertility, threatened by cancer treatment, is also a prominent issue. Semen cryopreservation is available for boys but there are no definitive preservation methods available for girls.[16]

Mood

One might assume that a severe stressor such as a diagnosis of cancer during childhood would overwhelm an individual's ability to cope emotionally and most if not all children would experience emotional difficulties. However, studies suggest that most children with cancer do not exhibit significant levels of depression or anxiety, although a significant minority do experience marked levels of psychological distress.[17–20] Some clinical observations have indicated that a subset of patients exhibit more problems, such as greater difficulty coping.[19] Other studies show the emotional well-being of children with cancer currently receiving chemotherapy to be remarkably similar to case-control classroom peers,[21] and initial studies of cancer survivors similarly failed to find increases in social and emotional problems in children with cancer,[22] although new data on survivors has challenged this view (see later discussion).

The type of cancer may play a role in the psychological effect on the child. Children with brain tumors are likely to experience more psychological distress, in large part because of the neurocognitive sequelae of their disease.[23] Similarly, those with severe medical late effects tend to have more depressive symptoms and poorer self-concept.[24]

The involvement of mental health professionals in addressing the psychosocial needs of patients and their families can mediate the overall distress they experience. Optimal psychosocial care for patients with cancer includes opportunities to assess functioning and separate transient distress from more serious and disruptive emotional difficulties. Identification of those children with mood and behavioral difficulties who will require additional services is essential in providing good oncologic care. In assessing a child's mood, the clinician must be knowledgeable about the side effects of the treatments, which may include fatigue, decreased appetite, and disturbed sleep. If a child does present with clinically significant depressive symptoms, the treatment follows the same course as it would in the physically well child; that is, with psychotherapy such as cognitive-behavioral therapy (CBT) and antidepressant medication as indicated.[25]

Although no large studies have been conducted in children with cancer, selective serotonin reuptake inhibitor (SSRI) medications are the pharmacologic antidepressant treatment of choice, as they are in the population at large.[26] In an uncontrolled pilot study of 15 children with cancer and depression or anxiety, fluvoxamine was well tolerated and effective.[27] Fifty percent of pediatric oncologists at Children's Hospital of Philadelphia reported prescribing SSRIs for their patients.[28] In another small study, 7% of children involved in National Institutes of Health (NIH) research trials for cancer were found to have been prescribed antidepressant medication.[29] The investigators of this study noted increasing acceptance for psychopharmacologic treatment of subthreshold psychiatric disorders to improve quality of life, and concluded that in addition to psychological support always being indicated in the setting of anxiety or depression, there is a role for the judicious use of psychotropic medications.[29]

Anxiety

Because of the need for frequent procedures and treatments (eg, blood draws and intravenous [IV] placements, as well as chemotherapy), the child with cancer often presents to mental health treatment with anticipatory anxiety and/or nausea and vomiting. Anticipatory anxiety without a nausea/vomiting component is initially addressed with behavioral interventions. Understanding the cause of the anxiety is helpful in determining what modifications will be most helpful. For preschool and school-age children, the worry may be about separation from a caregiver. They may demonstrate a greater resistance to being separated from parents or become more fearful of new people. They will want to know exactly where their parents will be before, during, and after. Distraction is a helpful and easy mechanism to alleviate anxiety. The use of handheld video games and watching videos has been shown to decrease anticipatory anxiety preoperatively for children and can be easily employed in the child's hospital room or waiting area.[30] Worries about pain are also foremost in a child's mind. Pain should be controlled or eliminated whenever possible, even when this may mean a delay in a procedure. The application of a topical anesthetic (EMLA cream) is standard practice in most pediatric oncology settings before venipuncture. In 1 recent study, the combination of EMLA with self-hypnosis further decreased the associated anticipatory anxiety.[31] Regularly scheduled lumbar punctures and bone marrow aspirates are part of many childhood cancer protocols. To minimize the pain associated with these procedures they are often done with conscious sedation. Parents and staff should explain procedures in simple terms including where and when a procedure will occur and, if there is pain associated with the procedure, how it will be addressed.

Anticipatory anxiety with nausea/vomiting (ANV) affects many children despite advances in antiemetic medication. The child may feel nauseated or vomit on arriving at the outpatient clinic or hospital. One study reports 59% of children experienced mild to severe anticipatory nausea and vomiting despite the use of ondansetron.[32] As with adults, ANV seems to fit the model of classic conditioning. The children with the most severe cases of ANV are those who experience postchemotherapy nausea and vomiting. However, there is a subset of children who do not experience postchemotherapy nausea and vomiting, but manifest ANV. In mild cases, effective behavioral approaches include thought stopping, hypnosis, distraction, and relaxation.[33] More severe cases of ANV in association with postchemotherapy nausea and vomiting may respond to increased use of antiemetics, including higher doses of ondansetron, corticosteroids, and benzodiazepines. There are also some data to support the use of acupuncture in this population.[34]

TREATMENT-RELATED ISSUES

In the psychiatric evaluation and treatment of children with cancer, several prominent areas of difficulty related to cancer treatment emerge, and include psychiatric effects of chemotherapeutic agents, neurocognitive effects of treatment from chemotherapy and cranial radiation, and issues related to adherence with treatment. Acute and chronic pain associated with cancer and cancer treatment can further compound psychological distress. Close attention to providing adequate pain control is essential and interventions that reduce pain will reduce suffering.[35] A review of pain management, however, is beyond the scope of this article.

Corticosteroids

Corticosteroids are routinely used for the treatment of childhood cancers and their sequelae. In many chemotherapy protocols, including leukemias and lymphomas, corticosteroids play a central role. The appearance of adverse psychiatric symptoms is common in children who are receiving high-dose corticosteroids. These symptoms include changes in mood, sleep, and appetite.

Research in the area of psychiatric adverse effects to corticosteroids is much more extensive in adults than in children. The adult literature supports the role of corticosteroids in causing behavioral changes including depression, mood elevation, irritability, anger, insomnia, and excess talkativeness.[36-42] Psychiatric sequelae are usually dose-dependent and studies have reported increased severity of psychiatric symptoms with higher doses of corticosteroids. Patients can become severely depressed, manic, psychotic and/or delirious. In the largest study of its type, severe psychiatric reactions were seen in 1.3% of patients receiving prednisone 40 mg per day or less; in 4% to 6% of patients receiving 41 to 80 mg per day; and in 18.4% of patient receiving more than 80 mg per day.[43]

The use of corticosteroids in children has been studied in children with renal, pulmonary, and gastrointestinal diseases more commonly than in children with cancer.[44-48] Effects seen in children with cancer are consistent with the behavioral changes seen in children with other illnesses and in the adult population. In children receiving prednisone at a dosage of 60 mg/m^2/d for leukemia and lymphoma, increased irritability, argumentativeness, tearfulness, reports of "talking too much," tiredness, low energy, and night waking were common symptoms, with a trend toward more symptoms in younger children.[49] In children with ALL, groups receiving prednisone 40 mg/m^2/d and 120 mg/m^2/d showed adverse changes in attention/hyperactivity, emotionality, sleep disturbance, depressed mood, listlessness, and peer relations, although there was no significant difference between the 2 steroid groups.[50]

Sleep is also significantly affected by the use of corticosteroids. In an unblinded study of children receiving dexamethasone as part of their treatment of ALL, fatigue was worsened, and total sleep, nighttime awakenings, and restlessness were increased.[51] Each child served as their own control by comparing 5-day periods on and off dexamethasone.

The child psychiatrist plays an important role in evaluating and managing corticosteroid-related psychiatric side effects during cancer. In mild cases, children may experience some sleep disturbance and irritability. Psychoeducation about the transient nature of symptoms and support of positive coping skills to adapt to these changes in the patient and family can be helpful. For more moderate cases in which the child's sleep is more impaired or their behavior and mood are more significantly changed, medication interventions can be extremely helpful. There are numerous case reports of symptom-targeted pharmacotherapy or attempts at prophylaxis with mood stabilizers, antidepressants, and antipsychotics, with varying results. A small open-label trial of olanzapine in adults with manic or mixed symptoms secondary to corticosteroids showed benefit, lending support to the role of atypical antipsychotics.[52] In our clinical practice, symptom-targeted medication interventions have been helpful in managing acute sleep difficulties, extreme irritability and sensitivity, and mood lability. Usually small doses of benzodiazepines or atypical antipsychotics for the duration of the corticosteroid dosing and a few days following are sufficient to manage the psychiatric sequelae of the corticosteroids. In a few cases, the severity of a child's depression or mania or the development of psychosis requires a reduction or discontinuation of the corticosteroids as well as acute psychopharmacologic intervention.

Interferon

Interferon-α (IFN-α), an immunomodulator, is used to treat some pediatric malignancies including chronic myelogenous leukemia, giant cell tumors, and malignant melanoma.[53–56] There is a paucity of data about IFN and depression in the pediatric population, and the assessment and treatment of children is based on the adult experience. Studies of interferons in adult patients, and particularly those with viral hepatitis, have shown evidence of psychiatric syndromes associated with treatment. Presentations include acute confusional states (delirium), depressive syndromes, and maniclike symptoms of irritability and agitation, and occasionally euphoria.[57–59] A depressive syndrome similar to major depression is the most common psychiatric sequela of IFN and has been described in adults being treated for hepatitis C and cancer.[60] Psychiatrists consulted to evaluate patients who are receiving IFN need to be aware that the treatment may be causing the depression.[61–65] It is also important to recognize that making the diagnosis of depression in a patient receiving IFN can be challenging as fatigue and decreased appetite are 2 of the most common side effects associated with IFN. In addition, thyroid function should be monitored with high-dose IFN, because autoimmune thyroiditis secondary to IFN can lead to hypothyroidism and complicate the clinical picture.[66]

Reports in the literature suggest that SSRI treatment of IFN-induced depression may be effective,[67–69] and may be considered as a prophylactic treatment in patients with severe premorbid psychopathology,[70] or a history of depression during past IFN treatment.[71] Although some studies have suggested wider prophylactic use in high-dose IFN patients,[72] it is more common to treat depression in patients who become symptomatic during treatment.[59] In our clinical experience, children diagnosed with depression while on IFN have benefited from the use of SSRIs. For mild forms of depression, psychotherapeutic strategies can be beneficial. Psychoeducation for patients and families that symptoms may be transient and biochemically mediated rather than the result of a sudden giving up or self-pity is essential.[64]

Neurocognitive Effects

Given the increased survival rates, a greater focus is being placed on the long-term sequelae of cancer treatment and in particular on the neurocognitive effects. More than 50% of children treated for a childhood malignancy are at risk for developing neurocognitive deficits.[2] Cranial radiation causes the most striking effects on the neurocognitive capabilities of the developing brain, as measured in long-term survivors; however, multiple aspects of treatment can contribute to neurocognitive decline including primary CNS tumor effects, neurosurgical sequelae, and systemic and CNS-focused chemotherapies. Damage to developing cortical and subcortical white matter has been implicated as a key mechanism in the neurocognitive changes.[73–76] In addition to the types of tumors and treatments, the following patient factors also play a role in who is at greatest risk of neurocognitive decline: female sex, younger age at treatment, genetic polymorphisms, and population and social risk factors.[77,78] The largest body of research focuses on children who were treated for CNS malignancies and leukemia.[9,73,75,79–83]

Cranial radiation therapy (CRT) causes the greatest damage to developing white matter and as a result has been shown to cause the greatest negative sequelae for the developing brain. Studies have shown a decrease in IQ of between 15 and 25 points in children with brain tumors who are treated with CRT.[84,85] Children with ALL who have CNS involvement are also treated with CRT, and this population also shows significant cognitive decline over time. New protocols have been implemented to maintain the improved cure rates, but minimize the exposure to cranial radiation given the significant effect on cognition.[86] Protocols are using lower doses of cranial radiation, decreasing the tissue target volume, and postponing radiation in the highest risk groups or using early focal radiotherapy to minimize the cognitive effects. Newer forms and techniques for delivering radiation are also being used. For example, proton beam radiotherapy, as opposed to standard photon radiotherapy, may decrease the likelihood of significant neurocognitive decline, because there is no exit radiation dose thereby decreasing the volume of white matter involved.

Although cranial radiation is probably the most important single factor, brain tumors can also affect vital brain structures by direct mass effect or through sequelae of neurosurgery. A recent follow-up analysis of 24 patients who only required surgical resection of cerebellar tumors showed that although IQ was normal, neuropsychological testing showed deficits in attention, memory, processing speed, and visuospatial processing, and a variety of behavioral problems.[87] An investigation of patients treated for medulloblastoma showed that adverse factors such as neurologic deficits, meningitis, shunt infections, or the need for repeat surgery increased the risk for IQ deterioration after treatment, indicating that radiation and chemotherapy are not the only relevant considerations.[88] Furthermore, children who develop posterior fossa syndrome, a triad of mutism, ataxia, and behavioral changes postoperatively, are at greater risk for neuropsychological and psychosocial sequelae.[89,90]

Long-term cognitive effects from chemotherapeutic agents are most closely associated with methotrexate, whereas cytarabine and corticosteroids are implicated less strongly.[77,81,83] CNS-directed therapy with methotrexate (administered intrathecally), a mainstay of leukemia treatment, has neurocognitive effects. These effects are hypothesized to be mediated by methotrexate interfering with the folate metabolic pathway, and may result in demyelination and other toxic effects.[91] Several studies have examined the cognitive sequelae of CNS-directed chemotherapy. Children with ALL (who received CNS-directed therapy with methotrexate, but not cranial radiation) were compared with children with Wilms tumor (who experienced cancer but received no CNS-directed therapy) and sibling controls (who did not experience cancer but experienced the emotional distress of cancer in the family).[92] Children with ALL showed problems with sustained attention, which correlated with teacher reports of poorer academic performance, particularly in mathematics. They also had increased internalizing behaviors on the Child Behavior Checklist, a parent report measure of social competence and behavior problems.[93] In this and other studies, the impairments are milder than are usually seen from cranial radiation, although intellectual and academic functioning is affected. The most common neurocognitive deficits from chemotherapy are found in visual processing, visual-motor functioning, and attention and executive functioning, with female gender and young age (particularly less than age 3 years) as risk factors. Other findings include problems with academic performance, verbal abilities, and memory.[94,95] Platinum-based chemotherapies (such as carboplatinum) affect hearing, and therefore can affect learning and academic performance.[77]

In addition to morbidity-limiting strategies to minimize the neurotoxic effects (particularly cranial radiation), some investigators have examined interventions for neurocognitive effects after they have occurred.[96,97] These have focused on cognitive remediation and psychopharmacologic interventions.

Cognitive remediation has been studied as a specific program combining techniques from the fields of brain injury rehabilitation, special education/educational psychology, and clinical psychology.[98] This program involves activities to strengthen attentional skills and information processing speed; metacognitive strategies to prepare for, approach, complete, and generalize tasks; and cognitive-behavioral strategies to target attention. A multisite, randomized, clinical trial of this program resulted in improved academic achievement and improved attention by parental report.[99] An alternative model of cognitive rehabilitation for patients who had stem cell transplantations failed to show a major effect compared with a control group.[100]

Studies of pharmacologic interventions to treat attentional problems resulting from cancer treatment have focused on methylphenidate, with some promising results.[101–104] Although stimulants are probably less efficacious in the childhood cancer survivor population than in the general attention-deficit hyperactivity disorder population (75% response rate),[105] a recent randomized, double-blind, placebo-controlled, crossover trial of childhood survivors of ALL and brain tumors showed a response rate of 45.28%.[106] Controlled studies, including 1 specifically geared to evaluate side effects, suggest that patients generally tolerate the medication well, with a subgroup who tolerate the medication less well demonstrating increased side effects.[102,107]

COG recommends that a neuropsychological evaluation be done as part of entry into long-term follow-up and as clinically indicated for all childhood cancer survivors who received neurotoxic therapies. A complete list of recommendations by COG is available at http://www.survivorshipguidelines.org.[108] As in any child with academic difficulties and cognitive impairments, mental health professionals working with survivors of cancer have a role in educating family members and schools about deficits seen in this population, and advocating for appropriate accommodations and services. Studies show that the decline in IQ may not be apparent initially and can be progressive over time, highlighting the importance of following children longitudinally.

Adherence

Adherence to treatment regimens is a prominent issue with adolescents. Adolescents consistently show higher rates of nonadherence compared with children and adults in the treatment of cancer and other life-threatening illnesses.[109–113] Risk factors for poor adherence with cancer treatment in adolescents have been identified, including low socioeconomic status of the family,[113–115] barriers to communication such as cultural and linguistic differences,[116] and mental illness, including depression in a parent and behavioral disturbances during the patient's childhood.[117] Clinically, poor communication between adolescents and their parents around treatment seems to be a significant contributor to poor adherence. It is important to identify nonadherence issues early in treatment. Blood levels of a drug or its metabolites have been used to monitor adherence with oral medication regimens, such as 6-mercaptopurine in the treatment of ALL.[114,115] A nonjudgmental inquiry about the patient's consistency in taking the medication may be just as effective.[113] Confusion about appropriate doses or about who is responsible for administering the medication may contribute to unintentional nonadherence.

SUPPORT

The role of the family is central in children with cancer. As a child struggles with the intense period of stress associated with diagnosis and treatment, family members are the greatest potential source of support and strength for the child, but are also vulnerable themselves to the effects of the stress. Overall, parents of children with cancer seem to be quite resilient. A consistent theme reported in the literature is that functioning is preserved in cohesive, expressive families who provide high levels of support to their children and are able to access increased social support.

It has been theorized that cohesive families who display positive modeling and rewarding of competencies despite stress reduce symptomatic behaviors in children with illness.[118] In a study following newly diagnosed children with cancer for 9 months, higher cohesion and expressiveness in families was correlated with lower psychological distress and higher social competence.[119] Similarly, a prospective study of children undergoing stem cell transplantation showed that family cohesion and expressiveness were protective against child distress, especially if the parents did not exhibit high levels of depressive symptomatology.[120]

In contrast, parents with poor social support are more likely to have lower emotional health scores[121] and mothers with less social support satisfaction have been shown to have more distress.[122,123] Poor social support has also been shown to be predictive of symptoms of posttraumatic stress in parents[124]; increased social support during diagnosis and treatment may be protective against stress-related problems.[125] It is not completely clear if the benefit of social support for parents also reduces distress in the children themselves; 1 cross-sectional study indicated that social support of parents does not moderate the association between parent and child distress.[126] However, a prospective study by the same investigators indicated that maternal distress has a significant effect on the child, suggesting that helping to manage a mother's stress will help the child.[127]

Siblings are often the forgotten members of the family while parents deal with the multiple demands of having a child with cancer. Many individual pediatric cancer centers have support groups to address this unmet need. An example of a sibling support program, accessible to all via the Internet, is the SuperSibs! program.[128] In studies looking at the experience of siblings, supportive relationships were cited as important,[129] and siblings who had better social support experienced fewer symptoms of depression and anxiety and fewer behavior problems than those with lower levels of support.[130]

Parents often refer to the oncology staff as extended family and derive strength and support from the nurses, social workers, and physicians involved in their child's care. Care providers play an important role in helping families anticipate the many challenges of cancer treatment and manage them as they encounter these challenges. In addition to the powerful effects of caring personal interactions, it may be possible to use more formalized methods to bolster resilience. Some clinical interventions to support the psychosocial functioning of family members, such as problem-solving therapy and stress reduction techniques, have shown promise.[131–134]

EDUCATION

School is one of the most important normalizing factors for children and adolescents. School provides structure and social contact as well as a place to gain the skills needed for successful functioning later in life. Therefore, disruptions in school attendance because of treatment of cancer and the subsequent reintegration into the school setting are critical to address. Studies have consistently found that children with cancer are absent from school frequently and absenteeism is a problem at all stages of illness.[135] Teachers report no significant differences in overall behavioral functioning in school; however, parents and teachers observe increased difficulties in social functioning compared with peers, with regard to sensitivity and isolation.[136–139]

Although it is anxiety provoking for many, returning to school after the diagnosis of cancer can promote healthy psychological functioning. One study showed that adolescents who returned to school compared with those who enrolled in home-based programs were happier and less socially isolated.[140] Many pediatric oncology centers provide support to children when they return to school, including school reentry programs. In our pediatric oncology center, a clinic nurse and social worker, with permission and guidance from the child and parents, will visit the school before the child's return. The team presents developmentally appropriate information about the child's illness and treatment and answers questions posed by the students and teachers. The child's classmates are given the opportunity to have an open discussion about childhood cancer and a chance to think about how best to treat their classmate when they return. Children, parents, and teachers find these visits helpful as they facilitate an educational discussion around cancer and decrease the burden on the child and family to explain the diagnosis and treatment. Reentry programs are helpful in increasing knowledge and confidence for teachers and improving self-esteem and mood in patients.[141–143]

SURVIVORS

The landscape of childhood cancer has changed significantly in the past few decades and now most children diagnosed with cancer will survive. In 1997, 1 in 1000 adults were childhood cancer survivors, and this number is expected to increase.[2] The increased rate of survivorship has led to greater recognition of the long-term issues facing survivors. Cohort studies in the United States[144] and internationally[145–147] have shed light on the many sequelae of childhood cancer, from second malignancies and organ toxicity to neurocognitive and psychological late effects. Understanding how to appropriately assess this population and effectively intervene when needed represents a burgeoning field. Long-term follow-up clinics for childhood cancer survivors are available in some cancer centers and are being developed in others. Multidisciplinary teams are needed to address the myriad of medical and psychological issues that arise. COG has published guidelines for appropriate care, available at http://www.survivorshipguidelines.org.[108] Mental health clinicians play a critical role in evaluating the psychosocial needs in the survivor population.

Several studies have looked at psychological functioning in childhood cancer survivors. Initial reports were encouraging and in a review by Eiser and colleagues[22] of 20 studies that compared survivors of childhood cancer with population norms or control groups, there was a lack of significant social and emotional dysfunction. However, more recent studies have raised some concern about the psychological functioning in childhood cancer survivors. Increased awareness of the occurrence of avoidance, hyperarousal, and intrusive thoughts in survivors of childhood cancer has brought attention to the role of posttraumatic stress symptomatology.[148] A Danish study showed that childhood brain tumor survivors had higher rates of psychiatric hospitalization for psychosis and somatic causes, but not depression, compared with the general public and other childhood cancer survivors.[149] There also seems to be an increased risk of suicidal ideation. In an uncontrolled sample of 226 childhood cancer survivors, Recklitis and colleagues[150] found a significantly increased lifetime risk of suicidal ideation in childhood cancer survivors compared with sibling controls.

The Childhood Cancer Survivorship Study (CCSS), a multisite study funded by the National Cancer Institute of a cohort of 20,276 patients and 3500 sibling controls provides the most comprehensive data about psychosocial outcomes.[2] Reports using these data have noted significant psychosocial issues in this population. Hudson and colleagues[144] found moderate to severe impairment existed in some aspect of mental health, with significantly higher levels of cancer-related anxiety observed in patients with Hodgkin disease, sarcomas, and bone tumors. Brain tumor survivors from the CCSS cohort showed increased distress and depression compared with siblings.[151] Survivors of a variety of other tumors, including leukemia, lymphoma, neuroblastoma, and bone tumors, were found to have increased depression, somatization, and distress compared with siblings.[152] The data from this cohort also supported Recklitis' earlier findings of increased suicidal ideation in the childhood cancer survivor population.[153] Surveillance of psychosocial outcomes in survivors is essential, especially as cancer treatments continue to evolve and the number and makeup of the survivorship population changes.

CARE AT THE END OF LIFE

Although most children with cancer survive, childhood cancer remains the leading cause of illness-related death in childhood and is the second leading cause of death in children, behind accidents.[2] The reality of cancer as a sometimes terminal illness affects patients, families, and caregivers alike. Oncology teams utilize the services of social workers, psychologists, psychiatrists, chaplains, and child life specialists to assist the child, family, and staff with the challenges faced at the end of life. These care providers can facilitate family conversations about death between parents and with the child.[154] Conversations about dying and end-of-life care are inherently difficult and often avoided, but data support having open conversations with children. Kreicbergs and colleagues[155] found that parents of children with severe malignant disease who had conversations with their children about dying did not regret these conversations.

Children with cancer experience significant physical and psychological symptoms and suffering at the end of life.[156] Despite this, palliative care services are available at only 58% of institutions caring for pediatric oncology patients, highlighting 1 obstacle to offering optimal care to all children treated for cancer.[157]

Many of the difficulties encountered in the terminal phase of children with cancer are common to all children at the end of life. See the article by Knapp and colleagues elsewhere in this issue for further exploration of this topic.

SUMMARY

Overall, children with cancer are resilient, but as shown in this article, there are confronted with several challenges adjusting to their illness, dealing with treatment-related effects, and for some facing end-of-life care. Recent decades have brought about tremendous improvements in survival outcomes for children with cancer. As a result, mental health clinicians not only need to understand the immediate psychosocial issues but also appreciate and anticipate the long-term sequelae for a child with cancer. Mental health clinicians play a critical role in providing the assessment, support, and treatment needed in the childhood cancer population. Continued research in this field is imperative.

REFERENCES

1. Horner MJ, Ries LAG, Krapcho M, et al, editors. SEER Cancer Statistics Review, 1975–2006. Based on November 2008 SEER data submission. Bethesda (MD): National Cancer Institute. Available at: http://seer.cancer.gov/csr/1975_2006/, posted to the SEER web site, 2009.
2. National Cancer Policy Board (U.S.), Weiner SL, Simone JV. Childhood cancer survivorship: improving care and quality of life. Washington, DC: National Academies Press; 2003.
3. Moorman JE, Rudd RA, Johnson CA, et al. Centers for Disease Control and Prevention (CDC). National surveillance for asthma–United States, 1980–2004. MMWR Surveill Summ 2007;56(SS08):1–54.
4. Writing Group for the SEARCH for Diabetes in Youth Study Group, Dabelea D, Bell RA, et al. Incidence of diabetes in youth in the United States. JAMA 2007;297(24):2716–24.
5. Linabery AM, Ross JA. Trends in childhood cancer incidence in the U.S. (1992–2004). Cancer 2008;112(2):416–32.
6. O'Leary M, Krailo M, Anderson JR, et al. Progress in childhood cancer: 50 years of research collaboration, a report from the Children's Oncology Group. Semin Oncol 2008;35(5):484–93.
7. Pieters R, Carroll WL. Biology and treatment of acute lymphoblastic leukemia. Pediatr Clin North Am 2008;55(1):1–20, ix.
8. Pui CH, Evans WE. Treatment of acute lymphoblastic leukemia. N Engl J Med 2006;354(2):166–78.
9. Ris MD, Beebe DW. Neurodevelopmental outcomes of children with low-grade gliomas. Dev Disabil Res Rev 2008;14(3):196–202.
10. Gottardo NG, Gajjar A. Chemotherapy for malignant brain tumors of childhood. J Child Neurol 2008;23(10):1149–59.
11. Abrams A, Rauch P. Child psychiatry consultation. In: Rutter M, Bishop D, Pine D, et al, editors. Rutter's textbook of child and adolescent psychiatry. 5th Edition. Oxford (UK): Blackwell; 2008. p. 1143–55.
12. Massachusetts General Hospital Cancer Center. Parent and family support. Available at: http://www.massgeneral.org/children/specialtiesandservices/hematology_oncology/parent_family.aspx. Accessed January 4, 2010.
13. Abrams AN, Hazen EP, Penson RT. Psychosocial issues in adolescents with cancer. Cancer Treat Rev 2007;33(7):622–30.
14. Hedström M, Ljungman G, von Essen L. Perceptions of distress among adolescents recently diagnosed with cancer. J Pediatr Hematol Oncol 2005;27(1):15–22.
15. Evan EE, Kaufman M, Cook AB, et al. Sexual health and self-esteem in adolescents and young adults with cancer. Cancer 2006;107(Suppl 7):1672–9.
16. Weintraub M, Gross E, Kadari A, et al. Should ovarian cryopreservation be offered to girls with cancer. Pediatr Blood Cancer 2007;48(1):4–9.
17. Kashani J, Hakami N. Depression in children and adolescents with malignancy. Can J Psychiatry 1982;27(6):474–7.
18. Allen L, Zigler E. Psychological adjustment of seriously ill children. J Am Acad Child Psychiatry 1986;25(5):708–12.
19. Patenaude AF, Kupst MJ. Psychosocial functioning in pediatric cancer. J Pediatr Psychol 2005;30(1):9–27.
20. Pai AL, Drotar D, Zebracki K, et al. A meta-analysis of the effects of psychological interventions in pediatric oncology on outcomes of psychological distress and adjustment. J Pediatr Psychol 2006;31(9):978–88.

21. Noll RB, Gartstein MA, Vannatta K, et al. Social, emotional, and behavioral functioning of children with cancer. Pediatrics 1999;103(1):71–8.

22. Eiser C, Hill JJ, Vance YH. Examining the psychological consequences of surviving childhood cancer: systematic review as a research method in pediatric psychology. J Pediatr Psychol 2000;25(6):449–60.

23. Zeltzer LK, Recklitis C, Buchbinder D, et al. Psychological status in childhood cancer survivors: a report from the Childhood Cancer Survivor Study. J Clin Oncol 2009;27(14):2396–404.

24. Greenberg HS, Kazak AE, Meadows AT. Psychologic functioning in 8- to 16-year-old cancer survivors and their parents. J Pediatr 1989;114(3):488–93.

25. March J, Silva S, Petrycki S, et al. Fluoxetine, cognitive-behavioral therapy, and their combination for adolescents with depression: Treatment for Adolescents With Depression Study (TADS) randomized controlled trial. JAMA 2004;292(7): 807–20.

26. Kersun LS, Elia J. Depressive symptoms and SSRI use in pediatric oncology patients. Pediatr Blood Cancer 2007;49(7):881–7.

27. Gothelf D, Rubinstein M, Shemesh E, et al. Pilot study: fluvoxamine treatment for depression and anxiety disorders in children and adolescents with cancer. J Am Acad Child Adolesc Psychiatry 2005;44(12):1258–62.

28. Kersun LS, Kazak AE. Prescribing practices of selective serotonin reuptake inhibitors (SSRIs) among pediatric oncologists: a single institution experience. Pediatr Blood Cancer 2006;47(3):339–42.

29. Pao M, Ballard ED, Rosenstein DL, et al. Psychotropic medication use in pediatric patients with cancer. Arch Pediatr Adolesc Med 2006;160(8):818–22.

30. Patel A, Schieble T, Davidson M, et al. Distraction with a hand-held video game reduces pediatric preoperative anxiety. Paediatr Anaesth 2006;16(10):1019–27.

31. Liossi C, White P, Hatira P. A randomized clinical trial of a brief hypnosis intervention to control venepuncture-related pain of paediatric cancer patients. Pain 2009;142(3):255–63.

32. Tyc VL, Mulhern RK, Barclay DR, et al. Variables associated with anticipatory nausea and vomiting in pediatric cancer patients receiving ondansetron antiemetic therapy. J Pediatr Psychol 1997;22(1):45–58.

33. Stockhorst U, Spennes-Saleh S, Körholz D, et al. Anticipatory symptoms and anticipatory immune responses in pediatric cancer patients receiving chemotherapy: features of a classically conditioned response? Brain Behav Immun 2000;14(3):198–218.

34. Gottschling S, Reindl TK, Meyer S, et al. Acupuncture to alleviate chemotherapy-induced nausea and vomiting in pediatric oncology – a randomized multicenter crossover pilot trial. Klin Padiatr 2008;220(6):365–70.

35. Friebert S. Pain management for children with cancer at the end of life: beginning steps toward a standard of care. Pediatr Blood Cancer 2009;52(7):749–50.

36. Lewis DA, Smith RE. Steroid-induced psychiatric syndromes. A report of 14 cases and a review of the literature. J Affect Disord 1983;5(4):319–32.

37. Kershner P, Wang-Cheng R. Psychiatric side effects of steroid therapy. Psychosomatics 1989;30(2):135–9.

38. Wolkowitz OM, Rubinow D, Doran AR, et al. Prednisone effects on neurochemistry and behavior. Preliminary findings. Arch Gen Psychiatry 1990;47(10): 963–8.

39. Wolkowitz OM. Prospective controlled studies of the behavioral and biological effects of exogenous corticosteroids. Psychoneuroendocrinology 1994;19(3): 233–55.

40. Brown ES, Suppes T. Mood symptoms during corticosteroid therapy: a review. Harv Rev Psychiatry 1998;5(5):239–46.
41. Patten SB, Neutel CI. Corticosteroid-induced adverse psychiatric effects: incidence, diagnosis and management. Drug Saf 2000;22(2):111–22.
42. Warrington TP, Bostwick JM. Psychiatric adverse effects of corticosteroids. Mayo Clin Proc 2006;81(10):1361–7.
43. The Boston Collaborative Drug Surveillance Program. Acute adverse reactions to prednisone in relation to dosage. Clin Pharmacol Ther 1972;13(5):694–8.
44. Bender BG, Lerner JA, Kollasch E. Mood and memory changes in asthmatic children receiving corticosteroids. J Am Acad Child Adolesc Psychiatry 1988; 27(6):720–5.
45. Satel SL. Mental status changes in children receiving glucocorticoids. Review of the literature. Clin Pediatr (Phila) 1990;29(7):383–8.
46. Bender BG, Lerner JA, Poland JE. Association between corticosteroids and psychologic change in hospitalized asthmatic children. Ann Allergy 1991; 66(5):414–9.
47. Hall AS, Thorley G, Houtman PN. The effects of corticosteroids on behavior in children with nephrotic syndrome. Pediatr Nephrol 2003;18(12):1220–3.
48. Stuart FA, Segal TY, Keady S. Adverse psychological effects of corticosteroids in children and adolescents. Arch Dis Child 2005;90(5):500–6.
49. Harris JC, Carel CA, Rosenberg LA, et al. Intermittent high dose corticosteroid treatment in childhood cancer: behavioral and emotional consequences. J Am Acad Child Psychiatry 1986;25(1):120–4.
50. Drigan R, Spirito A, Gelber RD. Behavioral effects of corticosteroids in children with acute lymphoblastic leukemia. Med Pediatr Oncol 1992;20(1):13–21.
51. Hinds PS, Hockenberry MJ, Gattuso JS, et al. Dexamethasone alters sleep and fatigue in pediatric patients with acute lymphoblastic leukemia. Cancer 2007; 110(10):2321–30.
52. Brown ES, Chamberlain W, Dhanani N, et al. An open-label trial of olanzapine for corticosteroid-induced mood symptoms. J Affect Disord 2004;83(2–3):277–81.
53. Pulsipher MA. Treatment of CML in pediatric patients: should imatinib mesylate (STI-571, Gleevec) or allogeneic hematopoietic cell transplant be front-line therapy? Pediatr Blood Cancer 2004;43(5):523–33.
54. Kaban LB, Mulliken JB, Ezekowitz RA, et al. Antiangiogenic therapy of a recurrent giant cell tumor of the mandible with interferon alfa-2a. Pediatrics 1999; 103(6 Pt 1):1145–9.
55. Dickerman JD. Interferon and giant cell tumors. Pediatrics 1999;103(6 Pt 1): 1282–3.
56. Navid F, Furman WL, Fleming M, et al. The feasibility of adjuvant interferon alpha-2b in children with high-risk melanoma. Cancer 2005;103(4):780–7.
57. Renault PF, Hoofnagle JH, Park Y, et al. Psychiatric complications of long-term interferon alfa therapy. Arch Intern Med 1987;147(9):1577–80.
58. Greenberg DB, Jonasch E, Gadd MA, et al. Adjuvant therapy of melanoma with interferon-alpha-2b is associated with mania and bipolar syndromes. Cancer 2000;89(2):356–62.
59. Raison CL, Demetrashvili M, Capuron L, et al. Neuropsychiatric adverse effects of interferon-alpha: recognition and management. CNS Drugs 2005;19(2):105–23.
60. Loftis JM, Hauser P. The phenomenology and treatment of interferon-induced depression. J Affect Disord 2004;82(2):175–90.
61. Pavol MA, Meyers CA, Rexer JL, et al. Pattern of neurobehavioral deficits associated with interferon alfa therapy for leukemia. Neurology 1995;45(5):947–50.

62. Valentine AD, Meyers CA, Kling MA, et al. Mood and cognitive side effects of interferon-alpha therapy. Semin Oncol 1998;25(1 Suppl 1):39–47.

63. Hensley ML, Peterson B, Silver RT, et al. Risk factors for severe neuropsychiatric toxicity in patients receiving interferon alfa-2b and low-dose cytarabine for chronic myelogenous leukemia: analysis of cancer and leukemia group B 9013. J Clin Oncol 2000;18(6):1301–8.

64. Schaefer M, Engelbrecht MA, Gut O, et al. Interferon alpha (IFNalpha) and psychiatric syndromes: a review. Prog Neuropsychopharmacol Biol Psychiatry 2002;26(4):731–46.

65. Heinze S, Egberts F, Rötzer S, et al. Depressive mood changes and psychiatric symptoms during 12-month low-dose interferon-alpha treatment in patients with malignant melanoma: results from the multicenter DeCOG trial. J Immunother 2010;33(1):106–14.

66. Kirkwood JM, Bender C, Agarwala S, et al. Mechanisms and management of toxicities associated with high-dose interferon alfa-2b therapy. J Clin Oncol 2002;20(17):3703–18.

67. Hauser P, Khosla J, Aurora H, et al. A prospective study of the incidence and open-label treatment of interferon-induced major depressive disorder in patients with hepatitis C. Mol Psychiatry 2002;7(9):942–7.

68. Kraus MR, Schäfer A, Faller H, et al. Paroxetine for the treatment of interferon-alpha-induced depression in chronic hepatitis C. Aliment Pharmacol Ther 2002;16(6):1091–9.

69. Dieperink E, Ho SB, Thuras P, et al. A prospective study of neuropsychiatric symptoms associated with interferon-alpha-2b and ribavirin therapy for patients with chronic hepatitis C. Psychosomatics 2003;44(2):104–12.

70. Schäfer M, Schmidt F, Amann B, et al. Adding low-dose antidepressants to interferon alpha treatment for chronic hepatitis C improved psychiatric tolerability in a patient with schizoaffective psychosis. Neuropsychobiology 2000;42(Suppl 1):43–5.

71. Hauser P, Soler R, Reed S, et al. Prophylactic treatment of depression induced by interferon-alpha. Psychosomatics 2000;41(5):439–41.

72. Musselman DL, Lawson DH, Gumnick JF, et al. Paroxetine for the prevention of depression induced by high-dose interferon alfa. N Engl J Med 2001;344(13):961–6.

73. Moore BD 3rd. Neurocognitive outcomes in survivors of childhood cancer. J Pediatr Psychol 2005;30(1):51–63.

74. Mulhern RK, White HA, Glass JO, et al. Attentional functioning and white matter integrity among survivors of malignant brain tumors of childhood. J Int Neuropsychol Soc 2004;10(2):180–9.

75. Mulhern RK, Merchant TE, Gajjar A, et al. Late neurocognitive sequelae in survivors of brain tumours in childhood. Lancet Oncol 2004;5(7):399–408.

76. Askins MA, Moore BD 3rd. Preventing neurocognitive late effects in childhood cancer survivors. J Child Neurol 2008;23(10):1160–71.

77. Nathan PC, Patel SK, Dilley K, et al. Guidelines for identification of, advocacy for, and intervention in neurocognitive problems in survivors of childhood cancer: a report from the Children's Oncology Group. Arch Pediatr Adolesc Med 2007;161(8):798–806.

78. Phipps S, Dunavant M, Srivastava DK, et al. Cognitive and academic functioning in survivors of pediatric bone marrow transplantation. J Clin Oncol 2000;18(5):1004–11.

79. Moleski M. Neuropsychological, neuroanatomical, and neurophysiological consequences of CNS chemotherapy for acute lymphoblastic leukemia. Arch Clin Neuropsychol 2000;15(7):603–30.

80. Bhatia S. Cancer survivorship–pediatric issues. Hematology Am Soc Hematol Educ Program 2005;507–15.

81. Butler RW, Haser JK. Neurocognitive effects of treatment for childhood cancer. Ment Retard Dev Disabil Res Rev 2006;12(3):184–91.

82. Palmer SL, Reddick WE, Gajjar A. Understanding the cognitive impact on children who are treated for medulloblastoma. J Pediatr Psychol 2007;32(9):1040–9.

83. Janzen LA, Spiegler BJ. Neurodevelopmental sequelae of pediatric acute lymphoblastic leukemia and its treatment. Dev Disabil Res Rev 2008;14(3): 185–95.

84. Mulhern RK, Kepner JL, Thomas PR, et al. Neuropsychologic functioning of survivors of childhood medulloblastoma randomized to receive conventional or reduced-dose craniospinal irradiation: a Pediatric Oncology Group Study. J Clin Oncol 1998;16(5):1723–8.

85. Ris MD, Packer R, Goldwein J, et al. Intellectual outcome after reduced-dose radiation therapy plus adjuvant chemotherapy for medulloblastoma: a Children's Cancer Group Study. J Clin Oncol 2001;19(15):3470–6.

86. Little AS, Sheean T, Manoharan R, et al. The management of completely resected childhood intracranial ependymoma: the argument for observation only. Childs Nerv Syst 2009;25(3):281–4.

87. Steinlin M, Imfeld S, Zulauf P, et al. Neuropsychological long-term sequelae after posterior fossa tumour resection during childhood. Brain 2003;126(Pt 9): 1998–2008.

88. Kao GD, Goldwein JW, Schultz DJ, et al. The impact of perioperative factors on subsequent intelligence quotient deficits in children treated for medulloblastoma/posterior fossa primitive neuroectodermal tumors. Cancer 1994;74(3): 965–71.

89. Levisohn L, Cronin-Golomb A, Schmahmann JD. Neuropsychological consequences of cerebellar tumour resection in children: cerebellar cognitive affective syndrome in a paediatric population. Brain 2000;123(Pt 5):1041–50.

90. Wolfe-Christensen C, Mullins LL, Scott JG, et al. Persistent psychosocial problems in children who develop posterior fossa syndrome after medulloblastoma resection. Pediatr Blood Cancer 2007;49(5):723–6.

91. Buizer AI, de Sonneville LM, Veerman AJ. Effects of chemotherapy on neurocognitive function in children with acute lymphoblastic leukemia: a critical review of the literature. Pediatr Blood Cancer 2009;52(4):447–54.

92. Buizer AI, de Sonneville LM, van den Heuvel-Eibrink MM, et al. Behavioral and educational limitations after chemotherapy for childhood acute lymphoblastic leukemia or Wilms tumor. Cancer 2006;106(9):2067–75.

93. Achenbach TM. Manual for the Child Behavior Checklist/4-18 and 1991 profiles. Burlington (VT): University of Vermont Department of Psychiatry; 1991.

94. Campbell LK, Scaduto M, Sharp W, et al. A meta-analysis of the neurocognitive sequelae of treatment for childhood acute lymphocytic leukemia. Pediatr Blood Cancer 2007;49(1):65–73.

95. Anderson FS, Kunin-Batson AS. Neurocognitive late effects of chemotherapy in children: the past 10 years of research on brain structure and function. Pediatr Blood Cancer 2009;52(2):159–64.

96. Butler RW, Mulhern RK. Neurocognitive interventions for children and adolescents surviving cancer. J Pediatr Psychol 2005;30(1):65–78.

97. Butler RW, Sahler OJ, Askins MA, et al. Interventions to improve neuropsychological functioning in childhood cancer survivors. Dev Disabil Res Rev 2008; 14(3):251–8.

98. Butler RW, Copeland DR. Attentional processes and their remediation in children treated for cancer: a literature review and the development of a therapeutic approach. J Int Neuropsychol Soc 2002;8(1):115–24.

99. Butler RW, Copeland DR, Fairclough DL, et al. A multicenter, randomized clinical trial of a cognitive remediation program for childhood survivors of a pediatric malignancy. J Consult Clin Psychol 2008;76(3):367–78.

100. Poppelreuter M, Weis J, Mumm A, et al. Rehabilitation of therapy-related cognitive deficits in patients after hematopoietic stem cell transplantation. Bone Marrow Transplant 2008;41(1):79–90.

101. Thompson SJ, Leigh L, Christensen R, et al. Immediate neurocognitive effects of methylphenidate on learning-impaired survivors of childhood cancer. J Clin Oncol 2001;19(6):1802–8.

102. Mulhern RK, Khan RB, Kaplan S, et al. Short-term efficacy of methylphenidate: a randomized, double-blind, placebo-controlled trial among survivors of childhood cancer. J Clin Oncol 2004;22(23):4795–803.

103. Conklin HM, Khan RB, Reddick WE, et al. Acute neurocognitive response to methylphenidate among survivors of childhood cancer: a randomized, double-blind, cross-over trial. J Pediatr Psychol 2007;32(9):1127–39.

104. Daly BP, Brown RT. Scholarly literature review: management of neurocognitive late effects with stimulant medication. J Pediatr Psychol 2007;32(9):1111–26.

105. Barkley RA. A review of stimulant drug research with hyperactive children. J Child Psychol Psychiatry 1977;18(2):137–65.

106. Conklin HM, Helton S, Ashford J, et al. Predicting methylphenidate response in long-term survivors of childhood cancer: a randomized, double-blind, placebo-controlled, crossover trial. J Pediatr Psychol 2010;35(2):144–55.

107. Conklin HM, Lawford J, Jasper BW, et al. Side effects of methylphenidate in childhood cancer survivors: a randomized placebo-controlled trial. Pediatrics 2009;124(1):226–33.

108. Children's Oncology Group. Long-term follow-up guidelines for survivors of childhood, adolescent and young adult cancers, Version 3.0. Arcadia (CA): Children's Oncology Group; October 2008. Available at: www.survivorshipguidelines.org. Accessed February 16, 2010.

109. Smith SD, Rosen D, Trueworthy RC, et al. A reliable method for evaluating drug compliance in children with cancer. Cancer 1979;43(1):169–73.

110. Lansky SB, Smith SD, Cairns NU, et al. Psychological correlates of compliance. Am J Pediatr Hematol Oncol 1983;5(1):87–92.

111. Tebbi CK, Cummings KM, Zevon MA, et al. Compliance of pediatric and adolescent cancer patients. Cancer 1986;58(5):1179–84.

112. Festa RS, Tamaroff MH, Chasalow F, et al. Therapeutic adherence to oral medication regimens by adolescents with cancer. I. Laboratory assessment. J Pediatr 1992;120(5):807–11.

113. Tebbi CK. Treatment compliance in childhood and adolescence. Cancer 1993; 71(Suppl 10):3441–9.

114. de Oliveira BM, Viana MB, Zani CL, et al. Clinical and laboratory evaluation of compliance in acute lymphoblastic leukaemia. Arch Dis Child 2004;89(8):785–8.

115. Lancaster D, Lennard L, Lilleyman JS. Profile of non-compliance in lymphoblastic leukaemia. Arch Dis Child 1997;76(4):365–6.

116. Spinetta JJ, Masera G, Eden T, et al. Refusal, non-compliance, and abandonment of treatment in children and adolescents with cancer: a report of the SIOP working committee on phychosocial issues in pediatric oncology. Med Pediatr Oncol 2002;38(2):114–7.

117. Die-Trill M, Stuber ML. Psychological problems of curative cancer treatment. In: Holland JC, editor. Psycho-oncology. New York: Oxford University Press; 1998. p. 897–906.

118. Holmes CS, Yu Z, Frentz J. Chronic and discrete stress as predictors of children's adjustment. J Consult Clin Psychol 1999;67(3):411–9.

119. Varni JW, Katz ER, Colegrove R Jr, et al. Family functioning predictors of adjustment in children with newly diagnosed cancer: a prospective analysis. J Child Psychol Psychiatry 1996;37(3):321–8.

120. Jobe-Shields L, Alderfer MA, Barrera M, et al. Parental depression and family environment predict distress in children before stem cell transplantation. J Dev Behav Pediatr 2009;30(2):140–6.

121. Dockerty JD, Williams SM, McGee R, et al. Impact of childhood cancer on the mental health of parents. Med Pediatr Oncol 2000;35(5):475–83.

122. Speechley KN, Noh S. Surviving childhood cancer, social support, and parents' psychological adjustment. J Pediatr Psychol 1992;17(1):15–31.

123. Sloper P. Predictors of distress in parents of children with cancer: a prospective study. J Pediatr Psychol 2000;25(2):79–91.

124. Rabineau KM, Mabe PA, Vega RA. Parenting stress in pediatric oncology populations. J Pediatr Hematol Oncol 2008;30(5):358–65.

125. Grootenhuis MA, Last BF. Adjustment and coping by parents of children with cancer: a review of the literature. Support Care Cancer 1997;5(6):466–84.

126. Robinson KE, Gerhardt CA, Vannatta K, et al. Parent and family factors associated with child adjustment to pediatric cancer. J Pediatr Psychol 2007;32(4):400–10.

127. Robinson KE, Gerhardt CA, Vannatta K, et al. Survivors of childhood cancer and comparison peers: the influence of early family factors on distress in emerging adulthood. J Fam Psychol 2009;23(1):23–31.

128. Goldish M. SuperSibs!. Available at: http://www.supersibs.org/. Accessed January 4, 2010.

129. Sloper P. Experiences and support needs of siblings of children with cancer. Health Soc Care Community 2000;8(5):298–306.

130. Barrera M, Fleming CF, Khan FS. The role of emotional social support in the psychological adjustment of siblings of children with cancer. Child Care Health Dev 2004;30(2):103–11.

131. Streisand R, Rodrigue JR, Houck C, et al. Brief report: parents of children undergoing bone marrow transplantation: documenting stress and piloting a psychological intervention program. J Pediatr Psychol 2000;25(5):331–7.

132. Sahler OJ, Varni JW, Fairclough DL, et al. Problem-solving skills training for mothers of children with newly diagnosed cancer: a randomized trial. J Dev Behav Pediatr 2002;23(2):77–86.

133. Sahler OJ, Fairclough DL, Phipps S, et al. Using problem-solving skills training to reduce negative affectivity in mothers of children with newly diagnosed cancer: report of a multisite randomized trial. J Consult Clin Psychol 2005;73(2):272–83.

134. Kazak AE. Evidence-based interventions for survivors of childhood cancer and their families. J Pediatr Psychol 2005;30(1):29–39.

135. Cairns NU, Klopovich P, Hearne E, et al. School attendance of children with cancer. J Sch Health 1982;52(3):152–5.

136. Vannatta K, Gartstein MA, Short A, et al. A controlled study of peer relationships of children surviving brain tumors: teacher, peer, and self ratings. J Pediatr Psychol 1998;23(5):279–87.

137. Vance YH, Eiser C. The school experience of the child with cancer. Child Care Health Dev 2002;28(1):5–19.

138. Noll RB, Bukowski WM, Rogosch FA, et al. Social interactions between children with cancer and their peers: teacher ratings. J Pediatr Psychol 1990;15(1): 43–56.

139. Noll RB, Ris MD, Davies WH, et al. Social interactions between children with cancer or sickle cell disease and their peers: teacher ratings. J Dev Behav Pediatr 1992;13(3):187–93.

140. Searle NS, Askins M, Bleyer WA. Homebound schooling is the least favorable option for continued education of adolescent cancer patients: a preliminary report. Med Pediatr Oncol 2003;40(6):380–4.

141. Larcombe I, Charlton A. Children's return to school after treatment for cancer: study days for teachers. J Cancer Educ 1996;11(2):102–5.

142. Pallmeyer TP, Saylor CF, Treiber FA, et al. Helping school personnel understand the student with cancer: workshop evaluation. Child Psychiatry Hum Dev 1986; 16(3):205–17.

143. Katz ER, Varni JW, Rubenstein CL, et al. Teacher, parent, and child evaluative ratings of a school reintegration intervention for children with newly diagnosed cancer. Child Health Care 1992;21(2):69–75.

144. Hudson MM, Mertens AC, Yasui Y, et al. Health status of adult long-term survivors of childhood cancer: a report from the Childhood Cancer Survivor Study. JAMA 2003;290(12):1583–92.

145. Garwicz S, Möller T, Olsen JH, et al. Association of the Nordic Cancer Registries; Nordic Society for Paediatric Haematology and Oncology. Nordic studies on late effects of treatment of cancer in childhood and adolescence. Acta Oncol 2004; 43(7):682–3.

146. Geenen MM, Cardous-Ubbink MC, Kremer LC, et al. Medical assessment of adverse health outcomes in long term survivors of childhood cancer. JAMA 2007;297(24):2705–15.

147. Olsen JH, Möller T, Anderson H, et al. Lifelong cancer incidence in 47,697 patients treated for childhood cancer in the Nordic countries. J Natl Cancer Inst 2009;101(11):806–13.

148. Bruce M. A systematic and conceptual review of posttraumatic stress in childhood cancer survivors and their parents. Clin Psychol Rev 2006;26(3): 233–56.

149. Ross L, Johansen C, Dalton SO, et al. Psychiatric hospitalizations among survivors of cancer in childhood or adolescence. N Engl J Med 2003;349(7):650–7.

150. Recklitis CJ, Lockwood RA, Rothwell MA, et al. Suicidal ideation and attempts in adult survivors of childhood cancer. J Clin Oncol 2006;24(24):3852–7.

151. Zebrack BJ, Gurney JG, Oeffinger K, et al. Psychological outcomes in long-term survivors of childhood brain cancer: a report from the childhood cancer survivor study. J Clin Oncol 2004;22(6):999–1006.

152. Zeltzer LK, Lu Q, Leisenring W, et al. Psychosocial outcomes and health-related quality of life in adult childhood cancer survivors: a report from the childhood cancer survivor study. Cancer Epidemiol Biomarkers Prev 2008;17(2):435–46.

153. Recklitis CJ, Diller LR, Li X, et al. Suicide ideation in adult survivors of childhood cancer: a report from the Childhood Cancer Survivor Study. J Clin Oncol 2010; 28(4):655–61.

154. Beale EA, Baile WF, Aaron J. Silence is not golden: communicating with children dying from cancer. J Clin Oncol 2005;23(15):3629–31.

155. Kreicbergs U, Valdimarsdóttir U, Onelöv E, et al. Talking about death with children who have severe malignant disease. N Engl J Med 2004;351(12): 1175–86.

156. Wolfe J, Grier HE, Klar N, et al. Symptoms and suffering at the end of life in children with cancer. N Engl J Med 2000;342(5):326–33.

157. Johnston DL, Nagel K, Friedman DL, et al. Availability and use of palliative care and end-of-life services for pediatric oncology patients. J Clin Oncol 2008; 26(28):4646–50.

Partnerships Between Pediatric Palliative Care and Psychiatry

Caprice Knapp, PhD[a],*, Vanessa Madden, BSc[a],
Daniel Button, MS, LCSW, ACHP-SW, Rebecca Brown, MDiv[b],
Barbara Hastie, PhD[c]

KEYWORDS

• Pediatric palliative care • Pediatric psychiatry
• Partners in Care: Together for Kids • Streetlight program

Children with life-threatening illnesses and their families may face physical, emotional, psychosocial, and spiritual challenges throughout the children's course of illness. Pediatric palliative care is a model of care that is designed to meet such challenges, and the number of programs available in the United States continues to increase. Given the psychosocial and emotional needs of children and their families it is clear that psychiatrists can, and do, play a role in delivering pediatric palliative care. In this article the partnership between pediatric palliative care and psychiatry is explored. The authors present an overview of pediatric palliative care followed by a summary of some of the roles for psychiatry. Next, 2 innovative pediatric palliative care programs that psychiatrists may or may not be aware of are described. Finally, the authors discuss some challenges that are faced in further developing this partnership and suggestions for future research.

OVERVIEW OF PEDIATRIC PALLIATIVE CARE

Annually in the United States about 53,000 children die from a variety of causes.[1] In addition, it has been estimated that there are about 500,000 children coping with

A version of this article was previously published in the *Child and Adolescent Psychiatric Clinics of North America, 19:2.*

[a] Departments of Epidemiology and Health Policy Research, University of Florida, 1329 SW 16th Street, Gainesville, FL 32610, USA
[b] Department of Pediatrics, University of Florida, 1329 SW 16th Street, Gainesville, FL 32610, USA
[c] Department of Community Dentistry & Behavioral Science, University of Florida, 1329 SW 16th Street, Gainesville, FL 32610, USA
* Corresponding author.
E-mail address: capricegaring@hotmail.com

life-threatening conditions and about 1 to 1.5 million children coping with complex, chronic conditions each year in the United States.[2,3] As advances in technology and medical interventions prolong the lives of seriously ill children, it becomes clear that many of these children could benefit from pediatric palliative care. Pediatric palliative care is defined by the World Health Organization (WHO) as "the active total care of the child's body, mind, and spirit, and also involves giving support to the family"[4] The WHO goes on to say that care should begin at diagnosis, should alleviate physical, psychological, and social distress, and should improve the child's quality of life.[4]

Pediatric palliative care is provided in several settings such as general and children's hospitals, skilled nursing facilities, long-term care facilities, hospices, and community settings. There is limited comprehensive information about the prevalence of pediatric palliative care in the United States. Local and national directories do exist, but these are often sponsored by national organizations, such as the National Hospice and Palliative Care Organization (NHPCO), Children's Hospice International (CHI), and International Association for Hospice and Palliative Care (IAHPC), and therefore only list members.[5,6] Another possible reason that there is not a national directory of pediatric palliative care services may be due to the lack of a common definition. For example, a pediatric oncology unit in a hospital may have a social worker and a physician with specialty training in providing psychosocial support or pain and symptom management for children, whereas a community day care center for children with life-threatening illnesses may only employ an expressive therapist. It is unclear whether both of these programs would be considered a pediatric palliative care program. Nonetheless, the number of pediatric palliative care providers has likely increased alongside the general increase in palliative care providers. In 1974 the first hospice legislation was introduced in the United States and today there are roughly 4500 hospices in the United States.[5] It is unclear how many hospices serve children, but a 2007 national survey completed by 378 hospices found that 294 are willing to serve pediatric patients.[7] Another study of 1527 deceased, publicly insured children in Florida found that 11% used hospice care in the last 6 months of life.[8] Regarding inpatient palliative care, 2 recent studies found that 20% to 25% of hospitals have a palliative care program[9,10] and 58% of organizations that participate in the Children's Oncology Group have a pediatric palliative care program.[11]

Provision of pediatric palliative care is limited by the availability of providers. Many studies have found that end of life or palliative training, particularly in pediatrics, is not addressed at all, or in a limited way, throughout medical education for physicians. Two-thirds of medical school administrators felt that not enough time in their programs was devoted to palliative care and only one-third reported that they had a formal course in palliative care.[12] Knowledge of palliative care is critical to primary care providers because they are often the referring physicians to palliative care programs. A 2009 study by Thompson and colleagues[13] of 303 pediatricians in Florida found that 49% had ever referred a child to palliative care, 29% did not know what palliative services were available in their area, and when asked about 11 diagnoses there was no consensus on whether children with those diagnoses should be referred. Lack of knowledge also affects pediatric nurses. A 2009 study by Knapp and colleagues[14] of 279 pediatric nurses in Florida found that being employed in an area where a pediatric palliative care program was offered and having worked in a hospice in the past were associated with higher levels of knowledge about palliative care. Although these studies primarily focus on physicians and nurses, it is likely that the lack of palliative care education and training also affects other members of the interdisciplinary team such as social workers, clinical psychologists, psychiatrists, chaplains, child life specialists, expressive therapists, and volunteers. There is a need for future research to understand the educational needs and preferences of educational methods for members of the interdisciplinary team. In 2006 the American Board of Medical Specialties (ABMS) formally recognized palliative care as a subspecialty. Recognition of this specialty also recently occurred in Australia, Canada, Ireland, and the United Kingdom.[15] Recognition by the ABMS may help to address some of the most commonly cited barriers to incorporating palliative care into medical education: lack of time, funding, and knowledgable faculty.

Once a pediatric palliative care program is developed and implemented, service provision may prove to be complicated. Children in pediatric palliative care programs have a variety of medical conditions, many of which are rare, making clinical guidance, prognostication, care planning, and staffing difficult. Not only are the physical needs of the children difficult to predict, their practical and psychological needs are also important and dynamic. Services provided to children include pain and symptom management, expressive therapies, support counseling, personal care, massage, nursing care, and nutritional counseling. Services provided to other family members include respite, counseling, bereavement, and sibling specific support. Service provision may be complicated by age. Studies have shown that 90% of neonates who die in a hospital spend their entire lives there and although the myth that infants do not manifest pain has widely been denounced, pain can nonetheless be difficult to assess.[16,17] Service provision may be complicated by diagnoses. In the Institute on Medicine's 2003 report, 4 prototypical trajectories of child's death were illustrated.[18] Yet, children's pediatric palliative care needs vary both within and across those trajectories and diagnoses. This variation is particularly problematic when pediatric palliative care is integrated, meaning that it is provided alongside curative or life-prolonging care. National experts, professional organizations, policy makers, clinicians, and researchers have all promoted integrated pediatric palliative care as an optimal model of care for children with life-threatening illnesses.[4,18–20] Unfortunately, there is limited information available on pediatric palliative care provision undertaken before the end of life. Service provision may be complicated by a lack in funding. Although reimbursement may be available from some third-party payers, many pediatric palliative care programs must rely on gifts, grants, and donations for financial support.

OPPORTUNITIES FOR PSYCHIATRY IN PEDIATRIC PALLIATIVE CARE

Psychiatrists can play an important role in the care of dying children and adolescents. There are many opportunities for psychiatry in pediatric palliative care, and several are described here.

Psychosocial Needs of Children

It is well known that adult patients at the end of life often have psychosocial needs related to loss, loss of functioning, loss of control, and loss of social interaction.[21] Potential issues associated with the end of life are depression, anxiety, delirium, post-traumaticstress disorder (PTSD), suicidal thoughts, personality disorders, neurologic disorders, decreased capacity to make informed decisions, grief, and impacts on health-related quality of life.[21] Caregivers also may suffer from depression, anxiety, PTSD, and prolonged grief. Prevalence of psychological disorders at the end of life for adults has been well studied. Studies, primarily of human immunodeficiency virus (HIV) and cancer patients, have shown that 10% to 50% of terminally ill adults have some symptoms of depression.[22,23] A 2008 chart review of 2716 patients found that hospice patients are 4 times as likely to be depressed as the general population and that depression was associated with female gender, being unmarried, having

a longer length of stay in hospice, HIV, and neurologic disorders.[15] It has been estimated that 44% of terminally ill adults have delirium and 50% to 70% have
anxiety.[24,25] Moreover, many of these psychological disorders are comorbid.

Although limited information exists, it is likely that children with life-threatening
illnesses face similar psychosocial and psychological issues. Understanding of their
illness influences children's psychological issues and how they make sense of the
world at that point in time.[26] Younger children are thought to have lower stress
because they are less likely to understand the full impact of their disease.[27] Children
with life-threatening illnesses are also thought to be more likely to have several risk
factors of PTSD because they may have been exposed to numerous life-threatening
treatments during their illness.[27] Moreover, when children are seriously ill it is believed
that they may regress developmentally and then regain milestones once they have
recovered.[28] Older children and adolescents may also have a difficult time with
body image, fertility, and sexuality.[26] Sexual identity is important for many adolescents; they should be allowed to progress through normal sexual milestones and staff
should be encouraged to candidly engage in conversations with adolescents.[26]
Parental functioning affects all of these psychosocial issues; parents act as caregiver,
transporter, decision maker, and provide other supportive functions for seriously ill
children and adolescents.

One reason that there is little evidence about the prevalence of psychosocial issues
with seriously ill children and adolescents is the interaction between psychological
and physical factors. These interactions make it difficult to diagnose psychological
factors. Symptoms such as weight loss, insomnia, anorexia, and social withdrawal
could be from the child's disease or from psychological factors.[25] Causality of the
psychological and physical factors is often unclear. For example, depression is
strongly associated with pain, and the patient's perception of pain may decrease after
being treated with antidepressants and psychotherapeutic interventions.[29] It is difficult
to tell if the pain causes depression or vice versa.

Psychiatrists can help to alleviate children's anxiety, depression, and stress,
promote psychological comfort, or help manage pain, but only if these can be accurately assessed. There are several barriers that psychiatrists face when seeing pediatric palliative care patients. Many children may be hesitant to engage with
psychiatrists because they do not understand what psychiatrists do or they may not
be comfortable with yet another medical team member. Adolescents especially may
be hesitant. Tools such as pain scales, pain diaries, and self-reports can be used to
assess psychosocial functioning, but the ability to use these tools is affected by the
physical and emotional development of the child.[29] Perhaps more problematic is
that many standardized tools were not developed for children and lack clinically meaningful cutoff scores. Once psychological functioning is assessed, there are several
types of interventions such as pain management, psychopharmacology, cognitive-
behavioral interventions, and psychodynamic therapy,[27] and the ability to use these
interventions depends on the development of the child, stage of illness, and family
dynamics. For example, the use of cognitive-behavioral interventions such as cognitive restructuring, activity-rest cycles, hypnosis, relaxation techniques, diaphragmatic
breathing, and progressive muscle relaxation may not be appropriate for very young
children or children with limited cognitive capacity.[30] Older children and adolescents
might be able to engage in group psychotherapy or existential psychotherapy that
help to identify the ways in which the child copes with his illness.[31] Interventions
can also be symptom specific. Children with fatigue can be instructed to perform
essential activities in the morning, avoid long periods of inactivity, perform mild exercise, and nap often.[30] Psychopharmacology can be used to treat symptoms, although

the effectiveness of many medications is not known for children. At the end of life medications should be chosen that react quickly because the child's estimated length of survival may be short. Potential medication interactions should also be monitored.[24] Regardless of the interventions chosen; the interdisciplinary team should be frequently updated on the child's treatment and progress.

Psychosocial Needs of Parents and Siblings

Children should not die but they do, and there can be no greater pain for a parent than their child's death. Kubler-Ross described 5 reactions to a life-threatening illness: denial, anger, bargaining, depression, and acceptance.[31] As parents experience these reactions, the probability of negative psychological impacts is high. Parents are subject to similar psychological disorders as children, such as depression, stress, anxiety, and PTSD. Studies of parents whose children have been diagnosed with cancer found high levels of stress, anxiety, depression, uncertainty, and loneliness, and these feelings can persist long after the child has completed treatment.[32] Evidence suggests that 25% to 33% of parents have difficulty returning to a state of emotional equilibrium after their children complete treatment.[32] In a study of 162 mothers and fathers of children diagnosed with cancer, the results showed that fathers were more distressed than mothers at the point of diagnosis and mothers were more distressed than fathers 12 months after diagnosis.[32] PTSD is also well studied in parents of pediatric oncology patients. Evidence suggests that about 10% of mothers and 7% of fathers have severe PTSD and 27% and 28% have moderate PTSD, respectively.[27] Studies have also noted PTSD in parents of children who have undergone transplants and parents of infants receiving care in a neonatal intensive care unit.[27] Predictors of PTSD in parents are anxiety, perception of the intensity of treatment, and social support.[27]

Parents use a variety of strategies to cope with their child's illness such as relying on religion, living one day at a time, having open communication, and acceptance. If parents are unable to cope with their children's illness on their own, or if they have psychological issues independent of their child's illness that are further exacerbated by their child's illness, psychiatric assistance may be needed. Open and ongoing conversations need to occur between parents and health care professionals to understand parents' goals, coping styles, family dynamics, and external support. Family problems unrelated to the child's illness such as substance abuse could exacerbate parents' psychological issues.[31] Family therapy can be used to assess roles within the family, resolve conflicts and dysfunction, address substance abuse and family relational processes, and understand ethnic factors.[23] Truth telling by parents is another area where psychiatrists may be able to intervene. Often a parent's hesitancy to tell their child the truth is manifested by their own pain and inability to cope with the child's illness,[26] both of which can be helped by psychotherapeutic methods.

Parents and providers must be vigilant to ensure that the needs of siblings are recognized and addressed. Siblings should be supported throughout the child's illness, and they should be helped to process grief after the child dies.[33] Several studies have shown that siblings have difficulty adjusting when parents are stressed and that siblings often feel guilty, angry, jealous, and anxious.[34–38] Siblings may also feel that the ill child is at center of family and they are in a minor role. Siblings of cancer patients had higher levels of depression and anxiety when their brother or sister was first diagnosed with cancer, but these differences petered out during follow-up as compared with healthy controls.[38] Despite all that is known about siblings and their needs, a recent study has suggested that those needs continue to be unmet. Contro and colleagues[39] found that when children are at the end of life their siblings still do not receive necessary services and that parents want the siblings to have access to support groups and playrooms. Interventions for siblings must carefully consider their developmental stage, past experiences with death, psychological health of the family, and the role that the sibling plays in the family. Bibliotherapy, photography, and art and music therapies are a few examples of interventions that can be used with siblings.[33]

Communication

Perhaps the most overlooked area of role of psychiatry in pediatric palliative care could be in regard to communication. Psychiatrists can play many roles in communication, such as delivering bad news, eliciting the patient's physical, emotional, and family history, determining a child or adolescents' capacity to engage in decision making, and having discussions about decision making ahead of time so that decisions are not impacted by stress. Communication about the end of life should happen early and often in the course of the child's illness.[23] In general, communication should start with open-ended questions to understand the child and parents' life values, views on illness and suffering, role of culture and religion, treatments, and death.[23] All communication should be empathetic and balance hopefulness with honesty.

Minors are not legally authorized to make medical decisions for themselves in the United States, yet health care professionals are encouraged to involve them in the decision-making process. Behaviorists believe that children and adolescents are capable of making medical decisions, yet neuroscientists have shown that the brain is not fully developed until early adulthood. Psychiatrists can help parents and the health care team to determine if children and adolescents can understand facts, appreciate the significance of the facts, and express a choice based on rational consideration. Psychiatrists can help facilitate discussions between all parties and reframe decisions about end of life and advance care planning.[23] Studies show that family members often want to have meetings with staff and want to be involved in decision making.[39–41]

Bereavement

Even when death is expected, a parent is never fully prepared for the death of their child. Among some of the issues that parents face are anger, guilt, fear, uncertainty, concern for other family members, and questioning the purpose or life or their religious beliefs.[42] Family members need to recover physically, emotionally, behaviorally, socially, intellectually, and spiritually, and several factors including coping ability, experience with death in the past, family support system, and religiosity may affect their grief.[43] As time goes on psychological functioning should increase, but in some cases treatment may be needed for prolonged or chronic grief. Studies have found that prolonged grief is associated with increased mortality and morbidity.[25] Psychiatrists may be needed to diagnose depression in parents that can be treated effectively without interfering with the normal grieving process. Group and individual therapies as well as psychopharmacological interventions have all been found to be effective in treating grief.[24] Future research needs to be conducted to determine the longitudinal effectiveness of these psychotherapeutic interventions with bereaved parents.

Members of the palliative care team, including psychiatrists, can help in the bereavement process. Continued contact by the palliative care team with the family can be beneficial after the child's death. It has been suggested that the pediatric palliative care team develop a bereavement plan for families that lasts at least 13 months and up to 2 years.[25] However, some programs provide services to parents in perpetuity. An example is the United Kingdom's Child Death Helpline operated in partnership between Great Ormond Street Hospital and Alder Centre at the Royal Liverpool Children's Hospital.[44] The helpline is manned by volunteer parents who have been bereaved for a minimum of 3.5 years and is open to the public. Knowledge of local services, such as bereavement help lines or bereavement groups, is important to assist families in the healing process.

Numerous studies have been conducted with bereaved siblings and on grief in children and adolescents in general. This focus is particularly important for pediatric palliative care because siblings have spent most of their lives with the deceased brother or sister and yet, they are often overlooked in the grieving process.[43] Children as young as 2 years have a concept of death and their concepts continue to evolve as they age. Reactions to the death of a sibling are widely varied according to age. Although a few bereavement studies have been conducted with siblings, most of these studies focus on the initial months after the death of the ill child. Longer-term studies are needed to better understand what factors are associated with the ability of siblings to process grief over time.

In addition to the needs of siblings after a child's death, psychiatrists may be needed to help address the emotional needs of the child's friends, schoolmates, and other individuals in the community. Interventions may need to be conducted with children and staff in preschools, schools, and community organizations. Resources such as the National Center for School Crisis and Bereavement are available.[45] It is important for the child's peers to have confirmed information about the child's death to prevent rumors, receive a written statement that can be taken home to their parents, and be directed to grief counselors or psychiatrists if needed. Group grief support meetings may also need to take place on school grounds to provide a comfortable environment for children and adolescents to express their thoughts, concerns, and feelings.

INNOVATIVE PEDIATRIC PALLIATIVE CARE PROGRAMS

The development, implementation, and early experiences of 2 innovative pediatric palliative care programs in Florida are presented here. These programs are described to highlight the challenges and opportunities that psychiatrists may or may not be aware of.

Partners in Care: Together for Kids

Pediatric palliative care programs traditionally have been focused on the end of a child's life. In the United States this focus manifested in part because of Medicare reimbursement regulations that only allowed providers to refer patients to hospice care when the patient was believed to be within the last 6 months of life. Referral to hospice care also requires the patient to forgo curative or life-prolonging treatments. Recognizing the difficulty in prognostication for children, and more importantly that no parent wants to forgo even the slightest opportunity to treat their child, several national organizations released policy statements or advocated for more appropriate regulations for children. In 1995, under the guidance of Congressman Jim Moran and CHI, $3.2 million in federal funds was earmarked for several states to enact integrated, pediatric palliative care demonstration programs for children with life-threatening conditions and their families.[46] Integrated programs strive to provide a continuum of care for children and their families from time of diagnosis, with hope for a cure, and through bereavement if a cure is not attained. Since that time, 2 of the states have started programs while several others are in various phases of implementation. Florida began its program in 2005 and Colorado followed in 2008. Florida's program is called Partners in Care: Together for Kids (PIC:TFK). The PIC:TFK program is a partnership between local hospices, the State's Title V agency Children's Medical Services Network (CMSN), and the Agency for Health Care Administration (AHCA). Nurse care coordinators employed by CMSN identify potentially eligible children with life-limiting illnesses from their caseloads of children with special health care needs. Children may be at any stage in their illness trajectory, from the point of diagnosis onward. A referral from the children's primary care physicians is sought for possible program enrollment. Parents are invited to voluntarily enroll their children in the PIC:TFK program. After an initial assessment by the hospice a care plan is developed for each child. Services denoted on the care plan are provided by local hospices that operate in several counties across the State. Copies of the care plan are sent to the children's primary care physicians and distributed to members of the interdisciplinary team. Routine interdisciplinary team meetings are held to address any issues, update the team on progress, and revise the care plan as needed. Services provided to Medicaid-eligible children are reimbursed by the AHCA, which is the State's Medicaid agency. Services provided to children eligible for the State Children's Health Insurance Program are reimbursed by CMSN.

Since its inception in 2005, the PIC:TFK program has provided services to more than 800 children with life-threatening illnesses and their families. The diagnoses of the children in the program are varied and often multidimensional. For example, children receiving PIC:TFK services represent more than 100 different primary diagnoses and many children have multiple diagnoses. Survey data show that a high percentage of parents are highly satisfied with the PIC:TFK program's benefits and that parents and siblings of the ill children use supportive counseling the most.[46] This result provides some evidence that family members do have psychosocial needs related to their children's illnesses. No information is available about the psychiatric needs, or unmet needs, of children and families in the PIC:TFK program, but the quote that follows demonstrates one mother's experiences.

> I just can't imagine going through all this without the PIC:TFK staff. I know that they will be there for us when things get rough. They've taken the time to get to know us now, when things are calm and I know they'll be there for him when he's ready to die. I feel like we are part of a network of support now and we know that they'll be there for us later, when we need it when the time comes.

Additional evidence that parents have psychological needs that could be addressed through the program was illustrated in a 2009 study of 85 parents whose children were enrolled in the PIC:TFK program.[47] Knapp and colleagues found in this study that 48% of parents had probable current depressive symptoms as measured by the Center for Epidemiologic Studies Depression (CES-D) scale, meaning that their CES-D score was equal to or greater than 16. Results from the multivariate analyses showed that having probable depressive symptoms was associated with a greater impact on the family, as measured by the Impact on Family instrument. More than 60% of parents agreed that their child's illness had financial and social impacts on their family, including limiting their travel out of the city, not having much time left over for other family members, and that traveling to the hospital caused a strain on the caregiver. More than 70% of parents agreed that their child's illness resulted in parental fatigue, giving up things, having to change plans at the last minute, difficulties finding a reliable caregiver; 90% reported that living with an ill child can sometimes feel like a rollercoaster ride.

The biggest issue has been the impact on the family, and then sometimes needing direction in the right area to find resources. I think they're out there, but they're not always easy to access ... I sometimes wonder which is worse: to have a healthy child who then is an accident all of a sudden, or to live with an ill child all the time and to live with the uncertainty all the time, thinking when will they get worse?

Streetlight

Because of the specific needs of adolescents, program administrators have recognized that separate palliative care programs should be developed for adolescents. Providing palliative care to adolescents as opposed to children can require a different set of skills, expectations, and goals. Freyer[48] and Freyer and colleagues[49] provide a comprehensive discussion on the needs of dying adolescents. Healthy adolescents are faced with developing the skills to become independent from their parents emotionally and financially. Adolescents with life-threatening illnesses also want to become more autonomous; however, they must rely on their parents for support at the very least because their parents are the legal decision makers for their health care. Adolescents with life-threatening illnesses may also be faced with social isolation, overprotective parents, social rejection, delayed puberty, body alterations such as hair loss, and lack of normal sexual exploration.[50] Adolescent programs may include special teen social programs, chat rooms, or an area specifically for adolescents. For example, the Children's Hospital in Los Angeles has a Teen Impact Program. Established in 1988, the program includes a support group, adventure therapy trips, and special events.[51] Providing a separate adolescent program is important, but above many other aspects, adolescents need peer support. An innovative program in Florida called *Streetlight* addresses the need for a separate adolescent program, while emphasizing peer support and the importance of provider training.

Created in 2006, *Streetlight* is an innovate model of palliative care provided to adolescents receiving inpatient care at the University of Florida/Shands Hospital. Clinicians at the hospital believed that adolescents with life-threatening illnesses have distinct needs, and they create hope and personal support through music, pop culture, and strong peer relationships. In addition, hospital faculty and staff understood that many physicians are lacking in end-of-life care education and experiences, and that exposing future physicians to these circumstances early in their careers may be beneficial. As a result, *Streetlight* emerged as a program that would match up premedical honors students with adolescents with life-threatening illnesses receiving care in the hospital. Adolescents are able to be a part of the program from the point of diagnosis onward.

In the fall of 2006 the *Streetlight* program was started with 17 students. In the first year of the program different interventions were tried and revisions were made based on feedback from the students and the ill adolescents. Eventually, the program evolved to its present structure whereby teams of 6 to 7 students cover afternoon and evening shifts in the hospital. Premedical students must apply to become a *Streetlight* team member, and they receive intensive initial training plus weekly education materials on the needs of dying adolescents and pediatric palliative care. During their shifts the students interact with the ill adolescents in their rooms, the lounge, or in a group setting. One-on-one interaction allows the students to forge individual relationships with the adolescents. In the group setting, adolescents are provided with an often-needed diversion from their illness and treatment, and a chance to meet with other adolescents. Students can provide respite care to parents during hospital stays through daily visitation with the adolescent. Although not required, if the adolescent dies, the students often offer meals and companionship to parents and siblings, as well as attending and helping with memorial services.

Over the past 3 years, 500 adolescents have received services from *Streetlight*. The most common diagnoses of these adolescents who are admitted to the hospital on multiple occasions are cancer, cystic fibrosis, sickle cell disease, and organ failure/transplant.

Qualitative interviews were conducted with 5 of the *Streetlight* students and several themes emerged. First, although all of the adolescents were undergoing difficult medical conditions, the effect of family and peer support, or lack thereof, profoundly affected the adolescents.

> *She was very, very angry and was angry to everyone who walked into her room—the people serving her food she'd yell at, the nurses she'd yell at and she was really only OK with me being in there ... Mostly it was my presence; sometimes we didn't have to say anything at all. She never had visitors, I never saw anyone there ... Being in the hospital for months at a time, I know she felt really alone, so I think, that me not giving up [was important]. I would come in and already act like we were friends, act comfortable, just sit down and say "What's up?" not ask her [permission] ... These patients are in the hospital for their physical needs, but I think that we [Streetlight] keep them going. I think that family support is extremely important and when they don't have family support, then they look to us for support and it really does make a difference.*

Second, the palliative care needs of adolescents vary widely by disease.

> *I've seen him at least 30 times going into the hospital. During that time I've only seen his grandfather once, and I've never seen his father and never seen his mother. ...Then one month his lungs tanked and he needed a transplant and so he texted me to say he was in the ICU [intensive care unit] and so I go at night, the one time I had gotten off work, and he's just sitting there and I walk in and he's got his head in his hands and he's in a lot of pain and the machines are beeping. It's dark. It hit me that that is his reality ... When he gets sick and he's in the hospital, that's night after night after night. Who's he going to see? His mother is not there. For two nights in a row I spent the night with him like I was his family member, I sat in the chair and slept and he'd wake up a few times. I don't think a lot of people would have done that, but I think he needed it. Now he's doing better and we can have a regular friendship like between two dudes, who play off each other, and make jokes and stuff.*

Third, psychosocial pain is just as debilitating as physical pain for adolescents with life-threatening illnesses.

> *...He taught me a lot about the fears of the disease, I really didn't know anything about it. Problems, like trust issues between those patients and the doctors. I had no idea, when they discuss just how much pain they are in and the nurses and doctors not believing them, or thinking that they are exaggerating. I was surprised that kind of stuff even existed. He's at a weird age, where you are no longer with your parents, moved away from them, but you still want that support. ... he doesn't have anyone, his family live far away and he's just always alone day after day. It affects his school, it affects his work, it affects absolutely everything. I learned that from ... all the patients that I meet, that they may not be able to graduate on time, or not being able to walk at graduation, or giving up a sport, giving up a club, giving up work. It's really hard. Even if you're not terminal, even if you're fine, but you have to regularly go to the hospital for check-ups or for testing, it still affects you.*

Fourth, *Streetlight* has also had a profound effect on the premedical students in regard of their career choices, bedside manner, communication skills, and coping mechanisms. Freyer notes that adolescents want to engage in communication that is candid, collaborative, and has mutual respect.[48]

As far as direct patient contact, actually walking into a room and getting to know a person and feeling like I am involved to some extent with their health care, Streetlight has been the most intense and it has easily been the most valuable for me. [In my previous experiences] watching doctors was fantastic and the time I spent in the emergency room was great and I got to do a little bit helping with patients, some hands on, but it was still very different as it was more of a cold interaction. There was a lot of watching and dealing with unconscious patients. I was never asked to do anything that would test my bedside manner. Streetlight has put me in the closest position that I've ever been to being a health care provider, and being able to see what that might feel like.

...I've also thought that maybe more hospitals need entities like Streetlight which are completely dedicated to this, because there is a point where you can only ask so much of doctors, and you can only ask so much of the nursing staff. A doctor can't go sit down in a patients' room for 2 hours and hear their life story and counsel them. ...Maybe we just need more manpower focused on the emotional needs of people who are hospitalized long term or who are dealing with chronic medical problems.

... It's hard [to talk to patients who are dying]. I can't say it's not a problem and that it doesn't bother me, it bothers me. It's hard and it sticks with me after I go home. I still think about whatever kid I was talking to still lying in the hospital. But it doesn't drive me away, if anything it only makes me want to go back. So it's let me know that I'm OK with it. I've gotten to know patients and see them die. I've listened to kids tell me some pretty awful things about what they're going through and I keep going back. I think it has strengthened my sense that I am going into the field that is right for me.

...I was nervous about going in at first because I wasn't sure how I'd be accepted. I think Streetlight has helped break down that barrier between the well and the sick. What is the difference between a sick person and a not sick person? It's a physical ailment. You still have all the same needs as everybody else does.

At present, there are 56 premedical students participating in *Streetlight* and they work in the program 5 days a week. The program has expanded its services to include a cystic fibrosis Web site, and the students routinely participate in community events to increase awareness and raise money for the adolescents and the program. Recently 18 laptops were purchased and given to the adolescents so that they could access the Internet in their rooms and participate in *Streetlight's* Facebook page. Funding is the biggest challenge to the program. Gifts, grants, and donations support *Streetlight*. The program does have strong faculty and administrative support. Another significant challenge is that the hospital serves a 17-county catchment area with a high proportion of adolescents from a rural and indigent population. It is difficult to reach out to adolescents when they are not in the hospital. As the program continues to evolve, it must consider the needs of these adolescents and provide appropriate services.

Streetlight is an innovative program that matches up adolescents with life-threatening illnesses with premedical students. Studies that have explored the palliative care education experiences of residents have found that more than any other educational method, residents prefer training done at the bedside.[52] A program similar to *Streetlight* could be used to train clinical psychology graduate students or residents in pediatric psychiatry.

SUMMARY

Partnerships between psychiatrists and pediatric palliative care programs are important. However, these partnerships present several unique challenges and opportunities.

All providers need to have adequate training on pediatric palliative care in the context of their own specialty and have an understanding of the roles of the other providers on the team. A survey of psychiatrists found that 97% indicated that they should receive end-of-life training.[24] An example of a comprehensive program for psychiatrists is the Palliative Care Psychiatric Program at San Diego Hospice.[53] The program provides consultation with providers in the community, disseminates information to national and international audiences, has a week-long palliative care psychiatry rotation for residents, and mentors trainees on conducting palliative care psychiatry research. Members of the palliative care team may also need training on the role of psychiatry. For example, the palliative care team may primarily enlist the help of psychiatrists when children or family members have moderate to severe symptoms indicating psychiatric disorders, but they may not be aware that psychiatrists can also help the team in other aspects of care such as breaking bad news. Without training, providers may miss opportunities to provide care in the most effective manner. Future research needs to be conducted to determine the educational needs, and preferred methods of receiving information, of child psychiatrists.

Professional boundaries must be discussed initially and often throughout the child's illness by the palliative care team. Pediatric palliative care providers are experts at meeting the physical, psychological, emotional, and supportive needs of children and families, and licensed social workers typically diagnose psychological issues in palliative care.[24] Upon diagnosis, social workers may collaborate with the child's pediatrician to treat the psychological issues. Yet in some situations the needs of the child and family may be better served by a psychiatrist. Determining when those situations occur should be determined by the entire palliative care team, and follow-up by the treating provider should be routinely provided back to the rest of the team.

A fundamental component of pediatric palliative care is that it treats the family as a unit. As such, family therapy is important. Treating parents, siblings, and ill children simultaneously may be difficult and require psychiatrists to have additional training in pediatrics and end-of-life care. Treatment often is required for individuals in the community. Psychiatrists may be called on to provide services to peers and staff at schools and community organizations.

Psychiatrists could also provide liaison services to pediatric palliative care staff to help them cope with the emotional burdens of caring for seriously ill children. Even the most seasoned staff members can be greatly affected by the death of a child they have cared for, and psychiatrists can help facilitate individual or group debriefing sessions.

Psychiatrists may have established relationships with the child and family through a referral from the primary care physician, not the palliative care provider. In this case the palliative care team may not be privy to care that has been provided, and it is important that providers communicate so that the child's palliative care treatment goals integrate psychiatric care. In practice, this may be difficult to do. Failure to have open, continual communication from all providers may result in duplication of services or even unmet needs if one provider mistakenly believes that the other is addressing a particular issue.

More research is needed to develop and validate tools to assess psychological factors in children with life-threatening illnesses. Meaningful cutoff points are also needed so that providers know how to interpret and incorporate these tools into practice. Research can then be conducted to identify the prevalence of psychological issues with children and adolescents in palliative care programs, and these issues can be addressed in a systematic manner.

Finally, there may be logistical barriers in treating the psychological needs of parents. Parents may need psychological care unrelated to the child's illness. In this circumstance it may be difficult for the palliative care team to treat the parent. Finding a provider to treat the parent may be dependent on insurance status and benefits.

It is important for psychiatrists to partner with pediatric palliative care teams. Ultimately, all children with life-threatening illnesses and their families should have their psychological needs met, which could in turn improve their quality of life and health outcomes.

REFERENCES

1. Martin JA, Kung HC, Mathews TJ, et al. Annual summary of vital statistics: 2006. Pediatrics 2008;121(4):788–801.
2. Levetown M. Compendium of pediatric palliative care. Alexandria (VA): National Hospice and Palliative Care Organization; 2000.
3. End of Life Nursing Education Consortium. ELNEC pediatric palliative care training program. Washington, DC: American Association of Colleges of Nurses; 2009.
4. World Health Organization. WHO definition of palliative care. Available at: http://www.who.int/cancer/palliative/definition/en/. Published 2009. Accessed January 14, 2010.
5. National Hospice and Palliative Care Organization. Find a hospice or palliative care program. Available at: http://iweb.nhpco.org/iweb/Membership/MemberDirectorySearch.aspx?pageid=3257&showTitle=1. Accessed January 14, 2010.
6. Children's Hospice International. Locate a provider. Available at: http://www.chionline.org/resources/locate.php. Accessed January 14, 2010.
7. Friebert S. NHPCO facts and figures: pediatric palliative and hospice care in America. NHPCO facts and figures. Alexandria (VA): National Hospice and Palliative Care Organization; 2009.
8. Knapp CA, Shenkman EA, Marcu MI, et al. Pediatric palliative care: describing hospice users and identifying factors that affect hospice expenditures. J Palliat Med 2009;12(3):223–9. 9.
9. Meier DE. Palliative care in hospitals. J Hosp Med 2006;1(1):21–8.
10. London MR, McSkimming S, Drew N, et al. Evaluation of a comprehensive, adaptable, life- affirming, longitudinal (CALL) palliative care project. J Palliat Med 2005; 8(6):1214–25.
11. Johnston DL, Nagel K, Friedman DL, et al. Availability and use of palliative care and end-of-life services for pediatric oncology patients. J Clin Oncol 2008;26(28): 4646–50.
12. Sullivan AM, Warren AG, Lakoma MD, et al. End-of-life care in the curriculum: a national study of medical education deans. Acad Med 2004;79(8):760–8.
13. Thompson LA, Knapp C, Madden V, et al. Pediatricians' perceptions of and preferred timing for pediatric palliative care. Pediatrics 2009;123(5):e777–82.
14. Knapp C, Madden V, Wang H, et al. Pediatric nurses' knowledge of palliative care in Florida: a quantitative study. Int J Palliat Nurs 2009;15(9):432–9.
15. Irwin SA, Rao S, Bower K, et al. Psychiatric issues in palliative care: recognition of depression in patients enrolled in hospice care. J Palliat Med 2008;11(2):158–63.

16. Feudtner C, Christakis DA, Zimmerman FJ, et al. Characteristics of deaths occurring in children's hospitals: implications for supportive care services. Pediatrics 2002;109(5):887–93.
17. Feudtner C, DiGiuseppe DL, Neff JM. Hospital care for children and young adults in the last year of life: a population-based study. BMC Med 2003;1:3.
18. Field MJ, Behrman RE, Institute of Medicine (U.S.) Committee on Palliative and End-of-Life Care for Children and Their Families. When children die: improving palliative and end-of-life care for children and their families. Washington, DC: National Academy Press; 2003.
19. American Academy of Pediatrics. American Academy of Pediatrics. Committee on Bioethics and Committee on Hospital Care. Palliative care for children. Pediatrics 2000;106(2 Pt 1):351–7.
20. Children's Hospice International. Children's Hospice International Program for All-Inclusive Care for Children and Their Families (CHI PACC®). Available at: http://www.chionline.org/programs/. Published 2009. Accessed January 14, 2010.
21. APM Ad Hoc Committee on End-of-Life Care. Psychiatric aspects of excellent end-of-life care: a position statement of the Academy of Psychosomatic Medicine. J Palliat Med 1998;1(2):113–5.
22. Ferrando SJ. Commentary: integrating consultation-liaison psychiatry and palliative care. J Pain Symptom Manage 2000;20(3):235–6.
23. Lyness JM. End-of-life care: issues relevant to the geriatric psychiatrist. Am J Geriatr Psychiatry 2004;12(5):457–72.
24. Irwin SA, Ferris FD. The opportunity for psychiatry in palliative care. Can J Psychiatry 2008;53(11):713–24.
25. Hultman T, Reder EA, Dahlin CM. Improving psychological and psychiatric aspects of palliative care: the national consensus project and the national quality forum preferred practices for palliative and hospice care. Omega (Westport) 2008;57(4):323–39.
26. Brown MR, Sourkes B. Psychotherapy in pediatric palliative care. Child Adolesc Psychiatr Clin N Am 2006;15(3):585–96, viii.
27. Stuber ML, Shemesh E. Post-traumatic stress response to life-threatening illnesses in children and their parents. Child Adolesc Psychiatr Clin N Am 2006;15(3):597–609.
28. Stoddard FJ, Usher CT, Abrams AN. Psychopharmacology in pediatric critical care. Child Adolesc Psychiatr Clin N Am 2006;15(3):611–55.
29. Edwards CL, Scales MT, Loughlin C, et al. A brief review of the pathophysiology, associated pain, and psychosocial issues in sickle cell disease. Int J Behav Med 2005;12(3):171–9.
30. Poltorak DY, Benore E. Cognitive-behavioral interventions for physical symptom management in pediatric palliative medicine. Child Adolesc Psychiatr Clin N Am 2006;15(3):683–91.
31. Dein S. Psychiatric liaison in palliative care. Adv Psychiatr Treat 2003;9:241–8.
32. Hoekstra-Weebers JE, Jaspers JP, Kamps WA, et al. Gender differences in psychological adaptation and coping in parents of pediatric cancer patients. Psychooncology 1998;7(1):26–36.
33. Duncan J, Joselow M, Hilden JM. Program interventions for children at the end of life and their siblings. Child Adolesc Psychiatr Clin N Am 2006;15(3):739–58.
34. Lobato DJ, Kao BT. Brief report: family-based group intervention for young siblings of children with chronic illness and developmental disability. J Pediatr Psychol 2005;30(8):678–82.

35. Bellin MH, Kovacs PJ, Sawin KJ. Risk and protective influences in the lives of siblings of youths with spina bifida. Health Soc Work 2008;33(3):199–209.

36. Jackson C, Richer J, Edge JA. Sibling psychological adjustment to type 1 diabetes mellitus. Pediatr Diabetes 2008;9(4 Pt 1):308–11.

37. Sourkes B, Frankel L, Brown M, et al. Food, toys, and love: pediatric palliative care. Curr Probl Pediatr Adolesc Health Care 2005;35(9):350–86.

38. Lahteenmaki PM, Sjoblom J, Korhonen T, et al. The siblings of childhood cancer patients need early support: a follow up study over the first year. Arch Dis Child 2004;89(11):1008–13.

39. Contro N, Larson J, Scofield S, et al. Family perspectives on the quality of pediatric palliative care. Arch Pediatr Adolesc Med 2002;156(1):14–9.

40. Bartel DA, Engler AJ, Natale JE, et al. Working with families of suddenly and critically ill children: physician experiences. Arch Pediatr Adolesc Med 2000; 154(11):1127–33.

41. Heller KS, Solomon MZ. Continuity of care and caring: what matters to parents of children with life-threatening conditions. J Pediatr Nurs 2005;20(5):335–46.

42. Block SD. Clinical and ethical issues in palliative care. FOCUS The Journal of Lifelong Learning in Psychiatry 2007;V(5):393–7. Available at: http://www.focus. psychiatryonline.org/cgi/content/abstract/5/4/393. Accessed November 15, 2009.

43. Carter BS, Levetown M. Palliative care for infants, children, and adolescents: a practical handbook. Baltimore (MD): The Johns Hopkins University Press; 2004.

44. Knapp C, Madden V, Marston J, et al. Innovative pediatric palliative care models in four countries. J Palliat Care 2009;25(2):56–60.

45. Cincinnati Children's Hospital. National Center for School Crisis and Bereavement. Available at: http://www.cincinnatichildrens.org/svc/alpha/s/school-crisis/ default.htm. Accessed January 14, 2010.

46. Knapp CA, Madden VL, Curtis CM, et al. Partners in care: together for kids: Florida's model of pediatric palliative care. J Palliat Med 2008;11(9):1212–20.

47. Knapp C, Madden V, Curtis CM, et al. Family support in pediatric palliative care: how are families impacted by their children's illnesses? J Palliat Med, in press.

48. Freyer DR. Care of the dying adolescent: special considerations. Pediatrics 2004; 113(2):381–8.

49. Freyer DR, Kuperberg A, Sterken DJ, et al. Multidisciplinary care of the dying adolescent. Child Adolesc Psychiatr Clin N Am 2006;15(3):693–715.

50. Easson WM. The seriously ill or dying adolescent. Special needs and challenges. Postgrad Med 1985;78(1):183–4, 187–9.

51. Children's Hospital Los Angeles. Teen impact program. Available at: http://www. chla.org/site/c.ipINKTOAJsG/b.3768089/k.930E/Teen_Impact.htm. Accessed January 14, 2010.

52. Baker JN, Torkildson C, Baillargeon JG, et al. National survey of pediatric residency program directors and residents regarding education in palliative medicine and end-of-life care. J Palliat Med 2007;10(2):420–9.

53. Integrating mental health services into hospice settings: the Palliative Care Psychiatric Program, San Diego Hospice and the Institute for Palliative Medicine, San Diego. Psychiatr Serv 2009;60(10):1395–7.

Index

Note: Page numbers of article titles are in **boldface** type.

A

Abdominal pain
    in inflammatory bowel disease, 904–905
    in obesity, 959
Acceptance, in cystic fibrosis, 875–876
Accreditation Association for Ambulatory Health Care, medical home standards of, 791–792
Acebutolol, for Smith-Magenis syndrome, 851
Acetylcarnitine, for fragile X syndrome, 843
Acquired immunodeficiency syndrome. *See* HIV/AIDS.
Adalimumab, for inflammatory bowel disease, 906
Addictive behavior, obesity in, 966
Adherence, with treatment
    for asthma, 927
    for cancer, 1011–1012
    for epilepsy, 977–978
    for HIV/AIDS, 997–998
    for inflammatory bowel disease, 908–909
    posttransplant, 894–896
Adjustment disorder
    in diabetes mellitus, 941
    in inflammatory bowel disease, 907–908
Adolescents
    born preterm, mental health in, 822–823
    cancer in, 1005–1006
    cystic fibrosis in, 874–877
    diabetes mellitus in, 946–947
    epilepsy in, 977–978
    HIV/AIDS in, 990, 992–994, 998
    obesity in, 956
    palliative care for, 1028, 1030, 1033–1035
Adulthood, transition to, in inflammatory bowel disease, 911
Affective disorders, in epilepsy, 977
Aggression
    in fragile X syndrome, 842–843
    in Williams syndrome, 848
Agitation
    in Down syndrome, 840
    in fragile X syndrome, 842–843
    in Rett syndrome, 844
AIDS. *See* HIV/AIDS.

Pediatr Clin N Am 58 (2011) 1041–1059
doi:10.1016/S0031-3955(11)00083-6
0031-3955/11/$ – see front matter © 2011 Elsevier Inc. All rights reserved.

M

Moving?

Make sure your subscription moves with you!

To notify us of your new address, find your **Clinics Account Number** (located on your mailing label above your name), and contact customer service at:

Email: journalscustomerservice-usa@elsevier.com

800-654-2452 (subscribers in the U.S. & Canada)
314-447-8871 (subscribers outside of the U.S. & Canada)

Fax number: 314-447-8029

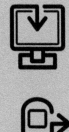

Elsevier Health Sciences Division
Subscription Customer Service
3251 Riverport Lane
Maryland Heights, MO 63043

*To ensure uninterrupted delivery of your subscription,
please notify us at least 4 weeks in advance of move.

Printed and bound by CPI Group (UK) Ltd, Croydon, CR0 4YY

03/10/2024

01040445-0007